FETAL ALCOHOL SYNDROME

From Mechanism to Prevention

FETAL ALCOHOL SYNDROME

From Mechanism to Prevention

Edited by

Ernest L. Abel, Ph.D.

Professor
Departments of Obstetrics/Gynecology and Psychology
Wayne State University
Detroit, Michigan

CRC Press
Boca Raton   New York   London   Tokyo

Library of Congress Cataloging-in-Publication Data

Catalog record is available from the Library of Congress.

International Standard Book Number 0-8493-7685-8
Printed in the United States of America 1 2 3 4 5 6 7 8 9 0
Printed on acid-free paper

INTRODUCTION

The contribution of maternal alcohol abuse during pregnancy to a variety of adverse prenatal outcomes known as *Fetal Alcohol Syndrome* and *Fetal Alcohol Effects* is now taken for granted. Widespread recognition of this relationship is reflected in the warning labels on every alcoholic beverage sold in the United States. Given the potential impact of alcohol abuse during pregnancy on the individual and on society as a whole, it is not surprising that research in this area covers many fronts.

This is the fourth volume CRC Press has specifically devoted to this topic. The three previous volumes, entitled Fetal Alcohol Syndrome, Volumes I, II and III, all appeared in the early 1980s. Since then, we have learned considerably more about this birth defect, and we are still continuing to discover more and more about its impact and how prenatal alcohol exposure produces such a gamut of effects.

The present book surveys a broad array of these topics by leading authorities in this area. Their research and the inferences they have drawn from that research have influenced our current understanding of fetal alcohol syndrome and related problems.

One of the questions that immediately came to mind in selecting topics for inclusion in this book was whether to focus on one particular site of damage, such as the central nervous system, or to present a broad overview of topics related to maternal alcohol abuse during pregnancy. As editor, I opted for the latter so as to emphasize the point that alcohol's effects on the developing embryo and fetus are very broad. No single area of the body is affected by alcohol abuse during pregnancy to the exclusion of all others. There is also no single time during development that is "safe" for the fetus when it comes to alcohol abuse during pregnancy; there is no single research strategy that can address all the questions that could or have been asked; and, there is certainly no "magic bullet" that will make the problem go away.

Accordingly, the first chapter in this book by Armant discusses the effects of alcohol exposure on the preimplantation embryo and indicates that its effects are far from what one might have anticipated: At relatively low levels, for instance, alcohol has surprising effects on the preimplantation embryo, including precocious implantation with no adverse effects on fetal development. Next, Maier and her coauthors discuss the "temporal windows" during which the embryo/fetus is especially vulnerable to alcohol-induced injury, and summarize evidence showing the timing of brain development is a critical factor in the brain's vulnerability to insult.

Anatomical and electrophysiological effects on the nervous system are examined in two chapters. Mattson and Riley review clinical autopsy studies and their more recent neuroimaging work. They contend that particular areas of the brain are more vulnerable to heavy alcohol exposure during gestation than others and that the pattern of brain damage appears to be distinguishable from that associated with other neurodevelopmental disorders. Berman and Krahl discuss the neurophysiological abnormalities seen in children and animals prenatally exposed to alcohol and attempt to relate them to abnormal anatomical findings described in the literature.

An in-depth review of the embryological development of the ear along with its structure and function is presented by Church, who then details how alcohol affects its development. In presenting this review of alcohol's effects, he makes the important point that hearing impairments at an early age of development are akin to sensory deprivation and that this sensory deprivation in an of itself may result in many of the behavioral problems association with FAS.

The chapters by Gottesfeld, and by Kim and coworkers, focus on alcohol's effects on the hypothalamic-pituitary-adrenal axis from different perspectives. Gottesfeld examines alcohol's effects on the immune system and how the hormones secreted by this axis modulate immune responsiveness. Kim *et al.* discuss the role of this axis in the response to stressors, and speculate on its possible involvement in alcohol's cognitive and behavioral effects. Next, Coles examines the effects of prenatal alcohol exposure on the behavior of children.

The next three chapters deal with alcohol's effects on neurochemical systems. Druse Manteuffel summarizes work dealing with the effects on neurotransmitter systems and second messenger systems. Hannigan and Randall examine the topic from the standpoint of reaction to pharmacological agents known to act on specific neurochemical transmitter systems. Subramanian examines the effects of alcohol on the neurochemical systems involved in lactation, and reviews possible effects on the newborn that may arise as a result of alcohol's effects on suckling behavior.

The following chapters deal with proposed mechanisms that may account for some of alcohol's effects. Saulnier and Randall present considerable evidence that several of alcohol's effects in the fetus are mediated through prostaglandins acting directly on the fetus or indirectly by altering utero-placental-umbilical blood flow. Fisher and Karl examine the role of nutritional factors in pregnancy and outline how these nutritional factors may mediate alcohol's effects on the fetus. Zimmerberg examines the role of disturbances in thermoregulation as a possible factor mediating the effects of prenatal alcohol exposure.

The final article by Hankin summarizes research on the impact of the alcohol warning label on drinking behavior of pregnant women and presents an analysis of her own data indicating that the label produced a modest reduction only for women under the age of 21.

....

What are some of the conclusions we can draw from these overviews? Certainly, it should be apparent that alcohol's effects on the developing embryo and fetus are very wide ranging. Although we are beginning to understand some of the ways alcohol impacts on the embryo and fetus, we are far from either attenuating that damage once it occurs, or preventing it from happening in the first place.

The simplistic idea that prevention only requires pregnant women to "just say no" undercuts what we know about alcoholism and addiction in general. If alcoholism is a medical disease comparable to other medical diseases such as diabetes, for example, one doesn't expect the problem to be controlled willfully. If it is not a disease but a "bad habit" which wouldn't happen if women just knew better, we would expect warning labels to have some impact, but as Hankin's chapter indicates, simple solutions don't work for complex problems.

A second conclusion is that neither fetal alcohol syndrome nor fetal alcohol effects arise from one or two drinks ingested at any time during pregnancy. Most of the contributors have deliberately emphasized that the adverse effects they are addressing arise from consumption of levels that would be considered "heavy" by most people -- levels generally associated with blood alcohol levels above, and in many cases far above 0.1 g% -- which coincidentally is the blood alcohol level legally associated with intoxication.

Although many studies have implied that problems can arise as a result of much lower levels of consumption, these inferences are based on an artifact related to averaging alcohol intakes over a week or a month. Consumption of seven drinks on a Saturday, for instance, is often reported as consumption of an average of one drink a day. As emphasized especially by West and his coworkers, the critical factor associated with drinking during pregnancy, as far as fetal damage is concerned, is the pattern of drinking. Researchers who disingenuously ignore or downplay this widely recognized fact in their press announcements about drinking and pregnancy in the belief that by frightening women they are helping them and their unborn children, must realize that such paternalism, even though altruistically motivated, only creates scepticism at best and distrust at worse.

A third conclusion is that implicit in many of these chapters is the recognition that many of the consequences of maternal alcohol abuse during pregnancy will not be recognized until children reach adolescence or adulthood when they will be challenged with problems and stresses not previously experienced. Some effects that seem short term may only become latent, arising once again and with greater intractability later on in life. Longitudinal studies are essential if we are to appreciate these potential problems. Studies in animals are just as important in these kinds of studies as they have been in elucidating earlier problems.

Even the wide-ranging issues presented in this book still fall far short of what could be presented. Little was said in any of these chapters, for instance, regarding genetic susceptibilities to alcohol's *in utero* effects, although dizygotic twins are known to be differentially affected by such exposure. Even less was said about socioeconomic factors related to the occurrence of fetal alcohol syndrome, although low socioeconomic status is almost always associated with fetal alcohol syndrome. Low socioeconomic status in turn is related to nutritional imbalances, which Fisher and Karl discuss, but only in the context of alcohol's effects. Whereas alcohol's effects on transport and availability of nutrients are obviously important, women do not become alcohol abusers the moment they become pregnant. Underlying nutritional deficiencies prior to pregnancy, whatever they may be, will be exacerbated by drinking, and these deficiencies are often relate to socioeconomic status. Other factors associated with low socioeconomic status that combine with alcohol abuse to exacerbate its effects include smoking, living in polluted environments, job stress, and availability and accessibility of medical care, to name only a few such factors.

These factors cannot be ignored in understanding how alcohol affects the developing embryo/fetus or in their prevention -- but that is the subject for another book.

THE EDITOR

DR. ERNEST L. ABEL is the Director of the Mott Center for Human Growth and Development and holds professorships within both the Departments of Obstetrics/Gynecology and Psychology at Wayne State University in Detroit, Michigan. He is the author of more than 30 books and 200 publications. He is also the Scientific Director of the federally funded Fetal Alcohol Research Center, the only one of its kind in the world exclusively devoted to research involving the effects of alcohol on the fetus. He is past President of the Behavioral Teratology Society and the Fetal Alcohol Study Group of the Research Society on Alcoholism. In 1989, he was awarded the Distinguished Faculty Fellowship Award by Wayne State University's Board of Governors.

CONTRIBUTING AUTHORS

D. Randall Armant, Ph.D.
Fetal Alcohol Research Center
Wayne State University School of Medicine
Departments of Obstetrics & Gynecology and Anatomy & Cell Biology
Detroit, Michigan   48201

Robert F. Berman, Ph.D. and Scott E. Krahl, Ph.D.
Fetal Alcohol Research Center
Wayne State University School of Medicine
Departments of Obstetrics & Gynecology and Psychology
Detroit, Michigan   48201

Michael W. Church, Ph.D.
Fetal Alcohol Research Center
Wayne State University School of Medicine
Department of Obstetrics & Gynecology
Detroit, MI   48201

Claire D. Coles, Ph.D.
Department of Psychiatry and Behavioral Science
Emory University School of Medicine
Atlanta, Georgia   30319

Mary Druse Manteuffel, Ph.D.
Department of Molecular & Cellular Biochemistry
Loyola University Chicago, Stritch School of Medicine
Maywood, Illinois   60153

Stanley E. Fisher, M.D. and Peter I. Karl, Ph.D.
Department of Pediatrics
New York University School of Medicine
North Shore University Hospital-NYU School of Medicine
Manhasset, New York 11030

Zehava Gottesfeld, Ph.D.
Department of Neurobiology & Anatomy
University of Texas - Houston Medical School
Houston, Texas   77225

Janet R. Hankin, Ph.D.
Department of Sociology
Wayne State University
Detroit, Michigan 48202

John H. Hannigan, Ph.D. and Surilla Randall, B.A., B.Sc.
Fetal Alcohol Research Center
Wayne State University School of Medicine
Departments of Obstetrics & Gynecology and Psychology
Detroit, Michigan 48201

C. Kwon Kim, M.A., Jill A. Osborn, B.Sc., and Joanne Weinberg, Ph.D.
Department of Anatomy, Faculty of Medicine
University of British Columbia
Vancouver, B.C., V6T 1Z3 Canada

**Susan E. Maier, Ph.D.,Wei-Jung A. Chen, Ph.D., and
James R. West, Ph.D.**
Alcohol and Brain Research Laboratory
Department of Human Anatomy & Neurobiology
Texas A&M University College of Medicine
College Station, Texas 77843

Sarah N. Mattson, Ph.D. and Edward P. Riley, Ph.D.
San Diego State University
Center for Behavioral Teratology
San Diego, California 92120

Jocelynn L. Saulnier, B.Sc. and Carrie L. Randall, Ph.D.
Center for Drug and Alcohol Programs
Department of Psychiatry
Medical University of South Carolina
Charleston, South Carolina 29425

Marappa G. Subramanian, Ph.D.
Fetal Alcohol Research Center
Wayne State University School of Medicine
Department of Obstetrics & Gynecology
Detroit, MI 48201

Betty Zimmerberg, Ph.D.
Department of Psychology and Program in Neuroscience
Williams College, Williamstown, MA 01267

TABLE OF CONTENTS

Chapter 1

ETHANOL-INDUCED ACCELERATION OF PREIMPLANTATION EMBRYONIC DEVELOPMENT

D. Randall Armant

I. ETHANOL USE NEAR THE TIME OF CONCEPTION

It is poorly understood how maternal alcohol consumption around the time of conception impacts on embryo survival and the establishment of pregnancy. This period is typically before there is an awareness that a pregnancy has been established and precautions to avoid alcohol consumption are adopted. It has long been assumed that drinking during the very early stages of pregnancy may account for significant levels of fetal wastage due to the toxicity of alcohol and its metabolites, particularly acetaldehyde.   However, data supporting this belief have not been readily obtained. Weekly administration of 1.8 g/kg ethanol during the first 3 weeks of pregnancy to the pig-tailed macaque, *Macaca nemistrina*, produces blood alcohol levels of 0.2 g%, but does not increase the risk of pregnancy loss during the first 30 days,[1] suggesting that ethanol toxicity is low during early primate embryogenesis. A recent prospective study of 500 women undergoing artificial insemination with donor sperm reveals that "moderate" alcohol intake has no significant effect on conception, as compared to non-drinking.[2] Controlling for a number of confounding factors, including smoking, coffee consumption and body fat distribution, their data actually show an increased pregnancy rate among alcohol drinkers, with a positive trend toward the group consuming the highest levels (> 10 glasses/week). These findings are surprising in light of studies of alcohol exposure during preimplantation development in mice that indicate detrimental effects.[3-4] However, very high dose levels are required to produce these effects. In the study of Checiu and Sandor,[3] mice injected i.v. on the third and fourth day of pregnancy with a 33% solution of ethanol to obtain a blood alcohol concentrations of 0.2 g% showed a reduced rate of implantation, impaired embryo transport in the oviduct, growth retardation, retardation of development, and abnormal morphological features in the resulting fetuses. A 25% ethanol-saline solution administered i.p. at a dose of 0.02 or 0.03 ml/g body wt (approximately 5 and 7.5 g/kg) reduces fetal weight only at the higher dose.[4] The relevance of exposure to these very high blood alcohol levels to the physiological effects of drinking by pregnant non-alcoholic women is unclear.

An investigation of implantation rates among rats exposed to "moderate" levels of alcohol during the preimplantation period may provide clues to what happened to the women studied by Zaadstra and coworkers.[2] Pregnant rats were given 2 or 4 g/kg body wt. of ethanol through a feeding tube on each of the first four days of pregnancy and the time of implantation on day 5 and fecundity at day 19 were determined.[5] These dosages should produce a peak blood alcohol level of approximately 0.13 g% at the lower dosage,[5-6] and about 0.15 g% at the higher dosage,[7] whereas the protocol used by Padmanabhan and Hameed[4] could produce blood alcohol levels four to six times higher.[8] Implantation occurs earlier in rats treated with 2 g/kg ethanol than in the control or 4 g/kg groups, and the total number of blastocysts that implant is the same in all groups. Fecundity is reduced only in the higher dose group (from 97% to 58%). Thus, exposure to "moderate" alcohol levels during early pregnancy is associated with precocious implantation and normal fetal development. Interestingly, placental weight is significantly elevated when mice are exposed to either 5 or 7.5 g/kg ethanol during the preimplantation period, and, at the lower dose, there is no observed fetal growth retardation.[4] The findings of these studies suggest that "moderate" levels of alcohol may enhance growth and development of the preimplantation embryo which is programmed primarily towards establishing the maternal-fetal interface that is crucial for placentation.

To better understand the biochemical and physiological basis of the influence of ethanol on early pregnancy, it is helpful to utilize *in vitro* models of preimplantation development. These experimental systems allow investigators to separate the direct effects of ethanol on embryonic development from confounding maternal influences, as well as to expose embryos to precise concentrations of ethanol or related chemicals during specific time periods. A description of the early stages of embryonic development and the experimental paradigms used to investigate them is provided in the following section.

II. EARLY EMBRYONIC DEVELOPMENT

A.   PREIMPLANTATION PERIOD

Mouse preimplantation development is characterized by a number of cell differentiation events in addition to a program of rapid, accelerating growth.[9-10] Examples of developing preimplantation embryos at several stages are provided in Figure 1. After a 24 h delay between fertilization and the first cell cleavage, cell number doubles every 12 h. The first morphogenetic event to take place is compaction, which occurs at the 8-cell stage on the third day of gestation (about 60 h post-coitum). The unpolarized, spherical blastomeres reorganize into epithelial-like cells, flatten against one another, become chemically coupled through gap junctions and form apical tight junctions.[11-13] The outer, polarized cells of this morula then begin to differentiate into trophectoderm cells, while the cells at internal positions contribute to the inner cell mass of the blastocyst that eventually forms.[9-10]

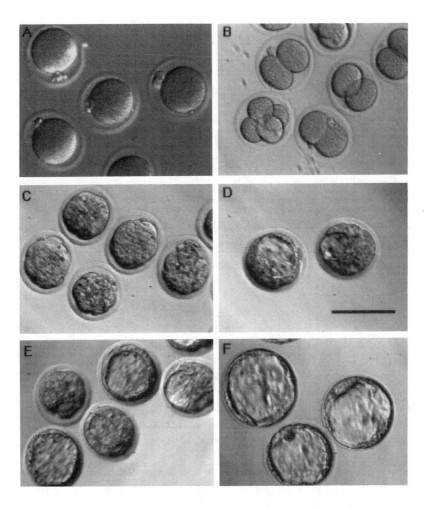

Figure 1. Preimplantation development of the mouse embryo. (A) Fertilized eggs surrounded by the zona pellucida, an extracellular matrix that contains the initial receptor for sperm at fertilization. Polar bodies, appearing in the perivitelline space between the oocyte plasma membrane and the zona pellucida, contain the two sets of chromosomes expelled during meiotic division. (B) Two-cell and four cell embryos, following the first and second cleavages. The cytoplasm is divided proportionally with each successive cleavage without any increase in the total mass of the embryo. (C) At the mid-eight-cell stage, the embryos undergo compaction. As the blastomeres become more tightly apposed and compacted, it becomes difficult to distinguish the individual cells of the morula. (D-E) After the embryo reaches the 16-cell stage, cavitation begins with the accumulation of small fluid-filled cavities that coalesce into a blastocoel. (F) With the continued expansion of the blastocoel, the inner cell mass and outer layer of trophectoderm cells can be clearly distinguished.

Late on the third day of development, the 16 to 32 cell embryo transits from the oviduct to the uterus where implantation will eventually occur. Owing to fluid accumulation between cells, the blastocyst forms through a process called cavitation and further expands during the fourth day of gestation. Cavitation is driven by the active transport of sodium and other solutes across the trophec-toderm, creating an osmotic gradient that promotes fluid accumulation.[14-15] The resultant blastocyst is composed of an outer layer of trophectoderm cells that ultimately form the placenta and fetal membranes of the conceptus, a fluid-filled blastocoel cavity that comprises most of the embryo volume, and a small inner cell mass composed of undifferentiated stem cells. Some extraembryonic tissues and all of the fetal tissues are derived from inner cell mass during the post-implantation phase of development. Thus, the majority of cells comprising the blastocyst are programmed for implantation and placentation, while a small number of embryonic stem cells are kept in reserve for later fetal development.

B.   BLASTOCYST IMPLANTATION

By the fifth day of gestation the blastocyst hatches from the surrounding extracellular matrix, or zona pellucida, and shortly thereafter implantation commences within a crypt formed by the folds of the uterine wall.[16] The ensuing multi-step process may be divided into several stages: 1) apposition of the blastocyst and the uterine wall, 2) adhesion of the trophectoderm to the uterine luminal epithelium, and 3) penetration of the luminal epithelium by the embryo, leading to invasion of the underlying stroma.[16] During this process, the blastocyst undergoes a developmental program whereby its non-adherent trophectoderm cells become adhesive trophoblast cells that are able to adhere to and penetrate the basement membrane of the uterine epithelium.[16-18] Implantation among mammalian species is diverse in terms of the extent of trophoblast invasion; however, it is haemochorial in both rodents and humans,[19] making the mouse a reasonable model of human trophoblast invasion.

Following the initial differentiation of trophectoderm and inner cell mass during preimplantation development, further differentiation occurs between the polar trophoblast that directly overlies the inner cell mass and the remaining mural trophoblast that, in mice, forms the invasive giant trophoblast cells.[20] In many other species, including humans, some of the trophoblast cells fuse to form a multinuclear syncytium.[16] Like the giant trophoblast cells of mice, these cells are capable of adhesion to the extracellular matrix, migration, phagocytosis and the release of matrix-degrading proteases.[17,20-23] Syncytiotrophoblasts in the human and giant trophoblast cells in the mouse are responsible for initiating the invasion of the endometrium during implantation.

C.   DEVELOPMENT *IN VITRO*

It is possible to fertilize mouse oocytes *in vitro* and culture them throughout preimplantation development using a chemically defined, simple medium.[24] This technique permits the assessment of embryogenesis in the presence of possible teratogens, including ethanol, under conditions that allow precise control over the dosage and length of exposure.[25] In addition to determining the rate at which embryos reach subsequent stages of development in culture, the rate of cavitation, can be determined by measuring the blastocoel volume morphometrically as blastocysts form from morulae and expand.[26] Quantitative measurement of the blastocoel volume has been automated using a computer with image analysis software.[27]

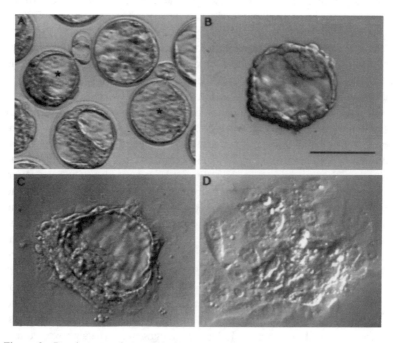

Figure 2. Development of mouse blastocysts *in vitro*, as described by Armant et al.[28] (A) Expanding blastocysts begin to hatch (hatching embryos are marked by asterisks) by penetrating the zona pellucida and squeezing itself through the opening. (B) Once free of the zona pellucida, the trophoblast cells of the intact blastocyst contact ECM proteins coated on the culture plate surface. (C) As the trophoblast cells begin to adhere to the substratum, they dissociate from the rest of the trophectoderm and assume a non-polarized, spread morphology. (D) The adhesive trophoblast cells migrate outward from the embryo. The area of migrating trophoblast cells increases steadily for several days, characteristic of the invasive phenotype of these cells.

The effect of ethanol on peri-implantation development may be studied, as well, using an *in vitro* model to eliminate influences of the maternal component of pregnancy. Aspects of mouse peri-implantation development are investigated using a defined culture system in which embryos recapitulate hatching, trophoblast adhesion to basement membrane proteins and trophoblast cell migration.[28] By precoating culture plates with adhesive proteins like fibronectin that are found in the endometrial extracellular matrix during trophoblast invasion, trophoblast cells adhere to the culture dish surface, dissociate from the blastocyst and migrate across the culture plate to form an outgrowth (Figure 2).   The rate of trophoblast differentiation can be determined by calculating the percentage of blastocysts undergoing outgrowth during culture, and the rate of trophoblast cell migration may be quantified by measuring the area of each blastocyst outgrowth using an image analysis system that has morphometry capabilities.[29] Blastocyst invasion has been modeled by following the invasion of purified endometrial extracellular matrix by blastocysts in culture.[30] The ontogeny of adhesiveness at the surface of the differentiating mural trophectoderm can be measured using a quantitative biochemical assay of fibronectin binding activity that utilizes intact blastocysts cultured *in vitro*.[31] The differentiation of blastocysts *in vitro*, culminating with outgrowth formation, reflects the developmental program responsible for the invasive phenotype of trophoblast cells that is necessary for implantation.

Embryonic development *in vivo* is approximately twice as fast as the rate *in vitro* under the best culture conditions, due to the maternal provision of optimal nutrient levels and growth factors. Efforts to culture embryos *in vitro* can be improved by carefully controlling the energy substrates that are provided in the medium.[24,32-35] Developmental progression during the preimplantation[36-41] and peri-implantation[42-51] phases has also been accelerated by the addition of growth factors. Morphological events that occur during early embryogenesis appear to be linked closely to the cell cycle,[52-56] making the growth rate of paramount importance to developing embryos.

III. THE DIRECT EFFECTS OF ETHANOL *IN VITRO*

The utility of an *in vitro* culture system to study the effects of alcohol on embryogenesis has been established using fetuses cultured during the developmental period when alcohol is most teratogenic. The ability to culture postimplantation mouse and rat fetuses undergoing organogenesis from gestation day 9.5 to 11.5 provides the technology to investigate the direct effects of ethanol, revealing growth retardation and altered differentiation at concentrations above 0.2 to 0.3%w/v.[57-60] These experiments produce many of the same developmental anomalies associated with fetal alcohol syndrome and support a role for the direct action of ethanol as a teratogen. Depending on the alcohol dose and route of administration, blood ethanol concentrations of intoxicated humans and animals attain peak levels that plateau for periods lasting from less than one to several hours.[6-8,61-63] Therefore, it is important to consider the limits of *in vivo* alcohol exposure when interpreting data from *in vitro* studies where a much higher concentration and a longer duration of exposure is possible. Indeed, acute, rather than long term, ethanol exposure *in vitro* may better mimic the conditions that embryos experience when pregnant animals are given alcohol. The principal advantage of *in vitro* embryo culture, of course, is that the alcohol exposure conditions may be varied precisely to determine the direct effects on embryonic development. It is also possible to specifically expose embryos to ethanol or one of its metabolites, such as acetaldehyde, to separate the effects of alcohol from those of other products that are generated after ethanol administration *in vivo*.

The potential role of acetaldehyde in alcohol toxicity during the preimplantation period must be considered, just as it has during fetal development. Exposure of mouse oocytes to ethanol, both *in vitro* and *in vivo*, is associated with non-disjunction of maternally-derived chromosomes and subsequent aneuploidy.[64] Acetaldehyde is mutagenic,[65] and could be partially responsible for the embryo toxicity of ethanol administered to pregnant animals. Alcohol can clearly be converted to acetaldehyde within the maternal system, but it is unclear whether the required enzymes are present in the preimplantation embryo, itself. Lau et al.[66] used *in vitro* culture to examine the direct effects of ethanol and acetaldehyde on mouse preimplantation embryos. Their study indicates that while ethanol induces chromosomal aberrations at concentrations above 0.03%, it does not alter embryonic growth at concentrations up to 1%. Acetaldehyde, on the other hand, is highly toxic at concentrations approximately three orders of magnitude below ethanol. Lau et al.[66] suggest that ethanol conversion to acetaldehyde by alcohol dehydrogenase in preimplantation embryos is responsible for alcohol toxicity based on the detection of alcohol dehydrogenase activity with a qualitative histochemical assay. The required concentrations of alcohol in this assay suggest a K_M for ethanol in excess of 400 mM, making it unlikely that the enzyme would function at alcohol levels attainable *in vivo*. Their conclusions contrast to the results of Nielsen and Pedersen[67] who used alcohol dehydrogenase as a reporter gene in transgenic preimplantation embryos and found untransfected embryos to be deficient in that enzyme when assayed histochemically.

If acetaldehyde production by preimplantation embryos is significant, its production in the absence of the maternal environment should be harmful to *in vitro* development. Two independent laboratories report normal blastocyst formation by preimplantation embryos cultured with ethanol concentrations as high as 0.8%.[68-69] Indeed, Wiebold and Becker [69] report improved development of 2-cell mouse embryos to the blastocyst stage when treated for three days with 0.1% ethanol (86%) as compared to controls (70%). Furthermore, implantation rates are significantly higher among the ethanol-treated embryos after their transfer to pseudopregnant dams. Therefore, the detrimental effects of maternal ethanol exposure during the preimplantation period, as reported by Checiu and Sandor,[3] may be due more to an impaired maternal support system than to the direct effects of ethanol on the embryo.

We have examined the hypothesis that exposure to ethanol during the preimplantation period is compatible with normal, indeed enhanced, embryonic development due to ethanol-induced physiological alterations that promote the growth and differentiation necessary for successful blastocyst implantation. The cells of the preimplantation embryo, although comprising several distinct populations, are homogeneous in their need for rapid growth. If ethanol partially reestablishes the *in vitro* growth rate closer to the *in vivo* rate, we would expect ethanol treatment at various stages of preimplantation development to uniformly accelerate development, improving the ability of blastocysts to implant when transferred back to the female reproductive tract. Several experiments in which embryos were directly exposed to ethanol *in vitro* are now described that support this hypothesis.

A.   DEVELOPMENT FROM ONE CELL TO BLASTOCYST

As pointed out above, an important issue in designing *in vitro* experiments with ethanol is to select alcohol concentrations that best mimic the exposure experienced by embryos from ethanol-treated mothers. *In vitro* fertilized embryos at the 1-cell, 2-cell, 4-cell or 8-cell stages were exposed for 24 h to 0.1%, 0.4% or 1.6% ethanol,[25] covering a range of concentrations from levels attainable in the blood of intoxicated animals to concentrations far exceeding a lethal dose. Depending upon the stage of development and concentration, ethanol exposure both inhibits and accelerates preimplantation development to the blastocyst stage.[25] Ethanol inhibits preimplantation development only at concentrations well above 0.1%, affecting the earliest stages to the greatest extent. One-cell and 2-cell embryos are inhibited in blastocyst formation by 1.6% ethanol and 1-cell embryos are also inhibited by 0.4%. However, the later stages are refractory to all levels of treatment and the percent embryos forming blastocysts is significantly increased when 1-cell or 2-cell embryos are exposed to 0.1% ethanol. Furthermore, exposure of 1-cell embryos to 0.1% ethanol stimulates their ability to hatch successfully from the zona pellucida, increases the rate of cell division and induces a precocious onset of trophoblast differentiation when the blastocysts that form are cultured on fibronectin. Thus, it appears that preimplantation embryos are not readily susceptible to alcohol toxicity, particularly at later stages, and their development is stimulated by exposure to 0.1% ethanol, which is in the physiologically appropriate region of the concentration range evaluated.

Improved development to the hatched blastocyst stage following ethanol exposure of 4-cell and 8-cell embryos was probably not detectable in this study[25] because control embryos at those stages already possess a very high level of developmental competence. To determine whether ethanol is also capable of stimulating development of preimplantation embryos at the 8-cell morula stage, morulae were collected on the third day of gestation and cultured for 48 h to monitor their rate of cavitation.[27] Morulae exposed to 0.1% ethanol for 24 h accumulate fluid at an elevated rate as they cavitate between 24 and 48 h of culture. It is particularly interesting that ethanol appears to potentiate a very rapid physiological change in the embryos. Treatment with 0.1% ethanol for either 5 min or 24 h will similarly induce an elevated rate of blastocoel formation.[27] The ability of a very acute exposure to produce this biological effect is highly significant, since peak blood alcohol levels *in vivo* persist for only a short time. Therefore, a 5 min exposure to 0.1 to 0.2% ethanol is more likely to duplicate embryo exposure during maternal alcohol consumption than would a longer exposure period. Because of the need for only a brief exposure, the observed stimulatory effects of ethanol do not appear to derive from the provision of an alternative carbon or energy source. Instead, it seems likely that ethanol produces a rapid biochemical perturbation that generates physiological changes in the embryo, ultimately accelerating the rate of development.

B.   BLASTOCYST DEVELOPMENT AND IMPLANTATION

Experiments employing the blastocyst outgrowth model demonstrate that the development of embryos already at the blastocyst stage is also accelerated by ethanol. Leach et al.[25] had noticed that embryos exposed to 0.1% ethanol at the 1-cell stage often began to form trophoblast outgrowths before hatching, whereas control embryos remained nonadhesive for about 10 h or longer following hatching. Stachecki et al.[70] clarified this observation by treating blastocysts with ethanol, then mechanically removing the zonae pellucidae to monitor blastocyst outgrowth independently of hatching. Blastocysts collected on gestation day 4 were treated with 0.05 to 1% ethanol for 5 min or 24 h. After 24 h of culture, the zonae were removed and culture was continued on plates coated with fibronectin. Blastocysts are optimally induced to differentiate after exposure to 0.1% ethanol for 5 min, as revealed by the rate of outgrowth formation and the area of trophoblast cells migrating around each embryo. It appears that all stages of preimplantation development benefit from ethanol exposure according to the criteria used in these experiments.[25,27,70]

To determine whether blastocysts induced to differentiate at an accelerated rate by ethanol are better able to undergo implantation *in utero*, Stachecki et al.[70] treated blastocysts for 5 min with 0 or 0.1% ethanol, cultured them for 24 h and transferred them to pseudopregnant dams. Ethanol-treated blastocysts implant at double the rate ($p < 0.05$) of control embryos. There are no detrimental effects of ethanol on development to term nor any enhancement of development after implantation. All ethanol treated embryos developing to term were alive and morphologically normal,[70] in agreement with the results of Wiebold and Becker.[69] Using an embryo transfer system, we found that the *in vitro* outgrowth model can provide information regarding embryo development that correlates with the *in vivo* implantation rate.[70] The findings of Stachecki et al.,[25,70] along with the earlier report of Wiebold and Becker,[69] document that ethanol significantly enhances embryo development *in vitro* and the potential for implantation after embryo transfer. These effects do not require an extended period of exposure to ethanol, as in the study of Wiebold and Becker,[69] but may be produced by a 5 min exposure. It is perhaps this ability of ethanol that is responsible for the intriguing results reported in studies of maternal alcohol exposure during preimplantation development in rats[5] and women.[2]

IV. ALTERATION OF SIGNAL TRANSDUCTION BY ETHANOL

The ability of ethanol to rapidly induce physiological changes in preimplantation embryos, leading to an elevated rate of growth and differentiation, suggests that ethanol may be altering signal transduction pathways that regulate the rate of embryogenesis. Growth factors accelerate the developmental progression of preimplantation embryos by activating signal transduction pathways.[36-41]   Perhaps ethanol sets off a chain of biochemical reactions in common with those initiated by growth factors. To test this hypothesis it is first necessary to consider the vast array of biochemical signals that can be generated within cells.

A.   SIGNAL TRANSDUCTION PATHWAYS IN GROWING CELLS

Growth factors are peptides that serve as endocrine (acting throughout the system), paracrine (acting on cells within local proximity), autocrine (acting on the same group of cells that produced them), or juxtacrine (acting through direct contact between adjacent cells) mediators of biological signals and are generally concerned with growth control.[71-72] As shown in Figure 3, growth factors act through a complex intracellular network of signal-transducing molecules that originates at the plasma membrane and modulates cell function, including the expression of specific genes. Growth factors stimulate target cells by binding to specific cell surface receptor proteins. A "signal" is then transmitted via a membrane-spanning domain of the receptor to an effector region (typically with protein tyrosine kinase (PTK) activity) that is located on the inside of the cell membrane. PTK catalyzes the phosphorylation of intracellular proteins and thereby alters their function. The altered activity of the PTK substrates provokes a cascade of molecular events that ultimately regulates cellular growth and, in some instances, differentiation. The regulatory cascades of growth factors frequently involve the activation of phospholipase C (PLC), either by tyrosine phosphorylation of the PLC gamma subunit or through the interaction of G proteins[73] with PLC.   PLC enzymatically generates two second messengers, diacylglycerol and inositol 1,4,5-trisphosphate (IP_3), by the hydrolysis of phosphatidylinositol 4,5-bisphosphate in the plasma membrane. Diacylglycerol is an activator of protein kinase C (PKC), and IP_3 stimulates the release of calcium, another important second messenger,[74-75] from intracellular storage sites into the cytoplasm. Calcium can then combine with calmodulin to activate a set of calmodulin-dependent protein kinases, which alters the activity of their particular set of substrate proteins.[76] The activity of calmodulin-dependent protein kinases is critical for the progression of the cell cycle,[76] and thereby regulates cell growth. There are also families of protein phosphatases[77] and other regulatory molecules that impact on these interdependent biochemical pathways. Through a mechanism that is beyond the scope of this article, the activity of protein kinases influences the expression of proto-oncogenes, such as c-myc, c-fos and c-jun, that activate specific genes.[78-80] This cascade ultimately impacts upon the physiological state of the cell and provides a universal regulatory strategy that is critical during the rapid growth and differentiation associated with embryogenesis.

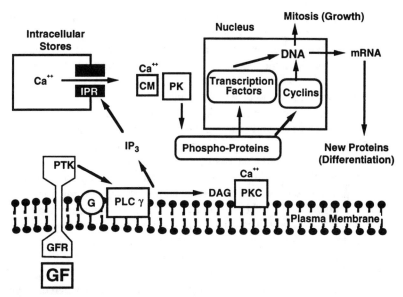

Figure 3. An illustration of the intracellular signalling pathways that regulate cell growth and differentiation by transducing chemical information from the plasma membrane to the nucleus. In this example, a growth factor (GF) binds to the extracellular domain of its receptor (GFR), altering the conformation of the GFR and activating a PTK site located in its intracellular domain. PLC becomes active when its gamma subunit is tyrosine phosphorylated, or through interaction with certain G proteins (G), to generate IP_3 and diacylglycerol (DAG). DAG activates PKC, a serine/threonine specific protein kinase. IP_3 binds to the IP_3 receptor (IPR), a ligand-gated calcium channel that releases calcium from intracellular storage sites into the cytoplasm where it can effect broad physiological changes by activating a plethora of enzymes (including PKC) and structural proteins. An important regulatory protein, calmodulin (CM), activates many enzymes upon binding calcium, including calmodulin-dependent protein kinases (PK). The phosphorylated substrates of these protein kinases are responsible for the activation of various transcription factors, leading to the expression of specific genes that mediate cell differentiation. Cell growth may also be stimulated in this pathway through cyclins that regulate the cell cycle.[76]

B. ETHANOL INDUCTION OF INTRACELLULAR CALCIUM TRANSIENTS

Ethanol has been long used at concentrations exceeding 5% to induce parthenogenetic activation of oocytes,[81-85] a phenomena that is attributed to the ability of ethanol to produce a transient rise in the intracellular calcium concentration ($[Ca^{2+}]_i$).[85-86] The injection of calcium directly into mouse oocytes induces germinal vesicle breakdown, cortical granule release, resumption of meiosis beyond metaphase II, and parthenogenetic cellular division, directly demonstrating that elevation of $[Ca^{2+}]_i$ will trigger oocyte maturation and egg activation.[87]   It is also clear that naturally occurring calcium oscillations regulate oocyte maturation, egg activation, and the acrosome reaction in sperm.[82,88-90]

The critical role of intracellular calcium in the events that immediately follow sperm-egg binding suggests that it could also play a role in the regulation of preimplantation embryonic growth and differentiation. Evidence from studies of parthenogenetic development suggests that the temporal pattern of $[Ca^{2+}]_i$ oscillations that occur at fertilization may influence the ability of embryos to complete preimplantation embryogenesis.[91-92] Therefore, ethanol-induced acceleration of preimplantation development may be derived from perturbation of second messenger molecules like calcium.

We have conducted a series of experiments to determine whether the mechanism of ethanol-induced acceleration of preimplantation development might involve calcium. While cavitation of murine morulae and outgrowth of blastocysts are accelerated by incubation with 0.1% ethanol for 5 min, the calcium ionophore A23187 produces similar enhancements of development.[27,70] This suggests that a brief exposure to ethanol may elevate $[Ca^{2+}]_i$ to stimulate development. Indeed, when the $[Ca^{2+}]_i$ levels of embryos are measured with the fluorescent indicator fluo 3-AM, an increase in $[Ca^{2+}]_i$ immediately follows ethanol exposure and returns to baseline levels after 10 min.[27] Ethanol induces a similar transient elevation of $[Ca^{2+}]_i$ when embryos are placed in calcium-free medium containing EGTA, demonstrating that the calcium is released from intracellular stores. It, therefore, appears that the direct introduction of ethanol during *in vitro* culture can accelerate preimplantation embryogenesis by altering the level of at least one important second messenger molecule, calcium.

Signal transduction by calcium can be blocked using the intracellular chelator BAPTA-AM.[88] Concentrations of BAPTA-AM above 1 μM will delay cavitation, and 100 μM completely inhibits development,[93] providing evidence that calcium signaling plays a critical role in preimplantation development. While 0.5 μM BAPTA-AM does not inhibit cavitation, it does block the rise in $[Ca^{2+}]_i$ caused by ethanol and attenuates the subsequent acceleration of cavitation. When the embryos are treated with ionomycin, which releases much more calcium than ethanol, the observed $[Ca^{2+}]_i$ rises and cavitation proceeds at the faster rate. Chelation of intracellular calcium by BAPTA-AM also inhibits cell division in preimplantation embryos, consistent with previous work demonstrating that the cell cycle is linked to calcium signaling.[76,94-95] These experiments reveal the central role of calcium in regulating early embryogenesis, perhaps through its ability to initiate mitosis, and further show that the action of ethanol is dependent on its ability to generate a calcium transient.

C. SIGNALING THROUGH THE SECOND MESSENGER, CALCIUM, IN PREIMPLANTATION EMBRYOS

The interaction of cells with growth factors[96-98] or the extracellular matrix[99-101] initiates signals that rapidly trigger calcium release from intracellular stores. Calcium, in turn, transduces intracellular signals that influence growth and differentiation. The ethanol-induced increase in $[Ca^{2+}]_i$ leads to oocyte activation through specific protein phosphorylations catalyzed by calcium activation of PKC or calmodulin-dependent protein kinases.[82] These protein phosphorylations modify the activity of other proteins, leading to altered gene expression.[102-104] Protein phosphorylation can also influence the activity of various enzymes and regulatory or structural proteins to produce profound changes in cellular activities. It is therefore important to understand how ethanol generates calcium oscillations in preimplantation embryos and the biochemical consequences of these events.

1. Mechanism of Calcium Release by Ethanol

How ethanol causes calcium release from intracellular stores is an open question. Physiologically, intracellular calcium release is regulated by calcium and IP_3 through their interaction with receptor-gated calcium channels that are associated with the membranes of calciosomes, the endoplasmic reticulum and other organelles that sequester calcium.[105] Ethanol could act directly on the membranes of those organelles to alter their biophysical state and compromise their ability to retain sequestered calcium since alcohols can physically disrupt cell membranes.[106] Alternatively, ethanol could interact with cellular regulatory proteins. For example, it could either interfere with the ability of the calcium channels to remain closed or alter the activity of proteins that modulate the level of IP_3.

Alcohols perturb cell membranes by inserting into the membrane bilayer, expanding the surface area and causing membrane fluidization.[107] The membrane fluidizing effect of alcohols is enhanced by their ability to interact with the hydrophobic region of the membrane lipid bilayer and increases with chain length and the polar placement of hydroxyl groups.[108] It could therefore be hypothesized that the carbon chain length and hydroxyl positioning of alcohols may correspondingly alter their ability to perturb lipids within embryonic cell membranes and initiate calcium signaling. However, the membrane disordering effect of ethanol does not account for its ability to alter $[Ca^{2+}]_i$ and accelerate preimplantation embryogenesis, since neither is stimulated by the structurally related alcohols, methanol, propanol, isopropanol or butanol.[109] These alcohols all inhibit embryo development and none of the alcohols at 0.1% are able to induce calcium transients in mouse morulae. At 1.0%, butanol raises the $[Ca^{2+}]_i$ to very high levels, perhaps because it, unlike ethanol or the other alcohols, is sufficiently hydrophobic to disrupt cell membranes and compromise the ability of the cell to retain sequestered calcium. The absence of a correlation between either developmental acceleration or elevation of $[Ca^{2+}]_i$ and the membrane disordering properties of alcohols suggests that ethanol is unique in its ability to transiently increase $[Ca^{2+}]_i$. The increase in calcium is most likely caused by the specific interaction of ethanol with regulatory proteins rather than a global disruption of cell membranes, suggesting that calcium is liberated from specific intracellular storage sites.

If ethanol elevates the $[Ca^{2+}]_i$ by inducing intracellular calcium channels to open, either directly or indirectly through the generation of IP_3, then it is first important to establish that these channels exist in preimplantation embryos, as they do in oocytes. The temporal release of calcium from intracellular stores varies with cell type and is regulated by (I) calcium-induced calcium release acting through the ryanodine receptor (e.g., skeletal muscle), (ii) the binding of IP_3 to the IP_3 receptor (e.g., *Xenopus* and mouse oocytes), or (iii) both mechanisms (e.g., atrial cells, neurons, sea urchin eggs).[110-117] The ryanodine and IP_3 receptors, although functionally distinct,[114,118-122] serve as calcium channels[111] that share both a structural and functional homology, reflecting their common origin during evolution.[105,123]

Identification of intracellular calcium receptors has been established in oocytes by microinjection of either IP_3 or ryanodine to determine whether a calcium transient is generated.[117] To infuse these molecules into multicellular preimplantation embryos, embryos are permeabilized to IP_3 or ryanodine by briefly pretreating the embryos with lysolecithin.[124] Using this method, Stachecki and Armant[93] found that mouse embryos generate intracellular calcium fluctuations predominantly through a calcium release mechanism involving the IP_3 receptor. This result was anticipated based on reports that mouse oocytes either lack or poorly utilize ryanodine receptors, but contain an IP_3-mediated calcium release mechanism.[116-117,125] Therefore, it is possible that ethanol releases calcium either by altering the ability of the IP_3 receptor to remain closed, or by modifying the activity of a protein involved in modulating IP_3 levels, such as PTK, PLC or a G protein capable of activating PLC.

2. Up-Regulation of c-myc Protein

Calcium initiates a cascade that alters the activity of calcium-dependent enzymes that can influence cell structure, other enzymatic activities and the circuitry of subsequent signal transduction events within the cell.[76] Calcium binds to calmodulin and together they activate calcium-calmodulin-dependent protein kinases. Activation of these enzymes or other protein kinases, such as PKC, may ultimately cause transcription factors to bind to specific sequences on DNA and induce new gene expression.

Calcium transients are required for the synthesis of DNA and other critical steps during the cell cycle.[76] An important transcription factor associated with rapidly dividing cells is c-myc.[126-127] Expression of c-myc can first be detected at the late 2-cell stage using the technique of reverse transcription and the polymerase chain reaction.[128] This is the time during preimplantation development when the mitotic rate is increasing. Prevention of c-myc expression with antisense oligonucleotides arrests further development,[129] demonstrating its critical role during preimplantation embryogenesis. Ethanol-induced calcium signaling could therefore up-regulate c-myc to promote the growth of embryonic cells.

We have investigated the expression of c-myc in ethanol-treated blastocysts using western blotting and quantitative immunohistochemistry.[130] Western blot staining of c-myc in blastocyst cell extracts with three different monoclonal antibodies indicates that c-myc levels increase up to 4-fold after exposure to 0.1% ethanol. Individual blastocysts stained with the antibodies reveal c-myc protein primarily within nuclei, as expected. Staining of c-myc increases beginning 1 min after ethanol treatment and continues to rise for 30 min. This transcription factor is associated with increased cell division,[127] a process central to preimplantation development. Cell number at the blastocyst stage is greater in cultured embryos treated with ethanol at the 1-cell stage[25] or 8-cell morula stage.[93] The ability of ethanol to accelerate development throughout the preimplantation period may be due to its effect on fundamental cell processes, such as mitosis, that regulate the rate of developmental events leading to blastocyst formation and implantation.

V. SUMMARY

While alcohol is associated with a variety of teratogenic effects,[57-60] it now appears clear that its toxicity during the earliest stages of pregnancy may be limited. Indeed, at "moderate" dose levels acute exposure to ethanol could be beneficial to conception. However, the strongest data in support of a beneficial role for ethanol have been obtained by treating embryos during *in vitro* culture. Maternal ethanol consumption could have associated risks that offset the beneficial effects of ethanol on the preimplantation embryo. Metabolism of ethanol by dehydrogenases within the mother's body could expose the conceptus to acetaldehyde toxicity. Alcohol may physiologically compromise the maternal support system, providing a suboptimal environment for embryo development. On the other hand, there have been several reports that "moderate" alcohol intake may be of physiological benefit to central nervous system function, cardiovascular disease and osteoporosis.[131-133] In regard to maternal support of embryonic development, alcohol promotes uterine decidualization and increases uterine blood flow and oxygen tension at the site of blastocyst implantation, possibly providing a milieu that increases the likelihood for successful implantation.[134-135] Further study is required to determine whether the beneficial effects of "moderate" ethanol exposure *in vivo* will outweigh the possible risks to preimplantation embryos.

The beneficial effects of ethanol during the preimplantation period and the teratogenic effects during later fetal development present an apparent paradox. One possible explanation for the observed dichotomy in the physiological response of embryonic cells to ethanol at these two developmental stages lies in the relative complexity of the conceptus. The preimplantation embryo is composed of a homogeneous population of embryonic cells that are engaged in rapid proliferation. Successful preimplantation development constitutes the production of a large number of trophectoderm cells to implant in the uterus and initiate placentation. During organogenesis, when alcohol is teratogenic, the fetus is composed of multiple cell populations engaged in forming the various organ systems. If ethanol promotes preimplantation development by driving the cell cycle ahead, as some data indicate,[25,93,130] then populations of fetal cells that are undergoing terminal differentiation could be adversely affected. For example, progenitor cells of the nervous system initially divide rapidly, but their terminal differentiation, which precedes axon extension and the formation of neural networks, occurs only after they exit from mitosis.[104,136] The proto-oncogene product, c-myc, which appears to be up-regulated by ethanol in embryonic cells,[130] prevents terminal differentiation in a host of cell types and can influence programmed cell death.[137-138] Thus, while a similar physiological mechanism (e.g., increased mitosis) may underlie the effects of alcohol during pre- and post-implantation embryogenesis, it is the developmental programming of the target cell populations that is critical. Most fetal cells are engaged in mitosis at any particular stage and, like preimplantation blastomeres, would not be adversely effected by ethanol. This hypothesis could account for diversity and non-lethality of fetal alcohol exposure.   It predicts that alcohol predominantly interferes with the development of cells that are exiting mitosis at the time of exposure, leaving the remaining cell populations unharmed. Fetal alcohol effects are, in fact, characterized by a large variety of structural and behavioral anomalies that range from the subtle to the serious.[139]

ACKNOWLEDGMENTS

This work was supported by the Wayne State University Fetal Alcohol Research Center grant, AA07606, from the National Institute on Alcohol Abuse and Alcoholism.

REFERENCES

1.   **Clarren, S. K. and Astley, S. J.,** Pregnancy outcomes after weekly oral administration of ethanol during gestation in the pig-tailed macaque: Comparing early gestational exposure to full gestational exposure, *Teratology*, 45, 1, 1992.

2. **Zaadstra, B.M., Looman, C.W., te Velde, E.R., Habbema, J.D., and Karbaat, J.,** Moderate drinking: No impact on female fecundity, *Fert. Steril.*, 62, 948, 1994.

3. **Checiu, M. and Sandor, S.,** The effect of ethanol upon early development in mice and rats. IX. Late effect of acute preimplantation intoxication in mice, *Morphol. Embryol.*, 32, 5, 1986.

4. **Padmanabhan, R. and Hameed, M.S.,** Effects of acute doses of ethanol administered at pre-implantation stages on fetal development in the mouse, *Drug Alcohol Depend.*, 22, 91, 1988.

5. **Mitchell, J.A.,** Effects of alcohol on blastocyst implantation and fecundity in the rat, *Alc. Clin. Exp. Res.*, 18, 29, 1994.

6. **Abel, E.L. and York, J.L.,** Absence of effect of prenatal ethanol on adult emotionality and ethanol consumption in rats, *J. Stud. Alcohol*, 40, 547, 1979.

7. **Abel, E.L., Greizerstein, H.B. and Siemens, A.J.,** Influence of lactation on rate of disappearance of ethanol in the rat, *Neurobehav. Toxicol.*, 1, 185, 1979.

8. **Ciociola, A.A. and Gautieri, R.F.,** Teratogenic and behavioral anomalies induced by acute exposure of mice to ethanol and their possible relation to fetal brain DNA synthesis, *Pharm. Res.*, 5, 447, 1988.

9. **Johnson, M.H.,** The molecular and cellular basis of preimplantation mouse development, *Biol. Rev. Cambridge Philosoph. Soc.*, 56, 463, 1981.

10. **Johnson, M.H.,** Membrane events associated with the generation of a blastocyst, *Int. Rev. Cytol. - Suppl.*, 12, 1, 1981.

11. **Fleming, T.P., Hay, M., Javed, Q., and Citi, S.,** Localisation of tight junction protein cingulin is temporally and spatially regulated during early mouse development, *Development*, 117, 1135, 1993.

12. **De Sousa, P.A., Valdimarsson, G., Nicholson, B.J., and Kidder, G. M.,** Connexin trafficking and the control of gap junction assembly in mouse preimplantation embryos, *Development*, 117, 1355, 1993.

13. **Fleming, T.P., Javed, Q., and Hay, M.,** Epithelial differentiation and intercellular junction formation in the mouse early embryo, *Development - Suppl.*, 105, 1992.

14. **Watson, A.J., Pape, C., Emanuel, J.R., Levenson, R., and Kidder, G.M.,** Expression of Na,K-ATPase alpha and beta subunit genes during preimplantation development of the mouse, *Dev. Genet.*, 11, 41, 1990.

15. **Biggers, J.D., Bell, J.E., and Benos, D.J.,** Mammalian blastocyst: Transport functions in a developing epithelium, *Am. J. Physiol.*, 255, C419, 1988.

16. **Schlafke, S. and Enders, A.C.,** Cellular basis of interaction between trophoblast and uterus at implantation, *Biol. Reprod.*, 12, 41, 1975.

17.   **Jenkinson, E.J. and Wilson, I.B.,** *In vitro* studies on the control of trophoblast outgrowth in the mouse, *J. Embryol. Exp. Morphol.*, 30, 21, 1973.

18.   **Sherman, M.I. and Atienza-Samols, S.B.,** *In vitro* studies on the surface adhesiveness of mouse blastocysts, in *Human Fertilization*, Ludwig, H. and Tauber, P.F., Eds., Georg Thieme Publishers, Stuttgart, Germany, 1978, 179.

19.   **Pijnenborg, R., Robertson, W.B., Brosens, I., and Dixon, G.,** Review article: Trophoblast invasion and the establishment of haemochorial placentation in man and laboratory animals, *Placenta*, 2, 71, 1981.

20.   **Gardner, R.L.,** Origin and differentiation of extraembryonic tissues in the mouse, *Int. Rev. Exp. Pathol.*, 24, 63, 1983.

21.   **Yagel, S., Parhar, R.S., Jeffrey, J.J., and Lala, P.K.,** Normal nonmetastatic human trophoblast cells share *in vitro* invasive properties of malignant cells, *J. Cell. Phys.*, 136, 455, 1988.

22.   **Glass, R.H., Aggeler, J., Spindle, A., Pedersen, R.A., and Werb, Z.,** Degradation of extracellular matrix by mouse trophoblast outgrowths: A model for implantation, *J. Cell Biol.*, 96, 1108, 1983.

23.   **Enders, A.C., Chavez, D.J., and Schlafke, S.,** Comparison of implantation *in utero* and *in vitro*, in *Cellular and Molecular Aspects of Implantation*, Glasser, S.R. and Bullock, D.W., Eds., Plenum Press, New York, NY, 1981, p. 365.

24.   **Summers, M.C., Bhatnagar, P.R., Lawitts, J.A., and Biggers, J.D.,** Fertilization *in vitro* of mouse ova from inbred and outbred strains: Complete preimplantation embryo development in glucose-supplemented KSOM, *Biol. Reprod.*, 53, 431, 1995.

25.   **Leach, R.E., Stachecki, J.J., and Armant, D.R.,** Development of *in vitro* fertilized mouse embryos exposed to ethanol during the preimplantation period: Accelerated embryogenesis at subtoxic levels, *Teratology*, 47, 57, 1993.

26.   **Manejwala, F., Kaji, E., and Schultz, R.M.,** Development of activatable adenylate cyclase in the preimplantation mouse embryo and a role for cyclic AMP in blastocoel formation, *Cell*, 46, 95, 1986.

27.   **Stachecki, J.J., Yelian, F.D., Schultz, J.F., Leach, R.E., and Armant, D.R.,** Blastocyst cavitation is accelerated by ethanol- or ionophore-induced elevation of intracellular calcium, *Biol. Reprod.*, 50, 1, 1994.

28.   **Armant, D.R., Kaplan, H.A., and Lennarz, W.J.,** Fibronectin and laminin promote *in vitro* attachment and outgrowth of mouse blastocysts, *Dev. Biol.*, 116, 519, 1986.

29. **Yelian, F.D., Edgeworth, N.A., Dong, L.J., Chung, A.E., and Armant, D.R.**, Recombinant entactin promotes mouse primary trophoblast cell adhesion and migration through the Arg-Gly-Asp (RGD) recognition sequence, *J. Cell Biol.*, 121, 923, 1993.

30. **Armant, D.R. and Kameda, S.**, Mouse trophoblast cell invasion of extracellular matrix purified from endometrial tissue: A model for peri-implantation development, *J. Exp. Zool.*, 269, 146, 1994.

31. **Schultz, J.F. and Armant, D.R.**, Beta-1 and beta-3 class integrins mediate fibronectin binding activity at the surface of developing mouse peri-implantation blastocysts. Regulation by ligand-induced mobilization of receptor, *J. Biol. Chem.*, 270, 11522, 1995.

32. **Brown, J.J. and Whittingham, D.G.**, The dynamic provision of different energy substrates improves development of one-cell random-bred mouse embryos *in vitro*, *J. Reprod. Fert.*, 95, 503, 1992.

33. **Chatot, C.L., Ziomek, C.A., Bavister, B.D., Lewis, J.L., and Torres, I.**, An improved culture medium supports development of random-bred 1-cell mouse embryos *in vitro*, *J. Reprod. Fert.*, 86, 679, 1989.

34. **Lawitts, J.A. and Biggers, J.D.**, Overcoming the 2-cell block by modifying standard components in a mouse embryo culture medium, *Biol. Reprod.*, 45, 245, 1991.

35. **Erbach, G.T., Lawitts, J.A., Papaioannou, V.E., and Biggers, J.D.**, Differential growth of the mouse preimplantation embryo in chemically defined media, *Biol. Reprod.*, 50, 1027, 1994.

36. **Harvey, M.B. and Kaye, P.L.**, Insulin-like growth factor-1 stimulates growth of mouse preimplantation embryos *in vitro*, *Mol. Reprod. Dev.*, 31, 195, 1992.

37. **Paria, B.C., Tsukamura, H., and Dey, S.K.**, Epidermal growth factor-specific protein tyrosine phosphorylation in preimplantation embryo development, *Biol. Reprod.*, 45, 711, 1991.

38. **Rao, L.V., Wikarczuk, M.L., and Heyner, S.**, Functional roles of insulin and insulinlike growth factors in preimplantation mouse embryo development, *In Vitro Cell. Dev. Biol.*, 26, 1043, 1990.

39. **Dardik, A. and Schultz, R.M.**, Blastocoel expansion in the preimplantation mouse embryo: Stimulatory effect of TGF-alpha and EGF, *Development*, 113, 919, 1991.

40. **Paria, B.C. and Dey, S.K.**, Preimplantation embryo development *in vitro*: Cooperative interactions among embryos and role of growth factors, *Proc. Natl. Acad. Sci. USA*, 87, 4756, 1990.

41. **Schultz, G.A. and Heyner, S.**, Growth factors in preimplantation mammalian embryos, *Oxford Rev. Reprod. Biol.*, 15, 43, 1993.

42. **Graham, C.H., Lysiak, J.J., McCrae, K.R., and Lala, P.K.**, Localization of transforming growth factor-beta at the human fetal-maternal interface: Role in trophoblast growth and differentiation, *Biol. Reprod.*, 46, 561, 1992.

43.   **Hunt, J.S.,** Immunobiology of pregnancy, *Curr. Opin. Immunol.,* 4, 591, 1992.

44.   **Kapur, S., Tamada, H., Dey, S.K., and Andrews, G.K.,** Expression of insulin-like growth factor-I (IGF-I) and its receptor in the peri-implantation mouse uterus, and cell-specific regulation of IGF-I gene expression by estradiol and progesterone, *Biol. Reprod.,* 46, 208, 1992.

45.   **Brice, A.L., Cheetham, J.E., Bolton, V.N., Hill, N.C., and Schofield, P.N.,** Temporal changes in the expression of the insulin-like growth factor II gene associated with tissue maturation in the human fetus, *Development,* 106, 543, 1989.

46.   **Jokhi, P.P., Chumbley, G., King, A., Gardner, L., and Loke, Y.W.,** Expression of the colony stimulating factor-1 receptor (c-fms product) by cells at the human uteroplacental interface, *Lab. Invest.,* 68, 308, 1993.

47.   **Hofmann, G.E., Horowitz, G.M., Scott, R.T., Jr., and Navot, D.,** Transforming growth factor-alpha in human implantation trophoblast: Immunohistochemical evidence for autocrine/paracrine function, *J. Clin. Endocrin. Met.,* 76, 781, 1993.

48.   **Haimovici, F. and Anderson, D.J.,** Effects of growth factors and growth factor-extracellular matrix interactions on mouse trophoblast outgrowth *in vitro, Biol. Reprod.,* 49, 124, 1993.

49.   **Paria, B.C., Das, S.K., Huet-Hudson, Y.M., and Dey, S.K.,** Distribution of transforming growth factor alpha precursors in the mouse uterus during the periimplantation period and after steroid hormone treatments, *Biol. Reprod.,* 50, 481, 1994.

50.   **Das, S.K., Tsukamura, H., Paria, B.C., Andrews, G.K., and Dey, S.K.,** Differential expression of epidermal growth factor receptor (EGF-R) gene and regulation of EGF-R bioactivity by progesterone and estrogen in the adult mouse uterus, *Endocrinology,* 134, 971, 1994.

51.   **Das, S.K., Wang, X.N., Paria, B.C., Damm, D., Abraham, J.A., Klagsbrun, M., Andrews, G.K., and Dey, S.K.,** Heparin-binding EGF-like growth factor gene is induced in the mouse uterus temporally by the blastocyst solely at the site of its apposition: A possible ligand for interaction with blastocyst EGF-receptor in implantation, *Development,* 120, 1071, 1994.

52.   **Holliday, R.,** Quantitative genetic variation and developmental clocks, *J. Theor. Biol.,* 151, 351, 1991.

53.   **Spindle, A., Nagano, H., and Pedersen, R.A.,** Inhibition of DNA replication in preimplantation mouse embryos by aphidicolin, *J. Exp. Zool.,* 235, 289, 1985.

54.   **Valdimarsson, G. and Kidder, G.M.,** Temporal control of gap junction assembly in preimplantation mouse embryos, *J. Cell Sci.,* 108, 1715, 1995.

55. **Smith, R.K. and Johnson, M.H.,** DNA replication and compaction in the cleaving embryo of the mouse, *J. Embryol. Exp. Morphol.,* 89, 133, 1985.

56. **Howlett, S.K.,** The effect of inhibiting DNA replication in the one-cell mouse embryo, *Roux's Arch. Dev. Biol.,* 195, 499, 1986.

57. **Brown, N.A., Goulding, E.H., and Fabro, S.,** Ethanol embryotoxicity: Direct effects on mammalian embryos *in vitro, Science,* 206, 573, 1979.

58. **Priscott, P.K.,** The effects of ethanol on rat embryos developing *in vitro, Biochem. Pharmacol.,* 31, 3641, 1982.

59. **Wynter, J.M., Walsh, D.A., Webster, W.S., McEwen, S.E., and Lipson, A.H.,** Teratogenesis after acute alcohol exposure in cultured rat embryos, *Teratogen. Carcinogen. Mutagen.,* 3, 421, 1983.

60. **Sulik, K.K., Johnston, M.C., and Webb, M.A.,** Fetal alcohol syndrome: Embryogenesis in a mouse model, *Science,* 214, 936, 1981.

61. **Phillips, T.J., Gilliam, D.M., and Dudek, B.C.,** An evaluation of the role of ethanol clearance rate in the differential response of long-sleep and short-sleep mice to ethanol, *Alcohol,* 1, 373, 1984.

62. **Batt, R.D.,** Absorption, distribution and elimination of alcohol, in *Human Metabolism of Alcohol,* Vol. I, Crow, K.E. and Batt, R.D., Eds., CRC Press, Inc., Boca Raton, FL, 1989, p. 3.

63. **Watson, P.E.,** Total body water and blood alcohol levels: Updating the fundamentals, in *Human Metabolism of Alcohol,* Vol. I, Crow, K.E. and Batt, R.D., Eds., CRC Press, Inc., Boca Raton, FL, 1989, p. 41.

64. **Kaufman, M.H.,** Ethanol-induced chromosomal abnormalities at conception, *Nature,* 302, 258, 1983.

65. **Obe, G., Jonas, R., and Schmidt, S.,** Metabolism of ethanol *in vitro* produces a compound which induces sister-chromatid exchanges in human peripheral lymphocytes *in vitro*: Acetaldehyde not ethanol is mutagenic, *Mutation Res.,* 174, 47, 1986.

66. **Lau, C.F., Vogel, R., Obe, G., and Spielmann, H.,** Embryologic and cytogenetic effects of ethanol on preimplantation mouse embryos *in vitro, Reprod. Toxicol.,* 5, 405, 1991.

67. **Nielsen, L.L. and Pedersen, R.A.,** Drosophila alcohol dehydrogenase: A novel reporter gene for use in mammalian embryos, *J. Exp. Zool.,* 257, 128, 1991.

68. **Kalmus, G.W. and Buckenmaier, C.C.,** Effects of ethanol and acetaldehyde on cultured pre-implantation mouse embryos, *Experientia,* 45, 484, 1989.

69. **Wiebold, J.L. and Becker, W.C.,** *In vivo* and *in vitro* effects of ethanol on mouse preimplantation embryos, *J. Reprod. Fert.,* 80, 49, 1987.

70.   **Stachecki, J.J., Yelian, F.D., Leach, R.E., and Armant, D.R.,** Mouse blastocyst outgrowth and implantation rates following exposure to ethanol or A23187 during culture *in vitro, J. Reprod. Fert.,* 101, 611, 1994.

71.   **Ullrich, A. and Schlessinger, J.,** Signal transduction by receptors with tyrosine kinase activity, *Cell,* 61, 203, 1990.

72.   **Massague, J. and Pandiella, A.,** Membrane-anchored growth factors, *Ann. Rev. Biochem.,* 62, 515, 1993.

73.   **Casey, P.J. and Gilman, A.G.,** G protein involvement in receptor-effector coupling, *J. Biol. Chem.,* 263, 2577, 1988.

74.   **Rink, T.J. and Merritt, J.E.,** Calcium signalling, *Curr. Opin. Cell Biol.,* 2, 198, 1990.

75.   **Berridge, M.J. and Irvine, R.F.,** Inositol phosphates and cell signalling, *Nature,* 341, 197, 1989.

76.   **Lu, K.P. and Means, A.R.,** Regulation of the cell cycle by calcium and calmodulin, *Endocrine Rev.,* 14, 40, 1993.

77.   **Cohen, P.,** The structure and regulation of protein phosphatases, *Ann. Rev. Biochem.,* 58, 453, 1989.

78.   **Gentz, R., Rauscher, F.J., Abate, C., and Curran, T.,** Parallel association of fos and jun leucine zippers juxtaposes DNA binding domains, *Science,* 243, 1695, 1989.

79.   **Blackwell, T.K., Kretzner, L., Blackwood, E.M., Eisenman, R.N., and Weintraub, H.,** Sequence-specific DNA binding by the c-myc protein, *Science,* 250, 1149, 1990.

80.   **Rosen, L.B., Ginty, D.D., and Greenberg, M.E.,** Calcium regulation of gene expression, *Adv. Second Messeng. Phosphoprot. Res.,* 30, 225, 1995.

81.   **Kaufman, M.H.,** The chromosome complement of single-pronuclear haploid mouse embryos following activation by ethanol treatment, *J. Embryol. Exp. Morphol.,* 71, 139, 1982.

82.   **Colonna, R., Tatone, C., Malgaroli, A., Eusebi, F., and Mangia, F.,** Effects of protein kinase C stimulation and free calcium rise in mammalian egg activation, *Gamete Res.,* 24, 171, 1989.

83.   **Cuthbertson, K.S. and Cobbold, P.H.,** Oscillations in cell calcium. Preface, *Cell Calcium,* 12, 61, 1991.

84.   **Surani, M.A., Barton, S.C., and Norris, M.L.,** Development of reconstituted mouse eggs suggests imprinting of the genome during gametogenesis, *Nature (Lond.),* 308, 548, 1984.

85.   **Cuthbertson, K.S. and Cobbold, P.H.,** Phorbol ester and sperm activate mouse oocytes by inducing sustained oscillations in cell calcium, *Nature,* 316, 541, 1985.

86.   **Cuthbertson, K.S., Whittingham, D.G., and Cobbold, P.H.,** Free calcium increases in exponential phases during mouse oocyte activation, *Nature,* 294, 754, 1981.

87. **Fulton, B.P. and Whittingham, D.G.,** Activation of mammalian oocytes by intracellular injection of calcium, *Nature*, 273, 149, 1978.

88. **Kline, D. and Kline, J.T.,** Repetitive calcium transients and the role of calcium in exocytosis and cell cycle activation in the mouse egg, *Dev. Biol.*, 149, 80, 1992.

89. **Florman, H.M., Corron, M.E., Kim, T.D., and Babcock, D.F.,** Activation of voltage-dependent calcium channels of mammalian sperm is required for zona pellucida-induced acrosomal exocytosis, *Dev. Biol.*, 152, 304, 1992.

90. **De Felici, M., Dolci, S., and Siracusa, G.,** An increase of intracellular free calcium is essential for spontaneous meiotic resumption by mouse oocytes, *J. Exp. Zool.*, 260, 401, 1991.

91. **Ozil, J.P.,** The parthenogenetic development of rabbit oocytes after repetitive pulsatile electrical stimulation, *Development*, 109, 117, 1990.

92. **Collas, P., Fissore, R., Robl, J.M., Sullivan, E.J., and Barnes, F.L.,** Electrically induced calcium elevation, activation, and parthenogenetic development of bovine oocytes, *Mol. Reprod. Dev.*, 34, 212, 1993.

93. **Stachecki, J.J. and Armant, D.R.,** Intracellular calcium transients induced through the inositol 1, 4,5-trisphosphate receptor regulate mouse blastocyst formation, *Biol. Reprod.*, 52 (Suppl.), 94 (Abstract), 1995.

94. **Lorca, T., Abrieu, A., Means, A., and Doree, M.,** Calcium is involved through type II calmodulin-dependent protein kinase in cyclin degradation and exit from metaphase, *Biochim. Biophys. Acta*, 1223, 325, 1994.

95. **Charbonneau, M. and Grandin, N.,** A hypothesis on p34cdc2 sequestration based on the existence of calcium-coordinated changes in H^+ and MPF activities during Xenopus egg activation, *Biol. Cell*, 75, 165, 1992.

96. **Mine, T., Kojima, I., Ogata, E., and Nakamura, T.,** Comparison of effects of HGF and EGF on cellular calcium in rat hepatocytes, *Biochem. Biophys. Res. Commun.*, 181, 1173, 1991.

97. **Kuriyama, S., Ohuchi, T., Yoshimura, N., and Honda, Y.,** Growth factor-induced cytosolic calcium ion transients in cultured human retinal pigment epithelial cells, *Invest. Ophthalmol. Vis. Sci.*, 32, 2882, 1991.

98. **Hirosumi, J., Ouchi, Y., Watanabe, M., Kusunoki, J., Nakamura, T., and Orimo, H.,** Effects of growth factors on cytosolic free calcium concentration and DNA synthesis in cultured rat aortic smooth muscle cells, *Tohoku J. Exp. Med.*, 157, 289, 1989.

99. **Jaconi, M.E., Theler, J.M., Schlegel, W., Appel, R.D., Wright, S.D., and Lew, P.D.,** Multiple elevations of cytosolic-free calcium in human neutrophils: Initiation by adherence receptors of the integrin family, *J. Cell Biol.*, 112, 1249, 1991.

100.   **Schwartz, M.A.,** Spreading of human endothelial cells on fibronectin or vitronectin triggers elevation of intracellular free calcium, *J. Cell Biol.*, 120, 1003, 1993.

101.   **Schwartz, M.A. and Denninghoff, K.,** Alpha v integrins mediate the rise in intracellular calcium in endothelial cells on fibronectin even though they play a minor role in adhesion, *J. Biol. Chem.*, 269, 11133, 1994.

102.   **Hoek, J.B. and Rubin, E.,** Alcohol and membrane-associated signal transduction, *Alcohol Alcohol.*, 25, 143, 1990.

103.   **Nishizuka, Y.,** The role of protein kinase C in cell surface signal transduction and tumour promotion, *Nature*, 308, 693, 1984.

104.   **Tixier-Vidal, A.,** Cell division and differentiation of central nervous system neurons, *Ann. N. Y. Acad. Sci.*, 733, 56, 1994.

105.   **Tsien, R.W. and Tsien, R.Y.,** Calcium channels, stores, and oscillations, *Annu. Rev. Cell Biol.*, 6, 715, 1990.

106.   **Littleton, J.M.,** Effects of ethanol on membranes and their associated functions, in *Human Metabolism of Alcohol,* Vol. III, Crow, K.E. and Batt, R.D., CRC Press, Inc., Boca Raton, FL, 1989, p. 161.

107.   **Sun, G.Y. and Sun, A.Y.,** Ethanol and membrane lipids, *Alc. Clin. Exp. Res.*, 9, 164, 1985.

108.   **Lyon, R.C., McComb, J.A., Schreurs, J., and Goldstein, D.B.,** A relationship between alcohol intoxication and the disordering of brain membranes by a series of short-chain alcohols, *J. Pharmacol. Exp. Ther.*, 218, 669, 1981.

109.   **Kowalczyk, C.L., Stachecki, J.J., Schultz, J.F., Leach, R.E., and Armant, D.R.,** The effects of alcohols on murine preimplantation development: Relation to relative membrane disordering potency, *Biol. Reprod.*, 51(Suppl.), 126 (Astract), 1994.

110.   **Berridge, M.J.,** Caffeine inhibits inositol-trisphosphate-induced membrane potential oscillations in Xenopus oocytes, *Proceedings of the Royal Society of London - Series B: Biological Sciences*, 244, 57, 1991.

111.   **Berridge, M.J.,** Inositol trisphosphate and calcium signalling, *Nature*, 361, 315, 1993.

112.   **Berridge, M.J. and Dupont, G.,** Spatial and temporal signalling by calcium, *Curr. Opin. Cell Biol.*, 6, 267, 1994.

113.   **Galione, A., McDougall, A., Busa, W.B., Willmott, N., Gillot, I., and Whitaker, M.,** Redundant mechanisms of calcium-induced calcium release underlying calcium waves during fertilization of sea urchin eggs, *Science*, 261, 348, 1993.

114.   **Lee, H.C., Aarhus, R., and Walseth, T.F.,** Calcium mobilization by dual receptors during fertilization of sea urchin eggs, *Science*, 261, 352, 1993.

115. **Miyazaki, S., Shirakawa, H., Nakada, K., and Honda, Y.,** Essential role of the inositol 1,4,5-trisphosphate receptor/calcium release channel in calcium waves and calcium oscillations at fertilization of mammalian eggs, *Dev. Biol.*, 158, 62, 1993.

116. **Xu, Z., Kopf, G.S., and Schultz, R.M.,** Involvement of inositol 1,4,5-trisphosphate-mediated calcium release in early and late events of mouse egg activation, *Development*, 120, 1851, 1994.

117. **Kline, J.T. and Kline, D.,** Regulation of intracellular calcium in the mouse egg: Evidence for inositol trisphosphate-induced calcium release, but not calcium-induced calcium release, *Biol. Reprod.*, 50, 193, 1994.

118. **Feng, L., Pereira, B., and Kraus-Friedmann, N.,** Different localization of inositol 1,4,5-trisphosphate and ryanodine binding sites in rat liver, *Cell Calcium*, 13, 79, 1992.

119. **Dargie, P.J., Agre, M.C., and Lee, H.C.,** Comparison of calcium mobilizing activities of cyclic ADP-ribose and inositol trisphosphate, *Cell Regulation*, 1, 279, 1990.

120. **Worley, P.F., Baraban, J.M., Supattapone, S., Wilson, V.S., and Snyder, S.H.,** Characterization of inositol trisphosphate receptor binding in brain. Regulation by pH and calcium, *J. Biol. Chem.*, 262, 12132, 1987.

121. **Clapper, D.L., Walseth, T.F., Dargie, P.J., and Lee, H.C.,** Pyridine nucleotide metabolites stimulate calcium release from sea urchin egg microsomes desensitized to inositol trisphosphate, *J. Biol. Chem.*, 262, 9561, 1987.

122. **Galione, A., Lee, H.C., and Busa, W.B.,** Calcium-induced calcium release in sea urchin egg homogenates: Modulation by cyclic ADP-ribose, *Science*, 253, 1143, 1991.

123. **Mignery, G.A., Sudhof, T.C., Takei, K., and De Camilli, P.,** Putative receptor for inositol 1,4,5-trisphosphate similar to ryanodine receptor, *Nature*, 342, 192, 1989.

124. **Khidir, M., Stachecki, J.J., Krawetz, S.A., and Armant, D.R.,** Rapid inhibition of mRNA synthesis during preimplantation embryo development: Vital permeabilization by lysolecithin potentiates the action of alpha-amanitin, *Exp. Cell Res.*, 219, 619, 1995.

125. **Ayabe, T., Kopf, G.S., and Schultz, R.M.,** Regulation of mouse egg activation: Presence of ryanodine receptors and effects of microinjected ryanodine and cyclic ADP ribose on uninseminated and inseminated eggs, *Development*, 121, 2233, 1995.

126. **Marcu, K.B., Bossone, S.A., and Patel, A.J.,** myc function and regulation, *Ann. Rev. Biochem.*, 61, 809, 1992.

127. **Evan, G.I. and Littlewood, T.D.,** The role of c-myc in cell growth, *Curr. Opin. Genet. Dev.*, 3, 44, 1993.

128. **Pal, S.K., Crowell, R., Kiessling, A.A., and Cooper, G.M.,** Expression of proto-oncogenes in mouse eggs and preimplantation embryos, *Mol. Reprod. Dev.*, 35, 8, 1993.

129. **Paria, B.C., Dey, S.K., and Andrews, G.K.,** Antisense c-myc effects on preimplantation mouse embryo development, *Proc. Natl. Acad. Sci. USA*, 89, 10051, 1992.

130. **Leach, R.E., Schultz, J.F., Saunders, D.E., and Armant, D.R.,** c-myc protein levels in murine blastocysts exposed to ethanol, *Fert. Steril.*, 62, S69 (Abstract), 1994.

131. **Govoni, S., Trabucchi, M., Cagiano, R., and Cuomo, V.,** Alcohol and the brain: Setting the benefit/risk balance, *Alcohol*, 11, 241, 1994.

132. **Gavaler, J.S. and Van Thiel, D.H.,** The association between moderate alcoholic beverage consumption and serum estradiol and testosterone levels in normal postmenopausal women: Relationship to the literature, *Alc. Clin. Exp. Res.*, 16, 87, 1992.

133. **Langer, R.D., Criqui, M.H., and Reed, D.M.,** Lipoproteins and blood pressure as biological pathways for effect of moderate alcohol consumption on coronary heart disease, *Circulation*, 85, 910, 1992.

134. **Mitchell, J.A. and Van Kainen, B.R.,** Effects of ethanol on the decidual cell reaction in rats, *J. Reprod. Fert.*, 95, 103, 1992.

135. **Mitchell, J.A. and Van Kainen, B.R.,** Effects of alcohol on intra-uterine oxygen tension in the rat, *Alc. Clin. Exp. Res.*, 16, 308, 1992.

136. **Cameron, R.S. and Rakic, P.,** Glial cell lineage in the cerebral cortex: A review and synthesis, *GLIA*, 4, 124, 1991.

137. **Penn, L.J., Laufer, E.M., and Land, H.,** c-myc: Evidence for multiple regulatory functions, *Sem. Cancer Biol.*, 1, 69, 1990.

138. **Koskinen, P.J. and Alitalo, K.,** Role of myc amplification and overexpression in cell growth, differentiation and death, *Sem. Cancer Biol.*, 4, 3, 1993.

139. **Day, N.L. and Richardson, G.A.,** Prenatal alcohol exposure: A continuum of effects, *Semin. Perinatol.*, 15, 271, 1991.

Chapter 2

THE EFFECTS OF TIMING AND DURATION OF ALCOHOL EXPOSURE ON DEVELOPMENT OF THE FETAL BRAIN

Susan E. Maier, Wei-Jung A. Chen and James R. West

I. INTRODUCTION

While the clinical syndrome characterized by prenatal alcohol abuse has been defined (Fetal Alcohol Syndrome or FAS), the precise nature of central nervous system (CNS) deficits specifically associated with the duration and timing of alcohol exposure during pregnancy is less well defined. This stems from a number of problems specific to clinical research, such as the unreliability of self report questionnaires regarding alcohol consumption patterns and duration, the variability in the timing of alcohol consumption during pregnancy, and an underestimate of the incidence of subtle effects of alcohol such as alcohol-related birth defects (ARBDs) and fetal alcohol effects (FAEs).[1] Notwithstanding, there is an unequivocal need to answer questions relating to select parameters of gestational alcohol exposure because not all women who consume alcohol during pregnancy deliver FAS babies. What is clear from the extensive literature on this topic is that alcohol abuse during gestation produces deficits in brain structure and function; what is not clear is a consensus regarding the periods during gestation that the conceptus is most susceptible to alcohol-induced brain injury, the brain regions most susceptible, and the threshold for such effects. Research questions such as these rely less on the clinical literature and case studies and more on the basic sciences where the use of animal model systems incorporating appropriate controls can be implemented so these questions can be addressed adequately.

Within this chapter, we identify evidence for critical temporal windows of vulnerability for alcohol-induced fetal brain injuries. On the other hand, it will become apparent that there is a significant gap in the literature with regard to the issue of temporal windows of vulnerability. There are a number of factors that may impact on the interpretation of results of experimental and clinical studies and these factors will be discussed.

II. TIMING OF EVENTS IN BRAIN DEVELOPMENT

A.   A COMPARATIVE ASPECT OF BRAIN DEVELOPMENT

The general stages of brain development, from neurulation to the formation of various brain regions, are similar among many mammalian species, although the timing of brain development relative to parturition can be quite different. For example, the period of the *brain growth spurt*,[2-3] a stage during brain development characterized by accelerated synaptogenesis, neuronal proliferation and myelination, commences prenatally during the third trimester in humans and continues into early postnatal life. On the other hand, the brain growth spurt in rats occurs entirely postnatally (Figure 1). Any comparisons made between species, in terms of the events occurring during brain development, requires a proper assessment and comprehensive understanding of the course and timing of brain development for each species.

The majority of the fetal alcohol studies examining brain development has relied on animal model systems, particularly rodents, due to ethical and practical justifications. Therefore, in order to extrapolate to humans the harmful consequences of maternal alcohol drinking during the brain growth spurt that has been identified using a rat model system, the administration of alcohol to the rats must occur postnatally to comprise the period of brain growth spurt, the "third trimester equivalent" (equivalent in terms of human brain development). Much of the research examining the effects of alcohol exposure during the third trimester equivalent has been accomplished by the technique known as artificial-rearing or "pup-in-the-cup"[4-5] which allows for control over many confounding effects of alcohol-related malnutrition in this postnatal model. Similarly, in a rat model system, the first and second halves of gestation are comparable to human first and second trimesters, and the studies aimed at examining the effects of alcohol during the first and second trimesters equivalent are conducted simply by administering the alcohol to the pregnant dams. In a later section, we will present and summarize some of the clinical and experimental evidence of alcohol exposure during each of the three trimesters (or trimesters equivalent) and demonstrate that the timing of the brain development is a crucial factor in determining temporal vulnerability to alcohol insults on developing brain.

B.   A REGIONAL PERSPECTIVE OF ASYNCHRONOUS BRAIN DEVELOPMENT

The time course of neurogenesis is distinctively different from a specific brain region or a group of homogeneous neurons to another. In the previous discussion, the period of brain growth spurt was defined from a standpoint of the entire brain development, however, "growth spurts" also occur for individual regions or neuronal populations (corresponding to the period of their genesis, hence the term neurogenesis), which contributes to the regional heterogeneity of the timing of brain development. For example, in the rat, neurogenesis for the locus coeruleus occurs between gestation days (GD) 11 and 13, with the peak occurring on GD12.[7]

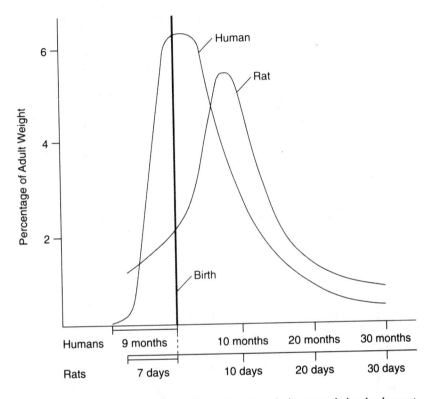

Figure 1. The *brain growth spurt* expressed as first order velocity curves during development in humans and rats. Growth is measured as the percentage of adult weight. In humans, the brain growth spurt commences during early gestation, peaks around birth and continues in early postnatal life. In rats, the growth curve ascends gradually during the latter part of gestation and peaks around the middle of the preweanling period. Unit scale: *months* in humans and *days* in rats. (From Coles, 1994, Alcohol Health and Research World.[6])

The neurogenesis for pyramidal cells in hippocampal fields CA1 and CA3 takes place between GD16-20; the peak of neurogenesis for pyramidal neurons in CA1 field is on GD18-19, while those in CA3 field the peak occurs on GD17.[8] Figure 2 illustrates the relative timing of neurogenesis of various brain regions and neuronal populations in rat brain.

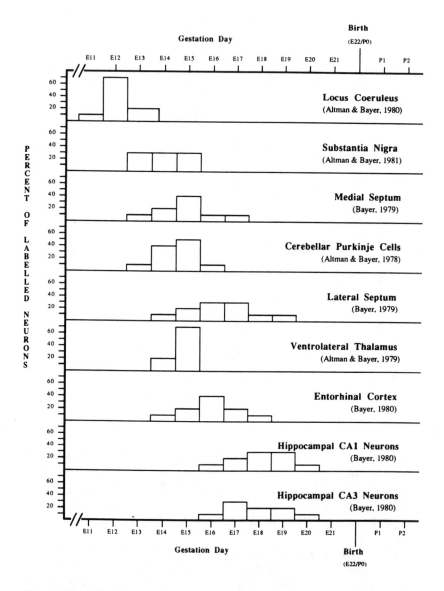

Figure 2. The timing of neurogenesis for various brain regions and neuronal populations in the rat relative to gestation age and birth, as determined by the number of neurons labeled by [³H]-thymidine autoradiography.[7-12]

Evidence indicates that the outcome of alcohol exposure during brain development may be influenced by regional vulnerability of alcohol and/or its interaction with temporal factors. Research from our laboratory demonstrates that, on a regional level, alcohol exposure during the third trimester equivalent produces a more severe depletion in cell numbers in the cerebellum[13] and olfactory bulb,[14] than in the hippocampus, [13] which supports the notion of regional vulnerability. Furthermore, within the cerebellum, Purkinje cells in lobules I and X, the early maturing regions, are more susceptible to alcohol insults than in lobules VI and VII, the late maturing regions,[15] which further demonstrates a region-specific effect and the correlation with the temporal continuity of the development and maturation of those lobules.

III. PRELIMINARY CONSIDERATIONS

A.   COMMON TERMINOLOGY
In the literature, there is a potential source of confusion in the discussion of fetal alcohol effects due to some vague terminology describing durations of alcohol exposure. The terms "acute" and "chronic" have been used to describe "short" and "long" (respectively) durations of alcohol exposure in experimental subjects. However, it is not always clear how these descriptors of alcohol exposure duration could be applied equally to studies of the conceptus, neonate or adult. For example, an acute study in the adult rat involving several days of alcohol exposure may not be interpreted as an acute study if performed on a neonatal rat with the similar duration of exposure. Thus, the operational definition of the terms "acute" and "chronic" within each individual experiment would likely lessen confusion associated with interpretation of duration of alcohol exposure on brain development.

B.   RISK FACTORS
1. Blood Alcohol Concentration
It is clear that blood alcohol concentration (BAC) is a reliable predictor of alcohol-induced fetal brain injury following third trimester equivalent alcohol exposure, thus any influence on peak BAC takes on considerable importance in the assessment of alcohol-induced fetal brain injury.[15]

Peak BAC is affected by several factors including the alcohol dose, pattern of alcohol administration (binge-like or continuous), alcohol concentration and repeated alcohol exposure. Increasing the alcohol dose under the same treatment conditions (binge-like or continuous) results in higher peak BACs than lower alcohol doses.[16-18] When alcohol is administered to rat pups in a condensed schedule, peak BAC is higher compared with a schedule where the alcohol is evenly spaced throughout a 24 hour period,[15] and this results in more severe brain injury even with a lower daily dose of alcohol. Administering alcohol to adult female rats in a highly concentrated solution (45%) resulted in a lower peak BAC than the identical dose given in lower concentrations (30%, 22.5%, 15%);[19] a phenomenon that has been found in both humans and rats[20] under various conditions. Furthermore, as adult rats are treated daily with alcohol in a binge-like paradigm, peak BAC is higher on the later days of treatment than on earlier treatment days, indicating that repeated alcohol exposure influences peak BAC in adult female rats.[19] Whether the influence of these two factors on peak BAC as determined in adult female rats could potentially affect fetal brain development remains to be determined, but the evidence to date demonstrating BAC-dependent effects in neonates on alcohol-induced brain injury certainly suggests that any influence on BAC remain important risk factors to be considered in animal model systems of alcohol exposure on fetal brain development.

2. Genetic Variation

Earlier clinical findings indicated that women of different races were unequally at risk for delivering an FAS or ARBD baby following gestational alcohol abuse.[21-22] One possible interpretation of those findings was that women of different races may metabolize alcohol differently.[23] However, a later report suggested that the findings of racial differences in the incidence of FAS babies were biased due to sampling error and discrepancy in normative data.[24] Miller et al.[25] examined the role of genotype in FAS by analyzing data collected from twins diagnosed as having FAS. They found that while some features of FAS were related to genotype, such as psychomotor retardation, posterior rotation of ears and scoliosis, the twins differed on measures of height, head circumference and interpupillary distance. Thus, while the findings on the issue of genetic variability in FAS in the clinical realm can be explained by differences in methodology, it remains an important question to address and animal model systems provide the framework for answering the question.

We have examined this issue using different inbred rat strains from the strains used to develop the NIH heterogeneous stock, two of which were the Maudsley Reactive (MR) and the Marshall (M520). When offspring from each strain were exposed to alcohol during the brain growth spurt, the MR strain was more severely affected than the M520 strain in terms of alcohol-induced cerebellar growth restrictions and cerebellar Purkinje cell loss.[26] These differences in susceptibility were not due to differences in alcohol pharmacokinetics[27] or BAC.[28]

In another study relating genetic influence to alcohol-induced brain injury, pregnant Long Sleep (LS) and Short Sleep (SS) mice were given alcohol from GD7-18, and their offspring were examined for alcohol-induced deficits.[28] Adult offspring from the alcohol-treated LS mothers were permanently affected by the gestational exposure to alcohol in terms of body and brain growth restrictions, while the SS mice were not affected by the prenatal alcohol treatment. Furthermore, an increase in embryo-lethality and severe alcohol-induced brain malformations were found in the C57BL/6J (inbred) mouse compared with the QS (Quackenbush Special; outbred) mouse strain[29] following a single intraperitoneal injection of alcohol on particular days of gestation. These findings, together with findings from the rat, show a compelling link between genotype and alcohol-induced brain injuries, and may be used to help to explain some of the individual differences in susceptibility to alcohol-induced deficits.

3. Polydrug Use

Polydrug use among pregnant women, both illicit and licit, has recently become a major concern in the field of teratology due to the potential interactive effects of these drugs on the developing fetus.[30-31] Several reports have indicated that alcohol is commonly used concurrently with other abused substances, such as cocaine and nicotine.[32-33] Experimental findings with regard to this issue have shown that concomitant exposure to alcohol and cocaine during gestation or early postnatal life predisposes the fetuses or neonates at a greater risk than exposure to each drug alone.[34-35] Similarly, exposure to alcohol and caffeine simultaneously during gestation (first two trimesters equivalent) produces an additive effect in reducing birth weight and a synergistic effect in drug associated mortality.[36]

Alcohol-induced deleterious effects may be potentiated by prescription or over-the-counter drugs, such as cimetidine (Tagamet®), ranitidine (Zantac®) and aspirin, which produce an elevation in BACs.[37-39] Not surprisingly, this polydrug-induced increase in BACs among pregnant women may subsequently result in more harm to the fetus. Recent evidence from our laboratory indicated that the elevation of BACs through polydrug use can cause detrimental effects on developing brain. Rat pups receiving an alcohol dehydrogenase inhibitor (4-methylpyrazole) in conjunction with alcohol during the brain growth spurt generated higher BACs and subsequently had more severe brain growth restrictions than those receiving alcohol alone, even though the alcohol doses administered to the rat pups were identical.[40]

IV. THE CLINICAL EVIDENCE

The consequences of fetal alcohol insults appear to be related to the timing and duration of alcohol exposure. Evidence supporting this notion is categorized and presented in the following sections based on three general characteristics of FAS; facial dysmorphology, growth retardation, microcephaly and neuropathology.

A. FACIAL DYSMORPHOLOGY

The first trimester is a period of susceptibility for the characteristic facial dysmorphology commonly observed in children diagnosed with FAS. Supporting evidence comes from various works showing that the facial dysmorphology was associated most closely with alcohol consumption during the first trimester or the period immediately prior to pregnancy.[41] Scores on the Anomalies Tally, especially the items relating directly to facial anomalies, were found to correlate significantly with the frequency of drinking, rather than the amount consumed during the first trimester.[42] Clarren *et al.*[43] found at autopsy that the FAS facial features were most prevalent in cases where the mother binge-drank throughout pregnancy. This suggests that different patterns of drinking can affect fetal outcome on this measure. In a subsequent report, Ernhart and coworkers[44] also reported that the time of conception is a critical period for alcohol-induced craniofacial anomalies. What is important about these physical facial anomalies being associated with first trimester exposure is that they were often related to difficulties in later cognitive development,[44] thus implying that the facial anomalies may indicate brain dysfunction. Although the threshold for these effects is not entirely clear, Day *et al.*[45] found that a minimum of one drink per day (0.5 ounce) for the first two months of pregnancy was sufficient to induce the characteristic facial dysmorphology. In contrast, Halmesmäki *et al.*[46] found no relation between the consumption of four drinks of alcohol weekly during the first trimester and adverse offspring outcome in their study of 530 pregnant Finnish women.

B. INTRAUTERINE   GROWTH   RETARDATION   AND MICROCEPHALY

The term intrauterine growth retardation (IUGR) has been used to describe the pattern of deficits in weight, height and head circumference at birth that are typically observed in neonates affected with FAS or FAE, as well as those who are known to have been exposed to alcohol *in utero* but have not presented with FAS or FAE.[42] IUGR caused by gestational alcohol abuse affects the individual for life; the effects are not transitory within a particular period during development and there is rarely a "catch-up" in growth to normal or near normal levels.[47] Head circumference, a component of IUGR, is the usual measure of microcephaly (definition: small head for body size). Women known to have consumed large quantities of alcohol during various portions of gestation typically have offspring affected with IUGR, including microcephaly.

While there are many studies showing effects of alcohol consumption throughout pregnancy on IUGR and microcephaly,[42,48] few have systematically attempted to determine critical periods or windows of vulnerability for these effects. From the clinical literature, it appears that IUGR is related to alcohol exposure in the latter part of gestation, rather than the early portion of fetal development. Specifically, Smith *et al.*[49] found that women who stopped drinking at midgestation (before the end of the second trimester) had babies that were no different in birth weight and head circumference from infants of women who never drank during pregnancy. Women who were identified as heavy drinkers, but who reduced their drinking during the last trimester, gave birth to infants who were similar in birth weight and head circumference to infants of women who never drank during pregnancy.[48] Furthermore, Jacobson *et al.*[50] found a significant correlation between measures of birth weight and microcephaly with alcohol consumption during the latter part of gestation, yet when those same infants were examined at 13 months of age, only body weight measures correlated significantly with latter gestation alcohol consumption. On the other hand, Coles[6] noted that microcephaly measures taken both at birth and school age (age 5-7 years) were less severe in offspring of mothers who discontinued drinking before the third trimester than offspring of mothers who continued to drink throughout pregnancy, even though weight and height measures were no longer different between these two groups of children at ages 5-7. This suggests that while the relationship between late gestation alcohol consumption and severity of body growth deficits are influenced by age (infant vs. 5-7 year old child), the severity of microcephaly occurring as a function of late gestation alcohol exposure is not changed as a result of maturation. In contrast to the results showing late gestation alcohol exposure and deficits in IUGR and microcephaly, Day et al.[45] found an association between first trimester exposure and low birth weight, and more of these babies were diagnosed as having FAS and FAE. When these same children were examined for IUGR at 18 months of age, Day et al.[47] found that the collective measures of IUGR taken at this age were related to alcohol exposure during the second and third trimesters. Thus, there appears to be difference between the manifestation of the deficit at different ages and the timing of the alcohol exposure.

C.   NEUROPATHOLOGY

The clinical evidence for fetal alcohol-induced neuropathology is sparse, mainly because most of the evidence comes from the few cases that have ended in autopsy. However, Clarren and his associates[43] published a report detailing gross morphology and histological examination of four brains from FAS children. They found scattered ectopic neurons in the white matter of all lobes of the cortex, extensive leptomeningeal neuroglial heterotopias, as well as significant absence of corpus callosum and anterior commissure. Another noteworthy study of three children and three fetuses with FAS showed extensive neuropathology at autopsy.[51] These researchers found neuropathology similar to that found by Clarren's group, including agenesis of corpus callosum, clumps of ectopic neurons both cerebellar and cerebral cortex, fused thalami (enlarged massa intermedia) and third ventricle, an absent or deformed vermis of the cerebellum, syringomyelia (enlargement of central canal of spinal cord) and defects in gyrification of the dentate gyrus and inferior olive. Furthermore, the cases at autopsy had characteristic FAS features of facial anomalies, reduced body and brain weights. These early clinical reports parallel the findings from animal experimentation on alcohol-induced alterations in neuronal circuitry.

Other evidence for neuropathology associated with alcohol exposure comes from studies exploiting the advances in neuroimaging. Using advanced Magnetic Resonance Imaging (MRI), Mattson et al.[52] found that children diagnosed with FAS have various degrees of disorganization within their brains. In the cases examined so far, they found absence or reduction in the size of the corpus callosum and reduced volumes of basal ganglia and diencephalon. Even when the overall decrease in the volume of the brain was controlled for, those structures were still smaller. Using the same imaging technique, Sowell et al.[53] found that the anterior vermal area of the cerebellum was smaller in FAS children than in age-matched controls. MRI is a useful technique for examining the brain development and structural outcomes of affected children. Part of the significance of the MRI technique, besides being a noninvasive method for visualization of brain structures, is that it provides a direction for focusing animal studies on issues related to other aspects of alcohol's effects, such as mechanisms of damage. In the past, experiments with animals provided a fruitful direction to human studies on FAS. For instance, deficits in hippocampus and cerebellum noted in animals suggested possible functional differences in learning and memory and fine motor control, respectively, in the FAS child. Hence the flow of ideas for future research now runs in both directions; the brain areas found to be affected from human MRI studies can be used by basic science researchers as a focal point to explore the nature of particular deficits in animal model systems.

V. THE EXPERIMENTAL EVIDENCE

Although the clinical literature documents examples of temporal windows of vulnerability for alcohol-induced fetal brain injury, it is still deficient in determining with any precision the full extent of the windows. In this regard, the findings from studies using animal model systems are more effective at pinpointing precise windows of vulnerability. While many experiments using animal model systems have examined alcohol-induced brain injuries resulting from exposure during one or perhaps two various major periods of brain development (e.g., early vs. late gestation), they failed to follow through and compare other periods of vulnerability using the same dependent measures and the same paradigm.[54] In this sense, the span of the known temporal windows is insufficient. In spite of this, there is some evidence for temporal windows and we peruse these findings in the following section.

A.   FACIAL ANOMALIES

The discovery of facial dysmorphology in animal models for the study of FAS came from experiments performed on mice,[55-56] nonhuman primates,[57] and beagles.[58] The facial anomalies in mice have been the product mostly of the administration of a single large dose of alcohol during a limited period within the first trimester equivalent (except see Chernoff[59] for observations of facial anomalies in mice with longer periods of exposure), while the facial anomalies in nonhuman primates and beagles occurred after lengthy gestational exposure to alcohol. Sulik and her associates[55-56] have consistently found facial anomalies in fetal offspring of C57BL/6J mice given a total of 5.8 g/kg alcohol in two intraperitoneal injections on GD7. The facial anomalies reported were remarkably similar to those found in FAS children including the characteristic decreased philtrial region, close set nasal pits, and cleft palate. Webster et al.[60] exposed pregnant C57BL/6J mice to alcohol on different days of gestation and found that facial deficits were the unique result of alcohol exposure limited to GD7 and GD8, but not GD9 or GD10 (where GD9-10 produced alcohol-induced deficits restricted to the limbs). In the QS strain of mice, Webster et al.[29] found that alcohol exposure on GD9 and GD11 had the most impact on facial anomalies and limb defects, although they remarked that these mice were more resistant to the teratogenic effects of alcohol than the C57BL/6J mouse strain.

On the other hand, Persaud and Sam[61] and Weston et al.[62] have not been able to replicate the alcohol-induced facial anomalies in the C57BL/6J, ICR (CD-1), Swiss-Webster or DBA/2J mouse strains using procedures similar to the Sulik group. Furthermore, the Weston group found spontaneous anomalies in the C57BL/6J mouse control animals, suggesting that perhaps that mouse strain is particularly susceptible to facial and ocular mutations.[63] Thus, in the absence of widespread alcohol-induced facial dysmorphology in animal model systems, the question of whether the facial mutations in animals are indicative of the clinical facial dysmorphology of FAS is still unanswered, even though its occurrence and critical period in the clinical realm is undeniable.

B. INTRAUTERINE GROWTH RETARDATION AND MICROENCEPHALY

Although there are problems associated with the interpretation of the craniofacial anomalies in animal model systems, especially related to the different mouse strains, issues relating to alcohol-induced IUGR including somatic growth deficits and microencephaly, are well studied. Nevertheless, the evidence for a deficit in body growth following alcohol exposure during the combined three trimesters equivalent is equivocal. Norton et al.[64] found a reduction in offspring body weights at postnatal day 8 (PD8) through PD38, while Borges and Lewis[65] did not. In both studies, the alcohol exposure began with the dam's consumption of an alcohol containing liquid diet from GD1 through at least PD10 (which is roughly equivalent to all three trimesters in the human). In terms of IUGR as indicated by fetal body weight or birth weight of a litter, several researchers have found a close association of this variable with alcohol exposure during primarily the second trimester equivalent. For example, Kotkoskie and Norton[66] found that pregnant rats intubated with varying doses of alcohol on GD14-15 produced fetuses with reduced body weights when examined on GD21. In addition, Blakley and Fedoroff[67] also found reduced fetal body weight on GD18 when pregnant mice were exposed to alcohol on GD11-17. In a retrospective analysis of several years worth of data, Hannigan et al.[68] showed the consistency of an alcohol-induced decrease in birth weight for alcohol treated rat pups from pregnant rats given continuous access to alcohol form GD6-20. While these various studies are important for revealing the nature of alcohol's effects on IUGR during select periods of gestation, they fail to make comparisons with other periods of gestation within the same experiment, thus are lacking in conclusiveness with regard to a critical period for alcohol-induced deficits on these particular measures.

Other studies comparing the effects of alcohol exposure during specific periods of gestation on measures of body growth have found significant alcohol-related growth deficits. Abel[69] found that alcohol exposure during the latter part of gestation in the rat (GD14-21, part of the second trimester equivalent) or throughout the entire gestation period (GD1-22) produced birth weight deficits in offspring, while exposure to an equivalent amount of alcohol during earlier portions (GD1-13) did not produce the same growth deficit. Phillips and Cragg[70] compared alcohol exposure during gestation (the second trimester equivalent) with exposure during part of the brain growth spurt (PD3-4) and found no change in body weights resulting from alcohol exposure. Using a murine model, Middaugh and Boggan[71] found that the latter stage of gestation (GD12-17) was the more critical period for alcohol-induced somatic growth deficits than earlier stages (GD5-10). However, these growth deficits were not observed at birth, but were found at later ages beginning at PD19-20, which underscores the importance of following the phenomenon through various stages of life.

Numerous experimental studies have found that alcohol exposure during the third trimester equivalent produces microencephaly (small brain for body size), even when somatic growth retardation occurs. Bonthius and West[72] found that alcohol exposure during a major portion of the brain growth spurt (PD4-9) produced microencephaly and this effect was related positively to blood alcohol concentration. Bonthius et al.[73] demonstrated further that a lower dose of alcohol during the brain growth spurt could produce more brain growth restrictions than a larger dose if it was administered in a condensed fashion, which resulted in higher peak BACs. Of greater interest is that alcohol exposure on a single day during the brain growth spurt (PD4) was found to be sufficient to induce microencephaly.[74] It is worth noting that animals with microencephaly following third trimester equivalent alcohol exposure did not suffer from body growth deficits, presumably because the artificial rearing negates the effects of alcohol on somatic growth. Noticeably, microencephaly occurs less frequently with alcohol exposure during the first two trimesters equivalent,[75-76] perhaps because brain growth is most rapid during the third trimester equivalent.

An important caveat bears on the interpretation of windows of vulnerability for body and brain growth deficits: research using animal model systems showing fetal body weight, birth weight of a litter or postnatal body growth deficits resulting from alcohol exposure during the have to be interpreted with care. From the ontogenetic development perspective, birth is the process that transforms a fetus from a "passive agent" that grows in a physically constrained uterus into an active organism.[77] Any direct comparisons of dependent measures between before and after birth require specific cautions due to the different environments that the fetus and the organism live in. Presently, the relative somatic growth rate of rat fetuses compared with the growth rate after birth is undocumented. Therefore, the utility of the trimesters equivalent term to describe discrete windows of vulnerability for alcohol-induced *body growth* deficits may be limited. As a consequence, the common use of the brain to body weight ratio indicating microencephaly may warrant the same caveat. The body and brain growth rates may be different at a specific developmental stage, given that the animal has undergone birth, where the restrictions on body growth have been significantly reduced. Thus, any discussion of issues relating to temporal windows of vulnerability for alcohol-induced effects on IUGR or microencephaly should reflect on this caution.

C.   ALTERED CIRCUITRY AND NEURONAL LOSS

It is important to recognize that alcohol-induced CNS dysfunction is not only a function of deficits in macro- or micro-neuroanatomical structures, but also the imbalance in neurochemical and other cellular functions. However, this discussion is limited to alcohol's detrimental effects on basic characteristics of neuronal migration, cytoarchitecture and neuronal loss.

Extensive studies on alcohol-induced changes in cortical neurogenesis[78-79] revealed that cortical neurogenesis was delayed by 1-2 days and that migration of cortical neurons was significantly altered in offspring of dams treated with alcohol during the second trimester equivalent.[78] Furthermore, Miller [80] found that the timing of alcohol relative to active proliferation of cortical precursor cells affects the number of surviving cells in the fetal and adult offspring. When dams were fed an alcohol-containing liquid diet during the active proliferation of either the ventricular zone (VZ; GD12-15) or subventricular zone (SZ; GD18-21), the final number of cells incorporating the marker changed as a function of timing. There was a decrease in the number of cells arising from VZ with alcohol exposure during GD12-15 and an increase in the number of cells arising from SZ with alcohol exposure during GD18-21. Thus the timing of alcohol exposure differentially affects the number of cortical cells in the adult offspring of alcohol consuming dams. Other evidence suggests that alcohol exposure during part of the second trimester equivalent (GD14-15) produces cortical brain malformations and disorganized cortical architecture in fetal (GD21) and adolescent rats.[66,81] Thus, the extent of mid-gestational alcohol exposure on cortical malformations and neuronal migration appears to be enduring.

Some of the evidence that normal patterns of brain circuitry can be altered by alcohol exposure during different periods of brain development was derived from data collected in our laboratory. The hippocampal formation is a brain structure well suited for the neuro-anatomical examination of alcohol's effects due to its orderly development, tri-lamination termination pattern of its afferents and the precise organization of various cells types within the structure, each with its own distinct period of neurogenesis. The hippocampal mossy fiber system was examined for evidence of altered circuitry, since this pathway normally arises as granule cell axons in the dentate gyrus and traverses a rather precise course making connections with pyramidal cell proximal apical dendrites as a narrow lamellar band in the *stratum lucidum* of field CA3 of the hippocampus. Alterations in this well established pathway can be detected easily. Exposure to alcohol during the third trimester equivalent not only produced an aberrant mossy fiber terminal field, but it had a greater impact on the mossy fiber organization than exposure to alcohol during the combined first and second trimesters equivalent.[82]   Importantly, alcohol exposure during either the first or second trimester equivalent alone had no detectable effect on the organization of the mossy fiber pathway.[83] Thus, it appears that not only timing (third *vs.* first or second trimester equivalent) of alcohol exposure can be harmful to this structure, but the duration of alcohol exposure also can have an impact on mossy fiber development; since no detrimental effects were found after exposure during either first or second trimester equivalent alone, but the extended duration of the combined first two trimesters equivalent produced an aberrant mossy fiber pattern. Interestingly, similar alcohol exposure had no effect on the organization of the commissural[84] or perforant pathway[85] terminal field lamellar patterns, demonstrating differential effects within the hippocampal formation.

Neuronal loss is another manifestation of alcohol's deleterious effects during different periods of brain development, and certain neurons in the hippocampus are differentially vulnerable to alcohol-induced injury. West *et al.*[86] demonstrated that continuous exposure to alcohol during the brain growth spurt resulted in no loss of hippocampal CA1 or CA3 cells, but a small significant increase in dentate gyrus granule cells. However, when the alcohol was given in a condensed schedule such that high peak BACs were achieved, the number of CA1 hippocampal cells were significantly reduced compared with the number of pyramidal cells in CA3, while the dentate granule cells were unaffected.[15] Although both studies demonstrated a loss of cells with exposure restricted to the third trimester equivalent, other research has demonstrated that the hippocampal CA1 cells were vulnerable to injury during the second trimester equivalent, a period of hippocampal pyramidal cell neurogenesis.[76]

The cerebellum shares some characteristics with the hippocampus in terms of features well suited to examine the effects of alcohol. Purkinje cells of the cerebellum are generated prenatally (GD14-18),[11] while cerebellar granule cells are generated primarily postnatally.[87] Marcussen *et al.*[88] compared the effects of alcohol during the period of Purkinje cell neurogenesis (part of the second trimester equivalent) with the period of Purkinje cell differentiation (part of the third trimester equivalent) and found that cerebellar Purkinje cells are more sensitive to alcohol insult during the period of early differentiation than the period of their neurogenesis. Using exposure to alcohol vapor, Phillips and Cragg[70] found the same pattern of Purkinje cell loss in the neonatal period compared with prenatal or adult exposure, where two days of alcohol exposure during the brain growth spurt (PD3-4) produced more Purkinje cell loss than two weeks of alcohol exposure given during a time encompassing Purkinje cell neurogenesis (GD7-21). The extent of Purkinje cell loss can be further narrowed to a single day of alcohol exposure during the third trimester equivalent, where Goodlett and his associates[74] found a significant loss of Purkinje cells in the brains of rat pups exposed to alcohol on PD4 and examined at PD10.

However, the loss of Purkinje cells as a function of PD4 alcohol exposure is not simply a function of when the brains were examined, since Hamre and West[89] found that Purkinje cell loss with third trimester equivalent exposure was observed at PD21. It is significant that the period of Purkinje cell neurogenesis is entirely prenatal, so there is no chance of recovery of normal Purkinje cell numbers under such conditions. In their noteworthy study, they found that alcohol exposure during PD4-5 resulted in the most severe Purkinje cell loss compared with other periods of alcohol exposure during the third trimester equivalent, such as PD6-7 and PD8-9, even though BACs were the same for the various times of alcohol exposure. While that paper demonstrated effects of timing of alcohol on loss of Purkinje cells in the vermal cerebellum, it focused on the density of Purkinje cells. Since density measures can be influenced by tissue shrinkage, other methods that incorporate the volume of the structure into the final estimate of cell number are an improvement. A more recent study has used unbiased stereological cell counting techniques to corroborate the Hamre and West study by showing that Purkinje cell loss arises with alcohol exposure on PD4-6, but not PD7-9 of the third trimester equivalent.[90] Unfortunately, neither study examined the period prior to PD4 for alcohol-induced Purkinje cell loss, thus a lower boundary for the period of susceptibility cannot be precisely determined.

VII. SUMMARY

Examples from the literature which indicate that there are particular periods during gestation when the fetus is most susceptible to certain CNS damage have been highlighted. Unfortunately, at present there are no definitive answers to the problem of temporal windows of vulnerability since there are too few studies in the literature that have systematically examined this question. While the accuracy of temporal windows is still vague, there are hints at critical periods for a few of the characteristics of FAS.

It is likely that the distinctive FAS facial dysmorphology is related to the time of conception or first trimester alcohol exposure. The clinical data are derived from cases of FAS in populations of women reporting heavy alcohol consumption during this period. This is alarming since a majority of women who abuse alcohol may not know they are pregnant for the first four to six weeks of gestation. Therefore, women contemplating pregnancy who are known to be heavy alcohol abusers should be counseled with regard to the risks of facial anomalies in their offspring should they continue their drinking habits into the first trimester.

In addition to the distinct facial anomalies of FAS, other hallmark features are IUGR and somatic growth deficits, and these deficits seem to be related to alcohol consumption during the latter part of gestation. In the clinical literature, this evidence is acquired by the comparison of women who consumed alcohol throughout the three trimesters of pregnancy with those who stopped consumption during the second trimester. Although this comparison shows a benefit of cessation of alcohol, it lacks experimental rigor. On the other hand, experiments using animal model systems have shown IUGR and somatic growth deficits following late gestation alcohol exposure only. Whether the late gestation period in the rat represents key developmental events related to the second trimester equivalent or simply the period immediately prior to parturition in terms of body growth is open to question. Even though the determination of a critical period of vulnerability for IUGR or somatic growth deficits in an animal model system may not be easily obtainable, the merits of terminating alcohol consumption as soon as possible after the determination of pregnancy seems to be the best counsel for women who are heavy drinkers in light of the available clinical data.

There is consistency within the clinical and experimental fields regarding the critical period of vulnerability for microcephaly in humans and microencephaly in animal model systems. The clinical literature shows microcephaly following alcohol consumption for the entire period of gestation (all three trimesters) and a beneficial effect of cessation of drinking after the second trimester on measures of head circumference, thus implicating the third trimester as a critical period for this measure. Nevertheless, the number of clinical studies that specifically examined microcephaly are sparse, and most of the data showing a critical period for microcephaly are derived from studies of IUGR. On the other hand, the experimental literature shows microencephaly most often occurs following alcohol exposure during the brain growth spurt, or third trimester equivalent. Given the striking results from the experimental data showing microencephaly with third trimester equivalent alcohol exposure, and the corresponding hint in the clinical literature with respect to benefits of cessation of drinking prior to the third trimester for measures of microcephaly, it is likely that the critical period is the third trimester for this measure.

The concordance with respect to critical periods for neuro-pathology between the clinical and experimental literature is less well defined. This likely stems from a lack of clinical cases that end in autopsy accompanied by adequate maternal drinking histories. The usefulness of MRI technique for addressing questions related to critical periods will undoubtedly be exploited, but the studies to date have not examined this research question and thus this literature is in its infancy. On the other hand, the experimental findings are laudatory in their precision with which critical periods of vulnerability have been found for selected neuronal populations, especially hippocampus, cerebellum and cerebral cortex. The quest for answers to temporal windows should not be considered complete until a broad spectrum of windows of vulnerability for various neuro-pathologies can be adequately identified. In this respect, the MRI technique used for detecting human neuropathology resulting from gestational alcohol exposure can help to drive the future directions of the experimental field.

Although it has been speculated there are multiple mechanisms for alcohol's injurious effects on fetal brain development, none have been examined thoroughly. There are several possibilities, and it is likely that alcohol acts through different mechanisms at different periods of development, accounting for the temporal vulnerability of fetal brain injury.[91] Experiments addressing the issue of temporal vulnerability will help address questions about mechanisms by narrowing the critical window for neuropathology to a particular period of susceptibility. Such advances could help in the identification of treatments that could reverse the cellular and molecular events that cause these neuropathologies during that particular window. Furthermore, knowing the precise timing of alcohol's most devastating effects on fetal brain development would obviously be of benefit for counseling women seeking pregnancy regarding the relative risks for fetal malformations with consumption of alcohol during certain periods of gestation. However, until we know with some degree of confidence when such windows of vulnerability occur, experiments addressing questions of mechanisms will have to continue unaided by this critical information.

(Preparation of this chapter was supported by NIAAA grant #10090 to JRW)

REFERENCES

1. **Day, N.L.,** Effects of prenatal alcohol exposure, in *Maternal Substance Abuse and the Developing Nervous System*, Zagon, I.S. and Slotkin, T.A., Academic Press, Boston, 1992, chap.3.
2. **Dobbing, J. and Sands, J.,** The quantitative growth and development of the human brain, *Arch. Dis. Child.*, 48, 757, 1973.
3. **Dobbing, J. and Sands, J.,** Comparative aspects of the brain growth spurt, *Early Hum. Dev.*, 3, 79, 1979.

4.   **Diaz, J.,** Experimental rearing of rat pups using chronic gastric fistulas, in *Developmental Psychobiology: New Methods and Changing concepts*, Shair, H.N., Barr, G.A. and Hofer, M.A., Eds., Oxford University Press, New York, 1991, chap.16.

5.   **West, J.R.,** Use of pup in the cup model to study brain development, *J. Nutr.*, 123, 382, 1993.

6.   **Coles, C.,** Critical periods for prenatal alcohol exposure: Evidence from animal and human studies. *Alcohol Health Res. World*, 18, 22, 1994.

7.   **Altman, J. and Bayer, S.A.,** Development of the brainstem of the rat. VI. Quantitative study of the time of origin of neurons in the brainstem tegmentum, *J. Comp. Neurol.*, 194, 905, 1980.

8.   **Bayer, S.A.,** Development of hippocampal region in the rat. I. Neurogenesis examined with [^{3}H]-thymidine autoradiography, *J. Comp. Neurol.*, 190, 87, 1980.

9.   **Altman, J. and Bayer, S.A.,** Development of the brainstem of the rat. VI. Quantitative study of the origin of neurons in the midbrain tegmentum. *J. Comp. Neurol.*, 198, 677, 1981.

10. **Bayer, S.A.,** The development of the septal region in the rat. I. Neurogenesis examined with [^{3}H]-thymidine autoradiography, *J. Comp. Neurol.*, 183, 89, 1979.

11. **Altman, J. and Bayer, S.A.,** Prenatal development of the cerebellar system in the rat. I. Cytogenesis and histogenesis of the deep nuclei and the cortex of the cerebellum, *J. Comp. Neurol.*, 179, 23, 1978.

12. **Altman, J. and Bayer, S.A.,** Development of the brainstem of the rat. IV. Quantitative study of the time of origin of neurons in the pontine region. *J. Comp. Neurol.*, 188, 455, 1979.

13. **Bonthius, D.J. and West, J.R.,** Acute and long-term neuronal deficits in the rat olfactory bulb following alcohol exposure during the brain growth spurt, *Neurotoxicol. Teratol.*, 13, 611, 1991.

14. **Bonthius, D.J. and West, J.R.,** Permanent neuronal deficits in rats exposed to alcohol during the brain growth spurt, *Teratology*, 44, 147, 1991.

15. **Bonthius, D.J. and West, J.R.,** Alcohol-induced neuronal loss in developing rats: increased brain damage with binge exposure, *Alc. Clin. Exp. Res.*, 14, 107, 1990.

16. **West, J.R., Black, A.C., Jr., Reimann, P.C., and Alkana, R.L.,** Polydactyly and polysyndactyly induced by prenatal exposure to ethanol, *Teratology*, 24, 13, 1981.

17. **Abel, E.L.,** Prenatal effects of alcohol on adult learning in rats, *Pharmacol. Biochem. Behav.*, 10, 239, 1979.

18. **Randall, C.L. and Taylor, W.J.,** Prenatal ethanol exposure in mice: teratogenic effects. *Teratology*, 19, 305, 1979.

19. **Maier, S.E., Strittmatter, M.A., Chen, W.-J.A., and West, J.R.,** Changes in blood alcohol levels as a function of alcohol concentration and repeated alcohol exposure in adult female rats: Potential risk factors for alcohol-induced fetal brain injury, *Alc. Clin. Exp. Res.,* in press.

20. **Roine, R.P., Gentry, R.T., Lim, R.T., Jr., Baraona, E., and Lieber, C.S.,** Effect of concentration of ingested ethanol on blood alcohol levels, *Alc. Clin. Exp. Res.,* 15, 734, 1991.

21. **Sokol, R.J., Ager, J., Martier, S., Debanne, S., Ernhart, C., Kuzma, J., and Miller, S.I.,** Significant determinants of susceptibility to alcohol teratogenicity. *Ann. N.Y. Acad. Sci.,* 477, 87, 1986.

22. **Chavez, G.F., Corder, J.F., and Becerra, J.E.,** Leading major congenital malformation among minority groups in the US, *MMWR,* 37, 17, 1988.

23. **Sokol, R.J., Smith, M., Ernhart, C.B., Baumann, R., Martier, S.S., Ager, J.W., and Morrow-Tlucak, M.,** A genetic basis for alcohol related birth defects (ARBD)? *Alc. Clin. Exp. Res.,* 13, 343, 1989.

24. **Abel, E.L. and Sokol, R.J.,** A revised conservative estimate of the incidence of FAS and its economic impact, *Alc. Clin. Exp. Res.,* 15, 514, 1991.

25. **Miller, M., Isreaal, J., and Cutton, J.,** Fetal alcohol syndrome, *J. Pediatr. Opthalom. Strab.,* 18, 6, 1981.

26. **Maier, S.E., Mahoney, J.C., Goodlett, C.R., and West, J.R.,** Strain differences in susceptibility to alcohol-induced Purkinje cell loss demonstrated using unbiased stereological counting methods, *Alc. Clin. Exp. Res.,* 18, 437, 1994.

27. **Goodlett, C.R., Nichols, J.M., and West, J.R.,** Strain differences in susceptibility to alcohol-induced brain growth restriction are not accounted for by differences in alcohol elimination rates, *Alc. Clin. Exp. Res.,* 15, 343, 1991.

28. **Goodlett, C.R., Gilliam, D.M., Nichols, J.M., and West, J.R.,** Genetic influences on brain growth restriction induced by developmental exposure to alcohol, *Neurotoxicology,* 10, 321, 1989.

29. **Webster, W.S., Walsh, D.A., Lipson, A.H., and McEwen, S.E.,** Teratogenesis after acute alcohol exposure in inbred and outbred mice, *Neurobehav. Toxicol.,* 2, 227, 1980.

30. **American Public Health Association,** Effects of *in utero* exposure to street drugs, *Am. J. Public Health,* 83 (suppl.), 1993.

31. **Day, N.L. and Richardson, G.A.,** Comparative teratogenicity of alcohol and other drugs, *Alcohol Health Res. World,* 18, 42, 1994.

32. **Chasnoff, I.J, Harvey, J., Landress, A.C.S.W., and Barrett, M.E.,** The prevalence of illicit-drug or alcohol use during pregnancy and discrepancies in mandatory reporting in Pinellas County, Florida, *N. Engl. J. Med.,* 322, 1202, 1990.

33.   Miller, N.S., The pharmacology of multiple drug and alcohol addiction, in *The Pharmacology of Alcohol and Drugs of Abuse and Addiction*, Miller, N.S., Ed., Springer-Verlag, New York, 1991.

34.   Chen, W.-J.A., Andersen, K.H., and West, J.R., Alcohol-induced brain growth restrictions (microencephaly) were not affected by concurrent exposure to cocaine during the brain growth spurt, *Teratology*, 50, 250, 1994.

35.   Church, M.W., Dintcheff, B.A., and Gessner, R.K., The interactive effects of alcohol and cocaine on maternal and fetal toxicity in Long-Evans rat, *Neurotoxicol. Teratol.*, 10, 355, 1988.

36.   Hannigan, J.H., Effects of prenatal exposure to alcohol plus caffeine in rats: Pregnancy outcome and early offspring development, *Alc. Clin. Exp. Res.*, 19, 238, 1995.

37.   Caballeria, J., Baraona, E., Rodamilans, M., and Lieber, C.S., Effects of cimetidine on gastric alcohol dehydrogenase activity and blood ethanol levels, *Gastroenterology*, 96, 388, 1989.

38.   Hernández-Munõz, R., Caballeria, J., Baraona, E., Uppal, R., Greenstein, R., and Lieber, C.S., Human gastric alcohol dehydrogenase: Its inhibition by H_2-receptor antagonists, and its effect on the bioavailability of ethanol, *Alc. Clin. Exp. Res.*, 14, 946, 1990.

39.   Roine, R.P., Gentry, R.T., Hernández-Munõz, R., Baraona, E., and Lieber, C.S., Aspirin increases blood alcohol concentrations in humans after ingestion of ethanol, *JAMA*, 264, 2406, 1990.

40.   Chen, W.-J.A., McAlhany Jr., R.E., and West, J.R., Alcohol dehydrogenase inhibitor, 4-methylpyrazole, augments ethanol-induced microencephaly in neonatal rats, *Alcohol*, in press.

41.   Graham, J.M., Hanson, J.W., Darby, B.L., Barr, H.M., and Streissguth, A.P., Independent dysmorphology evaluations at birth and 4 years of age for children exposed to varying amounts of alcohol *in utero*, *Pediatrics*, 81, 772, 1988.

42.   Ernhart, C.B., Wolf, A.W., Linn, P.L., Sokol, R.J., Kennard, M.J., and Filipovich, H.F., Alcohol-related birth defects: Syndromal anomalies, intrauterine growth retardation, and neonatal behavioral assessment, *Alc. Clin. Exp. Res.*, 9, 447, 1985.

43.   Clarren, S.K., Alvord, E.C., Jr., Sumi, S.M., Streissguth, A.P., and Smith, D.W., Brain malformations related to prenatal exposure to alcohol, *J. Pediatr.*, 92, 64, 1978.

44.   Ernhart, C.B., Sokol, R.J., Martier, S., Moron, P., Nadler, D., Ager, J.W., and Wolf, A., Alcohol teratogenicity in the human: A detailed assessment of specificity, critical period, and threshold, *Am. J. Obstet. Gynecol.*, 156, 33, 1987.

45. Day, N.L., Jasperse, D., Richardson, G., Robles, N., Sambamoorthi, U., Taylor, P., Scher, M., Stoffer, D., and Cornelius, M., Prenatal exposure to alcohol: Effect on infant growth and morphologic characteristics, *Pediatrics*, 84, 536, 1989.

46. Halmesmäki, E., Raivio, K.O., and Ylikorkala, O., Patterns of alcohol consumption during pregnancy, *Obstet. Gynecol.*, 69, 594, 1987.

47. Day, N.L., Goldschmidt, L., Robles, N., Richardson, G., Cornellius, M., Taylor, P., Geva, D., and Stoffer, D., Prenatal alcohol exposure and offspring growth at 18 months of age: The predictive validity of two measures of drinking, *Alc. Clin. Exp. Res.*, 15, 914, 1991.

48. Rosett, H.L., Weiner, L., Lee, A., Zuckerman, B., Dooling, E., and Oppenheimer, E., Patterns of alcohol consumption and fetal development, *Obstet. Gynecol.*, 61, 539, 1983.

49. Smith, I.E., Coles, C.D., Lancaster, J., Fernhoff, P.M., and Falek, A., The effect of volume and duration of prenatal ethanol exposure on neonatal physical and behavioral development, *Neurobehav. Toxicol. Teratol.*, 8, 375, 1986.

50. Jacobson, J.L., Jacobson, S.W., and Sokol, R.J., Effects of prenatal exposure to alcohol, smoking, and illicit drugs on postpartum somatic growth, *Alc. Clin. Exp. Res.*, 18, 317, 1994.

51. Pieffer, J., Majewski, F., Fischbach, H., Bierich, J.R., and Volk, B., Alcohol embryo- and feto-pathology, *J. Neurol. Sci.*, 41, 125, 1979.

52. Mattson, S.N., Riley, E.P., Jernigan, T.L., Garcia, A., Kaneko, W.M., Ehlers, C.L., and Jones, K.L., A decrease in the size of the basal ganglia following prenatal alcohol exposure: A preliminary report, *Neurotoxicol. Teratol.*, 16, 283, 1994.

53. Sowell, E.R., Mattson, S.N., Riley, E.R., and Jernigan, T.L., A reduction in the area of the anterior cerebellar vermis in children exposed to alcohol prenatally, *Alc. Clin. Exp. Res.*, 19 (Suppl.), 53A, 1995.

54. West, J.R., Fetal alcohol-induced brain damage and the problem of determining temporal vulnerability: A review, *Alc. Drug Res.*, 7, 423, 1987.

55. Sulik, K.K., Johnston, M.C., and Webb, M.A., Fetal alcohol syndrome: Embryogenesis in a mouse model, *Science*, 214, 936, 1981.

56. Sulik, K.K. and Johnston, M.C., Sequence of developmental alterations following acute ethanol exposure in mice: Craniofacial features of the fetal alcohol syndrome, *Am. J. Anat.*, 166, 257, 1983.

57. Clarren, S.K. and Bowden, D.M., Fetal alcohol syndrome: A new primate model for binge drinking and its relevance to human ethanol teratogenesis. *J. Pediatr.*, 101, 819, 1982.

58. Ellis, F.W. and Pick, J.R., An animal model of the fetal alcohol syndrome in beagles, *Alc. Clin. Exp. Res.*, 4, 123, 1980.

59.   **Chernoff, G.F.,** The fetal alcohol syndrome in mice: An animal model, *Teratology*, 15, 223, 1977.

60.   **Webster, W.S., Walsh, D.A., McEwen, S.E., and Lipson, A.H.,** Some teratogenic properties of ethanol and acetaldehyde in C57BL/6J mice: Implications for the study of the fetal alcohol syndrome, *Teratology,* 27, 231, 1983.

61.   **Persaud, T.V.N. and Sam, G.O.,** Prenatal influence of alcohol following a single exposure in two inbred strains of mice, *Ann. Anat.*, 174, 301, 1992.

62.   **Weston, W.M., Greene, R.M., Uberti, M., and Pisano, M.M.,** Ethanol effects on embryonic craniofacial growth and development: Implications for study of the fetal alcohol syndrome, *Alc. Clin. Exp. Res.*, 18, 177, 1994.

63.   **Robinson, M.L., Holmgren, A., and Dewey, M.J.,** Genetic control of ocular morphogenesis: Defective lens development associated with ocular anomalies in C57BL/6 mice, *Exp. Eye Res.*, 56, 7, 1993.

64.   **Norton, S., Terranova, P., Na, J.Y., and Sancho-Tello, M.,** Early motor development and cerebral cortical morphology in rats exposed perinatally to alcohol, *Alc. Clin. Exp. Res.*, 12, 130, 1988.

65.   **Borges, S. and Lewis, P.D.,** A study of alcohol effects on the brain during gestation and lactation, *Teratology*, 25, 283, 1982.

66.   **Kotkoskie, L.A. and Norton, S.,** Prenatal brain malformations following acute ethanol exposure in the rat, *Alc. Clin. Exp. Res.*, 12, 831, 1988.

67.   **Blakley, P.M. and Fedoroff, S.,** Effects of prenatal alcohol exposure on neural cells in mice, *Int. J. Dev. Neurosci.*, 3, 69, 1985.

68.   **Hannigan, J.H., Abel, E.L., and Kruger, M.L.,** "Population" characteristics of birthweight in an animal model of alcohol-related developmental effects, *Neurotoxicol. Teratol.*, 15, 97, 1993.

69.   **Abel, E.L.,** Effects of ethanol exposure during different gestation weeks of pregnancy on maternal weight gain and intrauterine growth retardation in the rat, *Neurobehav. Toxicol.*, 1, 145, 1979.

70.   **Phillips, S.C. and Cragg, B.G.,** A change in susceptibility of rat cerebellar Purkinje cells to damage by alcohol during fetal, neonatal and adult life, *Neuropathol. Appl. Neurobiol.*, 8, 441, 1982.

71.   **Middaugh, L.D. and Boggan, W.O.,** Postnatal growth deficits in prenatal ethanol exposed mice: Characteristics and critical periods, *Alc. Clin. Exp. Res.*, 15, 919, 1991.

72.   **Bonthius, D.J. and West, J.R.,** Blood alcohol concentration and microencephaly: A dose-response study in the neonatal rat. *Teratology,* 37, 223, 1988.

73.   **Bonthius, D.J., Goodlett, C.R., and West, J.R.,** Blood alcohol concentration and severity of microencephaly in neonatal rats depend on the pattern of alcohol administration, *Alcohol*, 5, 209, 1988.

74. **Goodlett, C.R., Marcussen, B.L., and West, J.R.,** A single day of alcohol exposure during the brain growth spurt induces brain weight restriction and cerebellar Purkinje cell loss, *Alcohol*, 7, 107, 1990.

75. **Hammer, R.P., Jr. and Scheibel, A.B.,** Morphologic evidence for a delay of neural maturation in fetal alcohol exposure, *Exp. Neurol.*, 74, 587, 1981.

76. **Barnes, D.E. and Walker, D.W.,** Prenatal alcohol exposure permanently reduces the number of pyramidal neurons in the rat hippocampus, *Dev. Brain Res.*, 1, 333, 1981.

77. **Oppenheim, R.W.,** Ontogenetic adaptations and retrogressive processes in the development of the nervous system and behavior: A neuroembryological perspective, in *Maturation and Development: Biological and Psychological Perspectives*, Connolly, K.J. and Prechtl, H.F.R., J.B. Lippincott Co., Philadelphia, 1981, chap.5.

78. **Miller, M.W.,** Effect of prenatal exposure to ethanol on the development of cerebral cortex: I. neuronal generation, *Alc. Clin. Exp. Res.*, 12, 440, 1988.

79. **Miller, M.W.,** Migration of cortical neurons is altered by gestational exposure to alcohol, *Alc. Clin. Exp. Res.*, 17, 304, 1993.

80. **Miller, M.W.,** Limited ethanol exposure selectively alters the proliferation of cortical precursor cells, *Alc. Clin. Exp. Res.*, 19 (suppl), 51A, 1995.

81. **Kotkoskie, L.A. and Norton, S.,** Cerebral cortical morphology and behavior in rats following acute prenatal ethanol exposure, *Alc. Clin. Exp. Res.*, 13, 776, 1989.

82. **West, J.R. and Hamre, K.M.,** Effects of alcohol exposure during different periods of development: Changes in hippocampal mossy fibers, *Dev. Brain Res.*, 17, 280, 1985.

83. **West, J.R., Hodges, C.A., and Black, A.C.,** Prenatal exposure to ethanol alters the organization of hippocampal mossy fibers in rats, *Science,* 211, 957, 1981.

84. **Dewey, S.L. and West, J.R.,** Perforant pathway lamination in the dentate gyrus is unaffected by prenatal ethanol exposure, *Alcohol,* 2, 221, 1985.

85. **Dewey, S.L. and West, J.R.,** Organization of the commissural projection to the dentate gyrus is unaltered by heavy ethanol exposure during gestation, *Alcohol*, 2, 617, 1985.

86. **West, J.R., Hamre, K.M., and Cassell, M.D.,** Effects of ethanol exposure during the third trimester equivalent on neuron number in rat hippocampus and dentate gyrus, *Alc. Clin. Exp. Res.,* 10, 190, 1986.

87. **Altman, J.,** Autoradiographic and histological studies of postnatal neurogenesis. III. Dating the time of production and onset of differentiation of cerebellar microneurons in rats, *J. Comp. Neurol.*, 136, 269, 1969.

88.   **Marcussen, B.L., Goodlett, C.R., Mahoney, J.C., and West, J.R.,**
       Developing rat Purkinje cells are more vulnerable to alcohol-induced
       depletion during differentiation than during neurogenesis, *Alcohol*, 11,
       147, 1994.
89.   **Hamre, K.M. and West, J.R.,** The effects of the timing of ethanol
       exposure during the brain growth spurt on the number of cerebellar
       Purkinje and granule cell nuclear profiles, *Alc. Clin. Exp. Res.*, 17, 610,
       1993.
90.   **Lundahl, K.R. and Goodlett, C.R.,** The extent of cerebellar Purkinje
       cell loss induced by binge-like alcohol exposure in neonatal rats
       depends on both the timing and duration of exposure, *Alc. Clin. Exp.
       Res.*, 19 (suppl), 52A, 1995.
91.   **West, J.R.,   Chen, W-J.A., and Pantazis, N.J.,** Fetal alcohol
       syndrome: The vulnerability of the developing brain and possible
       mechanisms of damage, *Metabol. Brain Dis.*, 9, 291, 1994.

Chapter 3

BRAIN ANOMALIES IN
FETAL ALCOHOL SYNDROME

Sarah N. Mattson and Edward P. Riley

Fetal alcohol syndrome (FAS) is characterized by a triad of features: (1) pre- and/or postnatal growth deficiency; (2) a specific pattern of craniofacial malformations; and (3) evidence of central nervous system dysfunction.[1] Although it is clear that alcohol is a physical and behavioral teratogen, its teratogenic effects on the developing brain have been difficult to quantify. Certainly, the multitude of behavioral and cognitive studies[2-6] should allow an inference about the state of the brain, but specific details about structural brain damage in humans are few. There is no question that prenatal exposure to high levels of alcohol affects the developing brain, however whether there is a specific pattern of brain damage is still in question. This chapter will address the brain anomalies that have been reported in individuals and groups with prenatal alcohol exposure and whether such a pattern or profile of brain damage exists. Early autopsy studies and more recent imaging studies will be discussed.

The first report of structural brain damage following prenatal alcohol exposure was in an infant with FAS who died shortly after birth.[7-9] The autopsy revealed extensive brain abnormalities including microcephaly, migration anomalies, callosal dysgenesis, and a "massive" neuroglial, leptomeningeal heterotopia covering the left hemisphere. A second infant, born to a binge drinker, was reported soon after the first.[9] This child died at 10 days of age and autopsy revealed severe hydrocephalus, as well as a thinned corpus callosum, extremely small cerebellum, and a large neuroglial, leptomeningeal heterotopia. Since then, other reports of structural central nervous system defects in children exposed to alcohol during gestation have included brainstem and cerebellar anomalies, migration errors, absent olfactory bulbs, and hydrocephalus, meningomyelocele, and porencephaly.[10-14] Clarren[14] summarized the results of 16 autopsies,[10,12-13,15] reporting a wide range of neuropathology, including evidence of severe CNS disorganization, agenesis of the corpus callosum and anterior commissure, neuroglial heterotopias, hydrocephalus, and microcephaly. Currently, reports of 25 autopsies appear in the literature and a summary of the results of 23 of these appears in Table 1. An additional autopsy report noted "no important abnormalities" of the brain[16] while another, mentioned by Clarren in a letter to the editor, notes an Italian case of anencephaly in a child with FAS.[17] Many[12,14] believe that the nature of the brain damage resulting from prenatal alcohol exposure is extremely variable, as no specific pattern of structural defect is typically found. However, more recent advances in brain imaging technology have provided data to the contrary by allowing a more systematic view of alcohol's teratogenicity.

Table 1

Summary of the neuropathology reported in children with fetal alcohol syndrome (FAS) or prenatal exposure to alcohol (PEA)

Abnormality	Method	Notes
Hydranencephaly	autopsy[12]	This report was questioned by Clarren, 1986
Anencephaly	autopsy[17] sonography[55]	2 cases
Holoprosencephaly	autopsy[56] autopsy[20] ultrasound/CT[20] ultrasound[20]	alobar semilobar semilobar
Cerebral dysgenesis	autopsy[10] autopsy[15] autopsy[13] autopsy[12] autopsy[57] MRI[19] MRI/autopsy[24] MRI[26]	2 cases 2 cases 4 cases "multifocal encephalopathy"
Abnormal neural/ glial migration	autopsy[10] autopsy[15] autopsy[13] autopsy[12] autopsy[57] autopsy[24]	3 cases 5 cases 3 cases
Hydrocephaly	autopsy[10] autopsy[12] n/a[55]	2 cases 2 cases
Microcephaly/ microencephaly	autopsy[10] autopsy[15] autopsy[13] autopsy[12] autopsy[32] autopsy[57] autopsy[20] MRI/autopsy[24] MRI[27] MRI[29] MRI[30]	5 cases 2 cases 2 cases/PEA group study

Abnormality	Method	Notes
Enlarged Ventricles	autopsy[10]	
	autopsy[15]	
	CT[11]	
	autopsy[12]	
	autopsy[57]	2 cases
	MRI[27]	
	MRI26	
Reduced/absent Ventricles	MRI/autopsy[24]	
	autopsy[12]	
Fused Ventricles	autopsy[12]	2 cases
Agenesis of corpus callosum	autopsy[10]	
	autopsy[13]	
	utopsy[12]	
	autopsy[32]	partial
	MRI/autopsy[24]	possible
	MRI[27]	
	MRI[31]	2 cases
Agenesis of anterior commissure	autopsy[10]	
	autopsy[12]	
	MRI[24]	
Basal ganglia	autopsy[12]	
	autopsy [13]	
	autopsy [20]	
	ultrasound/CT/[20]	2 cases
	ultrasound [20]	hypometabolism
	MRI/autopsy[24]	2 cases/PEA
	MRI[27]	group study
	PET[27]	
	MRI[29]	
	MRI[30]	
Diencephalon	autopsy[12]	4 cases
	autopsy[20]	
	ultrasound/CT[20]	
	ultrasound[20]	
	MRI/autopsy[24]	
	MRI[27]	2 cases
	MRI[29]	2 cases/PEA
	MRI[30]	group study
Cerebellar anomalies	autopsy[10]	3 cases
	autopsy[13]	
	autopsy[12]	5 cases
	MRI[27]	2 cases
	MRI[25]	Same case as Schaefer *et al.*, 1991
	MRI[29]	2 cases/PEA
	MRI[30]	group study
	PET[42]	hypometabolism

Table 1 (continued)

Summary of the neuropathology reported in children with fetal alcohol syndrome (FAS) or prenatal exposure to alcohol (PEA)

Abnormality	Method	Notes
Vermal dysgenesis	autopsy[13]	
	autopsy[12]	
	MRI[38]	group study
Brainstem dysgenesis	autopsy[10]	3 cases
	autopsy[12]	2 cases
	MRI[25]	Same case as Schaefer et al., 1991
Optic nerve	autopsy[12]	
	Ultrasound[20]	optic nerve pallor causing blindness
	autopsy[25]	Same case as Schaefer et al., 1991
Olfactory bulb/tract	autopsy[12]	
	MRI/autopsy[24]	
Hippocampus	MRI/autopsy[24]	
Pituitary	autopsy[25]	Same case as Schaefer et al., 1991
	MRI[28]	
Other neural tube defects	autopsy[11]	Sacral myelomeningocele
	n/a[55]	Lumbosacral meningomyelocele (2 cases)
	n/a[58]	Spina bifida (2 cases)
	autopsy[12]	Spina bifida
	n/a[17]	Lumbosacral meningomyelocele
	n/a[17]	Lumbosacral lipomeningocele

One of the concerns in using autopsy reports to delineate the effects of prenatal alcohol exposure is that those reports may not truly represent the majority of individuals with FAS. Rather, they may be among the most severely affected FAS cases and the severity of their brain damage may preclude an accurate picture of any pattern that may exist. By using modern brain imaging techniques, like magnetic resonance imaging (MRI), an evaluation of living children who are more likely to be representative of FAS can be accomplished. While there were some early case reports of FAS that contained results obtained with computerized tomography,[11,18] results of brain imaging techniques were not typically reported until much more recently. A summary of the existing reports utilizing MRI evaluations of children with FAS or PEA (prenatal exposure to alcohol) is presented in Table 2. As with the initial studies of FAS, the first descriptions of brain imaging results in children with FAS appeared in case reports. The first documentation of a brain MRI in a child with FAS appeared in a report on brain anomalies in children with malformative syndromes and mental retardation.[19] Results of the MRI were described as indicating "multifocal encephalopathy" in a one-year-old child, but no further details were provided. Soon after, three children of alcoholic women were described.[20] The CNS damage of these three children was consistent with the spectrum of holoprosencephaly. All three had a single "square-shaped" ventricle and midline fusions of the basal ganglia and thalami. One of the children, who also had microcephaly and median cleft lip and palate, typical of alobar holoprosencephaly, died early in life. The brains of the other two showed limited sagittal separation and were described as having semilobar holoprosencephaly. These two also had optic nerve abnormalities causing blindness, hypotonia, seizures, "neurodevelopmental arrest," and hydrocephalus. All three of these cases were born to mothers who reported heavy alcohol use only in the first trimester although chlordiazepoxide, imipramine, and nicotine exposures were also noted.

It has been proposed that in the most severe cases, FAS represents mild holoprosencephaly and the above three cases and others described here are certainly consistent with this suggestion. Holoprosencephaly is a spectrum of brain malformations in which the prosencephalon fails to cleave. This malformation complex varies in severity ranging from alobar (complete) through semilobar to lobar holoprosencephaly and is also associated with facial malformations including those characteristic of FAS, but also including cyclopia and cebocephaly.[21-22] Some of the neuroanatomical findings reported in this chapter (e.g., callosal agenesis and absent olfactory bulbs) may be related to the holoprosencephalic malformation complex. Holoprosencephaly was also observed in a fetal macaque whose mother had been given alcohol between gestational weeks two and nineteen[23] and in the mouse model of fetal alcohol syndrome, alcohol on the seventh day of gestation can produce brain and face malformations in the spectrum of holoprosencephaly.[22]

Table 2

Summary of the existing MRI reports concerning children with fetal alcohol syndrome (FAS) or prenatal exposure to alcohol (PEA)

Subjects/Design	Findings
Case report of a child with FAS[19]	Mulifocal encephalopathy
Case report of three children of alcoholic mothers[20]	All three children had brain damage on the spectrum of holoprosencephaly. One later died
Case report of one child with heavy alcohol exposure in the first trimester[24]	Significant brain damage including fusion of frontal lobes, caudate nuclei, and thalami; corpus callosum and ventricular abnormalities; small hippocampus, absent olfactory bulbs and tracts. Child later died
Clinical MRI readings and volumetric analysis of two children with FAS[27]	Both children showed reductions in the volume of the cerebral and cerebellar vaults, basal ganglia and diencephalon, and increases in cortical and subcortical fluid. Corpus callosum abnormalities were noted in both cases, with complete agenesis in one case
Clinical MRI readings of a group of children with FAS[28]	No abnormalities noted except hypoplastic pituitary in one case
Case report of a child exposed to both cocaine and alcohol *in utero*[26]	Enlargement of subarachnoid space and lateral ventricles; underoperculation of Sylvian fissure
Volumetric analysis of two children with PEA[29]	Both children showed reductions in cerebral and cerebellar vaults, and disproportionate reductions in basal ganglia
Assessment of area of corpus callosum in a group of 13 children with FAS/PEA[31]	Three cases of agenesis were noted. Excluding these cases, reductions were noted in the area of the corpus callosum as well as 4 of 5 equiangular regions
Assessment of area of cerebellar vermis in a group of 9 children with FAS/PEA[38]	Area reductions in the anterior cerebellar vermal region with relative sparing of the posterior vermal region
Volumetric analysis of a group of 6 children with FAS[30]	Volume reductions in the cerebral vault and basal ganglia

A child with FAS was included in a description of two children with partial callosal agenesis.[24] This female child was born to a 22-year-old woman who reportedly drank heavily in the first trimester, primarily in a binge pattern. At birth, microcephaly, mid-face hypoplasia, short palpebral fissures were noted as well as a small atrial septal defect. She suffered a variety of medical complications and died at 6.5 months of age. Computerized tomography at two days of age revealed "hypodense" cerebral white matter and fused frontal poles. At 5.5 months, an MRI revealed partial agenesis of the corpus callosum with no connection visible to the level of foramen of Monro and anterior thalamus. Fusion of the frontal lobes was again noted, as well as fusion of the caudate nuclei and thalami. The frontal horns of the lateral ventricle were not observed although the temporal and occipital horns of the lateral ventricles appeared normal. One month later, an autopsy revealed similar findings with the additional discovery of fibers of the anterior corpus callosum which were compressed by the fused frontal lobes and apparently hidden from view on MRI. Also, the hippocampal formations were small and there were no olfactory bulbs or tracts. The autopsy of this case was reported in more detail by Coulter et al.[25] In addition to the previously reported neuropathology, further notation was made of an abnormal pituitary gland without a hypophysial stalk, a single horizontal ventricle, fused cingulate gyri, and hypoplastic medullary pyramids. Microscopically, the temporal and frontal lobe cortical layers were poorly organized and there were small glial subarachnoid heterotopias and a large subarachnoid heterotopia. The dentate gyrus was thin and "deplete of neurons", the deep white matter was gliotic, and the third ventricle was small and "slitlike." There were abnormalities of the cerebellar Purkinje cells including cell loss, misorientation, disorganization, and dendritic abnormalities.

In 1994, a dysmorphologically unusual case was reported.[26] This 4-month-old male child was born to a 32-year old mother who was known to abuse alcohol and cocaine throughout the pregnancy. At birth (32 weeks gestation) his weight was at the 5th percentile. At five months, his head circumference was below the 5th percentile for three months, (corrected for prematurity), his height was at the 5th percentile, and his weight the 15th percentile. He had an abnormal face with some of the features of FAS (e.g., smooth philtrum, thin vermillion, short nose with flattened bridge, large intercanthal distance) as well as some of the features of prenatal cocaine exposure and features associated with the coincident exposure (e.g., low nasal bridge, long smooth philtrum, small toenails, periorbital edema, prominent glabella, short nose, thin upper lip, bitemporal narrowing, lateral nasal buildup, small mandible, flat supra-orbital ridges, posteriorly rotated/low-set ears). Although caution must be taken in attributing any brain abnormality solely to the alcohol-exposure, clinical reading of an MRI showed enlarged subarachnoid space and lateral ventricles, and underoperculation of the Sylvian fissure.

These case reports are similar to the previously reported autopsies in that no general pattern of brain damage can be noted, except possibly that associated with holoprosencephalic neuropathology. Although these case reports, like the autopsies, are interesting in that they provide relatively complete descriptions of individual cases, what they lack is a more detailed evaluation of individual brain structures and comparison with a control group. In addition, the evaluation of larger groups of children exposed to alcohol prenatally, rather than individual cases, can provide valuable information about alcohol-induced brain damage that may be generalized to the population of alcohol-exposed children.

In the first of a series of MRI reports, Mattson et al.[27] described two children with FAS. Both cases were boys, age 13 and 14 years, and were considered severely affected (IQs of 51 and 41, respectively). Both boys were evaluated using a detailed MRI protocol and the results were evaluated both clinically and with volumetric analysis. Clinically, the MRI for the first case showed only asymmetrical but otherwise normal ventricles, and a moderately hypoplastic corpus callosum. For the second case, clinical evaluation revealed agenesis of the corpus callosum and enlargement of the atrial and temporal horns of the lateral ventricles (see Figure 1). Morphometric analyses of the MR images for these two subjects were conducted and compared to nine normal controls matched for age as well as three age-matched children with Down syndrome. These analyses revealed that when compared to the normal controls, the volumes of the cerebral and cerebellar vaults, diencephalon, and basal ganglia were smaller in the children with FAS. In addition, in comparison to the children with Down syndrome, who were equivalently microcephalic (similar cranial vault volume), the children with FAS had smaller basal ganglia and diencephalic volumes. The children with FAS also had an increased amount of ventricular and subarachnoid fluid, suggesting a volume loss of brain tissue.

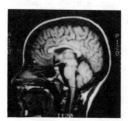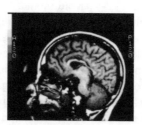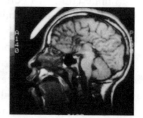

Figure 1. Mid-sagittal MR images of three children. Left: 14-year-old normal control; Center: 12-year-old child with FAS; Right: 14-year-old with FAS. Note callosal abnormalities in both children with FAS, including agenesis. (From Mattson, S. N., Jernigan, T. L., and Riley, E. P., MRI and Prenatal alcohol exposure, *Alcohol Health & Research World*, 18, 49, 1994.)

Shortly after this report, Knight et al.[28] reported the results of an MRI evaluation of a group of high functioning (IQs > 70) children with FAS. Unfortunately, only clinical evaluation was utilized and no abnormalities were noted except for one case with a hypoplastic pituitary. As suggested by Mattson et al.,[27] clinical evaluation of MRI is not likely to detect specific volumetric decreases unless they are extremely large.

Subsequently, Mattson *et al.*[29] reported additional MRI results in two children with prenatal exposure to alcohol (PEA). These two children, both age 16 years, had histories of heavy prenatal alcohol exposure and behavioral and cognitive difficulties (IQs = 64 and 69) but did not have the facial features necessary for a diagnosis of FAS. Similar to the previously described children with FAS, these two PEA children had reductions in the volumes of the cerebral and cerebellar vaults. Because of these overall reductions in brain size, subsequent comparisons were done using proportional volumes. When controlling overall brain size in this manner, only the volume of the basal ganglia was reduced as compared to the control group; the mean proportional volumes of the diencephalon, cortical and subcortical fluid, cortical gray matter, and the limbic and nonlimbic cortex did not differ from controls. Taken together with the previous report,[27] these results suggest that the basal ganglia are especially sensitive to the teratogenic effects of alcohol while other structures are relatively spared.

In a follow-up to this preliminary report, the MRIs of six children with FAS were evaluated.[30] These children were less affected than those in the previous reports, although all met the traditional criteria for FAS. They ranged in age from eight to 19 years and had IQs between <40 and 87. Five of the six had IQs ≥ 69. Morphometric analyses were conducted and the volumes of the cerebral and cerebellar vaults, basal ganglia, and diencephalon were compared to a group of seven age-matched normal controls. Once again, the FAS subjects' cerebral vault volume was smaller than that of the normal controls. The volume of the cerebellar vault was not quite as consistent. Although in four of the six subjects with FAS, the cerebellar vault was smaller than the controls, only a trend was noted statistically. When age and sex were statistically controlled, however, the cerebellar vault was significantly smaller in the FAS group than the controls. In total, of the ten children evaluated, eight showed reductions of the cerebellum, suggesting that this structure is, in fact, affected by prenatal alcohol exposure.

As in the previous reports, the basal ganglia and diencephalon volumes were reduced when compared to the control group. Furthermore, in this study, the components of the basal ganglia, the caudate and lenticular nuclei were also evaluated and were reduced in volume in the FAS group. When overall brain size was controlled, by using proportional values, the volume of the basal ganglia, but not the diencephalon was reduced (see Figure 2). In this analysis, however, reductions in the caudate nucleus appeared to account for most of the reduction in the volume of the basal ganglia.

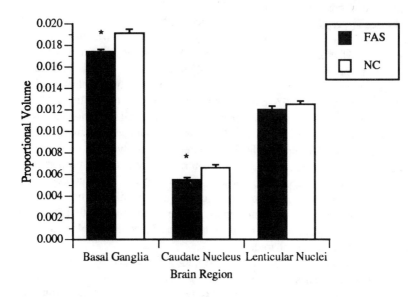

Figure 2. Proportional volume of the basal ganglia and the caudate and lenticular nuclei in six children with fetal alcohol syndrome (FAS) and seven normal controls (NC). $* = p < 0.05$; $** = p < 0.01$.

Another area of the brain that may be especially sensitive to prenatal alcohol exposure is the corpus callosum. Given that the first documented autopsy of a child with FAS displayed agenesis of the corpus callosum, the report of callosal agenesis in a living child[27] was interesting. Since that time additional reports of callosal anomalies have come to light. In total, 12 cases of callosal agenesis have been reported.[7,12-13,27,31] In addition, partial agenesis[32] and callosal abnormalities[24] have also been noted. An assessment of the total area of the corpus callosum was conducted in a group of 12 children with histories of significant prenatal alcohol exposure.[31] Ten (83%) of the exposed children met the traditional criteria for FAS. Using the mid-sagittal section, the area of the corpus callosum was measured using a computer-assisted digitizing system. In addition to the overall area, five equiangular regions were determined for each corpus callosum. When compared to a group of normal control children, the alcohol-exposed children had significantly smaller overall corpus callosum areas, as well as smaller regional areas for four of the five callosal regions. Specifically, regions 1, 3, 4, and 5 (numbered from the anterior to the posterior region) were smaller in the alcohol-exposed group than in the normal controls. Furthermore, when overall brain size was accounted for, similar results were obtained (see Figure 3). Interestingly, Hynd et al.[33] reported a similar study in children with attention deficit hyperactivity disorder (ADHD). Although the method of analysis was not identical, a similar pattern of results was uncovered. This is an extremely interesting similarity given the high prevalence of attentional deficits in children with FAS.[34]

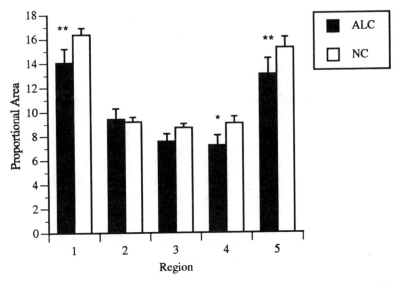

Figure 3. Proportional area of five equiangular regions of the corpus callosum in 10 children with prenatal exposure to alcohol (ALC) and 11 normal controls (NC). $* = p < 0.05$; $** = p < 0.01$. (From Riley *et al.*, Abnormalities of the corpus callosum in children prenatally exposed to alcohol, *Alcoholism: Clinical and Experimental Research*, in press. With Permission.)

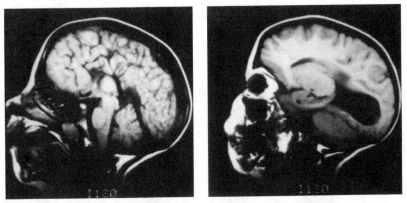

Figure 4. Two MR images of a nine-year-old girl with FAS showing agenesis (left) and colpocephaly (right). (From Riley *et al.*, Abnormalities of the corpus callosum in children prenatally exposed to alcohol, *Alcoholism: Clinical and Experimental Research*, in press. With Permission.)

Also of note in this study,[31] is the documentation of three cases of agenesis of the corpus callosum in this small sample of children exposed to alcohol prenatally (see Figures 1 and 4). The incidence of this abnormality was conservatively estimated as 3/44 or 6.8%. This is considerably higher than the rate of 0.3% in the general population and even the rate of 2.3% in developmentally disabled populations.[35-36] The high incidence of agenesis of the corpus callosum in alcohol-exposed populations has prompted the suggestion that FAS may become the most common syndrome associated with this brain anomaly.[37]

The most recent brain region assessed following prenatal alcohol exposure was the cerebellar vermis.[38] Using MRI, nine alcohol-exposed subjects between the ages of eight and 22 years were compared to 24 matched controls. Six of these individuals had FAS while the remaining three had PEA. Using the midsagittal section, three vermal regions were defined: anterior vermis (vermal lobules I-V); posterior vermis (vermal lobules VI-VII) and the remaining vermal region (including vermal lobules VIII-X). When compared to the age-matched normal controls, the area of the anterior vermal region was smaller in the alcohol-exposed subjects, although the overall vermal area, the posterior region and remaining vermal regions were similar in size between the groups (see Figure 5). These results suggest that, similar to findings in the animal literature,[39-40] the anterior vermis may be more sensitive to the effect of alcohol than the other vermal regions. This pattern of reduction in some areas and relative sparing in others suggests that regionally specific Purkinje cell death occurs in children as well as animals exposed to alcohol prenatally.

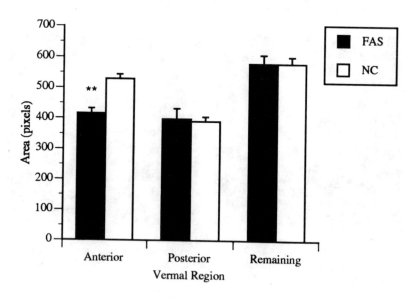

Figure 5. Area of the cerebellar vermis in 9 children with fetal alcohol syndrome (FAS) and 24 normal controls (NC). The vermis is divided into the anterior vermal region (vermal lobules I - V), posterior vermal region (vermal lobules VI - VII) and the remaining vermal region. $* = p < 0.05$; $** = p < 0.01$.

One final area of assessment concerns the functional aspects of these brain anomalies in FAS. Although little direct information is available, two recent reports are relevant. A 16-year-old female with FAS was evaluated using Positron Emission Tomography (PET) to evaluate glucose metabolism.[41] The mean cortical metabolism rate was two standard deviations above normal but the metabolism rate for the caudate, a part of the basal ganglia, was significantly below normal. The basal ganglia, and in particular the caudate, were previously shown to be reduced in volume following prenatal alcohol exposure.[29-30] The Loock et al.[41] study is important because these irregularities in glucose metabolism occurred in an individual who had a normal clinical MRI, again emphasizing the need for detailed brain analysis techniques. A small group of four children with FAS, ages 3-5, were recently evaluated using PET.[42] In this study, the results suggested general hypometabolism along with a dramatic decrease in glucose metabolism in the cerebellum. There was some suggestion of a decrease in the caudate nucleus. Although there are inconsistencies between these two reports, the reports of abnormal glucose metabolism in the basal ganglia and the cerebellum are consistent with previous reports of structural abnormalities in these brain regions.

Electrophysiological evaluations of children with FAS also indicate functional abnormalities associated with prenatal alcohol exposure. Case reports of alcohol-exposed children have been mixed, with both normal[43-44] and abnormal[11,27,45] findings on electrophysiological testing. Group studies, however, have proven to be more consistent (e.g.,[46]). In infants with FAS, electroencephalographic (EEG) studies have reported increased power, especially in the delta frequency band.[47-48] This increase in EEG power occurred in all three stages of sleep (quiet, indeterminate, and REM). In a study by the same authors where maternal smoking was also assessed, similar findings were reported and were independent of other maternal risk factors, including nicotine exposure.[49] The authors proposed that the EEG might be the most sensitive indicator of fetal alcohol effects, since the effects were present even in the absence of facial dysmorphology. Over the last 20 years, these authors have shown that EEG abnormalities exhibited by alcohol-exposed infants are not due to coincident nicotine exposure,[49] premature birth, or alcohol withdrawal,[50] but rather are specific to alcohol exposure,[49] more sensitive to binge than chronic drinking patterns,[51] and predict later motor and mental abnormalities.[52]

Recently, older children with FAS were evaluated using EEG and auditory event related potentials (ERPs). Children with FAS displayed reductions in the mean power of alpha frequencies in the left hemisphere, whereas a comparison group of children with Down Syndrome displayed reductions in alpha in the posterior cortical regions.[53] In addition, the FAS children had significantly longer P300 latencies in the parietal cortical region than normal controls on a passive auditory "oddball-plus-noise" paradigm.[54] These data suggest that specific brain regions are affected by a prenatal alcohol insult and that electrophysiological studies can be used to differentiate between different types of developmentally disabled groups.

In summary, although early descriptions of fetal alcohol syndrome presented a rather inconsistent picture of the neuropathology associated with prenatal alcohol exposure, later, more detailed analyses have revealed a clearer pattern of brain anomalies. While there remains much to be done, certain brain areas appear to be specifically affected by the alcohol insult while others are relatively spared. The brain as a whole is typically reduced in volume following prenatal alcohol exposure and some areas, like the diencephalon and the posterior vermis, are reduced proportionately. Other areas, namely the basal ganglia, some regions of the corpus callosum, and the anterior vermis of the cerebellum, show a disproportionate reduction given overall brain size. In addition, the brain abnormalities of children with FAS were structurally and functionally different from comparison groups of developmentally disabled children who were equally microcephalic and at least as functionally impaired. Taken together, the results suggest that there is a distinct pattern of brain damage that results from heavy prenatal alcohol exposure, that it may be distinguishable from other neurodevelopmental disorders, and that it is independent of the microcephaly typically associated with FAS.

REFERENCES

1. **Jones, K.L., Smith, D.W., Ulleland, C.N., and Streissguth, A.P.,** Pattern of malformation in offspring of chronic alcoholic mothers, *Lancet*, 1, 1267, 1973.

2. **Streissguth, A.P.,** The behavioral teratology of alcohol: Performance, behavioral, and intellectual deficits in prenatally exposed children, in *Alcohol and Brain Development*, West, J.R., Ed., Oxford, New York, 1986, chap. 1.

3. **Conry, J.,** Neuropsychological deficits in fetal alcohol syndrome and fetal alcohol effects, *Alc. Clin. Exp. Res.*, 14, 650, 1990.

4. **Streissguth, A.P., Barr, H.M., Olson, H.C., Sampson, P.D., Bookstein, F.L., and Burgess, D.M.,** Drinking during pregnancy decreases word attack and arithmetic scores on standardized tests: Adolescent data from a population-based prospective study, *Alc. Clin. Exp. Res.*, 18, 248, 1994.

5. **Streissguth, A.P., Sampson, P.D., Olson, H.C., Bookstein, F.L., Barr, H.M., Scott, M., Feldman, J., and Mirsky, A.F.,** Maternal drinking during pregnancy: Attention and short-term memory in 14-year old offspring--a longitudinal prospective study, *Alc. Clin. Exp. Res.*, 18, 202, 1994.

6. Janzen, L.A., Nanson, J.L., and Block, G.W., Neuropsychological evaluation of preschoolers with fetal alcohol syndrome, *Neurotoxicol. Teratol.*, 17, 273, 1995.

7. Jones, K.L. and Smith, D.W., Recognition of the fetal alcohol syndrome in early infancy, *Lancet,* 2, 999, 1973.

8. Jones, K.L. and Smith, D.W., The fetal alcohol syndrome, *Teratology*, 12, 1, 1975.

9. Clarren, S.K., Central nervous system malformations in two offspring of alcoholic women, *Birth Defects*, 13, 151, 1977.

10. Clarren, S.K., Alvord, E.C., Sumi, S.M., Streissguth, A.P., and Smith, D.W., Brain malformations related to prenatal exposure to ethanol, *J. Pediatr.*, 92, 64, 1978.

11. Goldstein, G. and Arulanantham, K., Neural tube defect and renal anomalies in a child with fetal alcohol syndrome, *J. Pediatr.*, 93, 636, 1978.

12. Peiffer, J., Majewski, F., Fischbach, H., Bierich, J.R., and Volk, B., Alcohol embryo- and fetopathy: Neuropathology of 3 children and 3 fetuses, *J. Neurol. Sci.*, 41, 125, 1979.

13. Wisniewski, K., Dambska, M., Sher, J.H., and Qazi, Q., A clinical neuropathological study of the fetal alcohol syndrome, *Neuropediatrics*, 14, 197, 1983.

14. Clarren, S.K., Neuropathology in fetal alcohol syndrome, in *Alcohol and Brain Development*, West, J.R., Ed., Oxford, New York, 1986, chap. 6.

15. Clarren, S.K., Recognition of the fetal alcohol syndrome, *J. Am. Med. Assoc.*, 245, 2436, 1981.

16. Habbick, B.F., Zaleski, W.A., Casey, R., and Murphy, F., Liver abnormalities in three patients with fetal alcohol syndrome, *Lancet*, 1, 580, 1979.

17. Clarren, S.K., Neural tube defects and fetal alcohol syndrome, *J. Pediatr.*, 95, 328, 1979.

18. DeBeukelaer, M.M., Randall, C, L., and Stroud, D.R., Renal anomalies in the fetal alcohol syndrome, *J. Pediatr.*, 91, 759, 1977.

19. Gabrielli, O., Salvolini, U., Coppa, G.V., Catassi, C., Rossi, R., Manca, A., Lanza, R., and Giorgi, P.L., Magnetic resonance imaging in the malformative syndromes with mental retardation, *Pediatr. Radiol.*, 21, 16, 1990.

20. Ronen, G.M. and Andrews, W.L., Holoprosencephaly as a possible embryonic alcohol effect, *Am. J. Med. Genet.*, 40, 151, 1991.

21. Sulik, K.K., Johnston, M.C., and Webb, M.A., Fetal alcohol syndrome: Embryogenesis in a mouse model, *Science*, 214, 936, 1981.

22. Sulik, K.K. and Johnston, M.C., Embryonic origin of holoprosencephaly: Interrelationship of the developing brain and face, *Scanning Electron Microscopy*, 1, 309, 1982.

23. **Siebert, J.R., Astley, S.J., and Clarren, S.K.,** Holoprosencephaly in a fetal macaque (*Macaca nemestrina*) following weekly exposure to ethanol, *Teratology,* 44, 29, 1991.

24. **Schaefer, G.B., Shuman, R.M., Wilson, D.A., Saleeb, S., Domek, D.B., Johnson, S.F., and Bodensteiner, J.B.,** Partial agenesis of the anterior corpus callosum: Correlation between appearance, imaging, and neuropathology, *Pediatr. Neurol.,* 7, 39, 1991.

25. **Coulter, C.L., Leech, R.W., Schaefer, G.B., Scheithauer, B.W., and Brumback, R.A.,** Midline cerebral dysgenesis, dysfunction of the hypothalamic-pituitary axis, and fetal alcohol effects, *Arch. Neurol.,* 50, 771, 1993.

26. **Robin, N.H. and Zackai, E.H.,** Unusual craniofacial dysmorphia due to prenatal alcohol and cocaine exposure, *Teratology,* 50, 160, 1994.

27. **Mattson, S.N., Riley, E.P., Jernigan, T.L., Ehlers, C.L., Delis, D.C., Jones, K.L., Stern, C., Johnson, K.A., Hesselink, J.R., and Bellugi, U.,** Fetal alcohol syndrome: A case report of neuropsychological, MRI, and EEG assessment of two children, *Alc. Clin. Exp. Res.,* 16, 1001, 1992.

28. **Knight, J.E., Kodituwakku, P.W., Orrison, W.W., Lewine, J.D., Maclin, E.L., Weathersby, E.K., Cutler, S.K., McClain, C.H., Handmaker, N.S., and Handmaker, S.D.,** Magnetic resonance imaging in high-functioning children with fetal alcohol syndrome who exhibit specific neuropsychological deficits, *Alc. Clin. Exp. Res.,* 17, 485, 1993.

29. **Mattson, S.N., Riley, E.P., Jernigan, T.L., Garcia, A., Kaneko, W.M., Ehlers, C.L., and Jones, K.L.,** A decrease in the size of the basal ganglia following prenatal alcohol exposure: A preliminary report, *Neurotoxicol. Teratol.,* 16, 283, 1994.

30. **Mattson, S.N., Sowell, E.R., Jernigan, T.L., Sobel, D.F., Jones, K.L., and Riley, E.P.,** A decrease in the size of the basal ganglia following prenatal alcohol exposure: A follow-up report (in press).

31. **Riley, E.P., Mattson, S.N., Sowell, E.R., Jernigan, T.L., Sobel, D.F., and Jones, K.L.,** Abnormalities of the corpus callosum in children prenatally exposed to alcohol, *Alc. Clin. Exp. Res.* (in press).

32. **Kinney, H., Faix, R., and Brazy, J.,** The fetal alcohol syndrome and neuroblastoma, *Pediatrics,* 66, 130, 1980.

33. **Hynd, G.W., Semrud-Clikeman, M., Lorys, A.R., Novey, E.S., Eliopulos, D., and Lyytinen, H.,** Corpus callosum morphology in attention deficit-hyperactivity disorder: Morphometric analysis of MRI, *J. Learn. Disabil.,* 24, 141, 1991.

34. **Nanson, J.L. and Hiscock, M.,** Attention deficits in children exposed to alcohol prenatally, *Alc. Clin. Exp. Res.,* 14, 656, 1990.

35. Jeret, J.S., Serur, D., Wisniewski, K., and Fisch, C., Frequency of agenesis of the corpus callosum in the developmentally disabled population as determined by computerized tomography, *Pediatr. Neurosci.*, 12, 101, 1986.

36. Jeret, J.S., Serur, D., Wisniewski, K.E., and Lubin, R.A., Clinicopathological findings associated with agenesis of the corpus callosum, *Brain Dev.*, 9, 255, 1987.

37. Jeret, J.S. and Serur, D., Fetal alcohol syndrome in adolescents and adults, *J. Am. Med. Assoc.*, 266, 1077, 1991.

38. Sowell, E.R., Jernigan, T.L., Mattson, S.N., Riley, E.P., Sobel, D.F., and Jones, K.L., Abnormal development of the cerebellar vermis in children prenatally exposed to alcohol: Size reduction in Lobules I through V(in press).

39. Goodlett, C.R., Marcussen, B.L., and West, J.R., A single day of alcohol exposure during the brain growth spurt induces brain weight restriction and cerebellar Purkinje cell loss, *Alcohol*, 7, 107, 1990.

40. West, J.R., Goodlett, C.R., Bonthius, D.J., Hamre, K.M., and Marcussen, B.L., Cell population depletion associated with fetal alcohol brain damage: Mechanisms of BAC-dependent cell loss, *Alc. Clin. Exp. Res.*, 14, 813, 1990.

41. Loock, C.A., Conry, J.L., Li, D.B.K., and Clark, C.M., Disregulation of caudate/cortical metabolism in FAS: A case study, *Alc. Clin. Exp. Res.*, 17, 485, 1993.

42. Hannigan, J.H., Martier, S.S., Chugani, H.T., and Sokol, R.J., Brain metabolism in children with fetal alcohol syndrome (FAS): A positron emission tomography study, *Alc. Clin. Exp. Res.*, 19, 53A, 1995.

43. Slavney, P.R. and Grau, J.G., Fetal alcohol damage and schizophrenia, *J. Clin. Psychiatry.*, 39, 782, 1978.

44. Marcus, J.C., Neurological findings in the fetal alcohol syndrome, *Neuropediatrics*, 18, 158, 1987.

45. Rasmussen, F., Gustavson, K.-H., and Bille, B., Familial minor neurodevelopmental disorders, *Clin. Genet.*, 25, 148, 1984.

46. Olegård, R., Sabel, K.-G., Aronsson, M., Sandin, B., Johansson, P.R., Carlsson, C., Kyllerman, M., Iversen, K., and Hrbek, A., Effects on the child of alcohol abuse during pregnancy, *Acta Pædiatr. Scand.*, 275, 112, 1979.

47. Havlicek, V. and Childiaeva, R., EEG component of fetal alcohol syndrome, *Lancet*, 1, 477, 1976.

48. Havlicek, V., Childiaeva, R., and Chernick, V., EEG frequency spectrum characteristics of sleep states in infants of alcoholic mothers, *Neuropädiatrie*, 8, 360, 1977.

49.   **Chernick, V., Childiaeva, R., and Ioffe, S.,** Effects of maternal alcohol intake and smoking on neonatal electroencephalogram and anthropometric measurements, *Am. J. Obstet. Gynecol.*, 146, 41, 1983.

50.   **Ioffe, S., Childiaeva, R., and Chernick, V.,** Prolonged effects of maternal alcohol ingestion on the neonatal electroencephalogram, *Pediatrics*, 74, 330, 1984.

51.   **Ioffe, S, and Chernick, V.,** Development of the EEG between 30 and 40 weeks gestation in normal and alcohol-exposed infants, *Dev. Med. Child Neurol.*, 30, 797, 1988.

52.   **Ioffe, S. and Chernick, V.,** Prediction of subsequent motor and mental retardation in newborn infants exposed to alcohol in utero by computerized EEG analysis, *Neuropediatrics*, 21, 11, 1990.

53.   **Kaneko, W.M., Phillips, E.L., Riley, E.P., and Ehlers, C.L.,** EEG findings in fetal alcohol syndrome and down syndrome children, Electroencephalogr. Clin. Neurophysiol., (in press).

54.   **Kaneko, W.M., Ehlers, C.L., Phillips, E.L., and Riley, E.P.,** Auditory event-related potentials in fetal alcohol syndrome and down syndrome children, *Alc. Clin. Exp. Res.*, (in press).

55.   **Friedman, J.M.,** Can maternal alcohol ingestion cause neural tube defects? *J. Pediatr.*, 101, 232, 1982.

56.   **Jellinger, K., Gross, H., Kaltenbäck, E., and Grisold, W.,** Holoprosencephaly and agenesis of the corpus callosum: Frequency of associated malformations, *Acta Neuropathol.*, 55, 1, 1981.

57.   **Ferrer, I. and Galofré, E.,** Dendritic spine anomalies in fetal alcohol syndrome, *Neuropediatrics*, 18, 161, 1987.

58.   **Majewski, F.,** Alcohol embryopathy: Some facts and speculations about pathogenesis, *Neurobehav. Toxicol. Teratol.*, 3, 129, 1981.

59.   **Mattson, S.N., Jernigan, T.L., and Riley, E.P.,** MRI and Prenatal alcohol exposure, *Alcohol Health Res. World,* 18, 49, 1994.

Chapter 4

NEUROPHYSIOLOGICAL CORRELATES OF
FETAL ALCOHOL SYNDROME

Robert F. Berman and Scott E. Krahl

I. INTRODUCTION

Clinical and experimental data collected over the last three decades have shown that the maternal consumption of alcohol during pregnancy can have profound teratological effects on the developing human fetus. The enduring manifestations of prenatal alcohol exposure, collectively termed *fetal alcohol syndrome* (FAS),[1] can include facial dysmorphologies, growth deficiencies, and a host of behavioral and cognitive dysfunctions. The latter are arguably the most detrimental to the individual and are typically expressed as hyperactivity, attentional deficits, and intellectual impairment.

Numerous studies have demonstrated that animals exposed prenatally to alcohol exhibit similar dysfunctions. These animal models of FAS allow researchers to systematically manipulate exposure parameters and to probe the brains of afflicted animals in an attempt to characterize the deleterious effects of alcohol on neural development. Our current understanding of these effects on the neurophysiology of both humans and animals will be reviewed in this chapter, along with an attempt to correlate these findings with relevant anatomical and pharmacological information.

II. HUMAN STUDIES

A.   EEG DATA

A number of electroencephalographic (EEG) studies of children exposed prenatally to alcohol have been carried out over the past twenty years. The initial report of EEG disturbances in such children was in 1976 by Havlicek and Childiaeva[2] at the University of Manitoba. They reported abnormal EEG sleep patterns in 15 children born to mothers who were either chronic alcoholics or who had consumed alcohol regularly during pregnancy. A more complete report by these authors followed in 1977.[3] In this study, EEG recordings were taken from 26 babies of alcoholic mothers and compared to those of 26 babies of healthy, non-alcoholic mothers. Half of the infants born to alcoholic mothers were pre-term and had significantly lower body weight (2,653 ± 115 g) compared to controls (3,257 ± 115 g). They were also described as restless and irritable in response to somatosensory or acoustic stimulation. Sleep EEGs were taken at least 3 days after birth, after it could be determined that no alcohol or other medications were still in the infants' systems. They reported that EEG activity during quiet sleep in infants of alcoholic mothers could be discriminated from control EEGs even by visual inspection, with high-amplitude electrical activity often superimposed on slow delta rhythms (i.e., from 0.1–0.2 Hz). Spectral analysis showed a pattern of increased power in most EEG frequency bands indicating EEG hypersynchrony. Hypersynchrony was seen during quiet sleep, transient indeterminate sleep, and active rapid-eye-movement sleep (REM). In addition, the difference in EEG power between quiet sleep and REM sleep, expressed as the quiet sleep:REM sleep ratio, was large in normal full-term babies, but not evident in alcohol-exposed infants. In a subsequent study, Chernick et al.[4] compared the offspring of alcoholic mothers to those from mothers who smoked during pregnancy. EEG recordings were taken at postnatal day (PD) 3. Both prenatal alcohol intake (> 2 oz absolute alcohol/day) and prenatal smoking (> 1 pack/day) resulted in lower birth weights and body lengths in both groups compared to controls, but only the alcohol-exposed infants showed smaller average head circumference. Again, the sleep EEG showed hypersynchrony in alcohol-exposed infants, but not in normal controls or in infants of smoking mothers. They concluded that smoking was not linked to the EEG effects observed after alcohol exposure, and that abnormal EEG patterns may be more sensitive indicators of prenatal alcohol exposure than the dysmorphology associated with FAS. These effects of prenatal alcohol on EEG power during quiet sleep, indeterminate sleep, and REM sleep persisted in alcohol-exposed infants 4–6 weeks after birth compared to control infants, suggesting prolonged effects of prenatal alcohol exposure on electrical activity of the brain.[5] Majewski[6] also reported abnormal EEGs in 38% of a group of FAS patients. Hypersynchrony and dysrhythmia were particularly evident.

Spohr and Steinhausen[7] reported on a longitudinal, neurological study of children previously diagnosed with FAS. At follow-up, approximately 3–4 years after the initial evaluation, the children were approximately 8–9 years of age. Repeated EEG recordings were available on 45 of the original 72 children with FAS. In general, the severity of morphological damage in these children, including epicanthal folds, blepharophimosis, ptosis, cleft palate, and cardiac defects, was reduced at follow-up. In addition, repeated EEG recordings for individuals were less pathological when compared to their initial evaluations. Interestingly, epileptic seizures were reported in four cases. Unfortunately, little detail is provided concerning the nature of the abnormal EEG patterns, so these results are difficult to compare with the earlier studies reporting hypersynchrony.

Scher et al.[8] examined neonatal EEG and sleep patterns in infants exposed prenatally to either alcohol or marijuana. Alcohol consumption during the first and second trimesters was associated with abnormal sleep patterns. Specifically, there was an increase in the number of arousals. Low-voltage irregular active sleep and trace alternate quiet sleep were both decreased, and indeterminate sleep was increased by first trimester alcohol use. In general, these findings confirm EEG sleep-state disturbances among neonates exposed to alcohol prenatally. It was suggested that alcohol may affect the development of serotonergic systems. This was based on the assumption that serotonergic neurons play an important role in the development of arousal mechanisms and in the maintenance of wakefulness. Unfortunately, this study did not report quantitative data concerning EEG patterns or frequency spectra.

In utero alcohol exposure can also affect the development of the neonatal EEG measured from 30–40 weeks of gestation in pre-term infants. Ioffe and Chernick[9] carried out EEG studies on 441 newborn infants of mothers who had ingested varying quantities of alcohol during pregnancy. Infants were studied at 36–48 hours of age. As in earlier studies by this group, infants of binge drinkers and alcoholic mothers showed higher total power of the EEG during REM-sleep and quiet-sleep periods compared to pre-term infants of abstainers. Furthermore, the effects on EEG power during REM and quiet sleep were greater in women who were binge drinkers, compared to chronic alcoholic women. They concluded that binge drinking may be more damaging to the fetus than continuous drinking of smaller amounts of alcohol. Ioffe and Chernick[10] recently examined the sleep EEGs of infants of abstainers, occasional drinkers, social drinkers, binge drinkers, or frankly alcoholic women. The EEG power, integrated across 1.56–25 Hz during REM sleep and quiet sleep, was then correlated with Bayley mental and motor developmental scores measured between 1.5 and 10 months of age. They found that the total power of the EEG during REM sleep was inversely related to subsequent motor development, and that the total EEG power during quiet sleep was inversely related to mental development. It was suggested that EEG power during REM sleep and quiet sleep at birth (40 weeks post-conceptional age) may be a sensitive index of prenatal alcohol effects on motor and cognitive development, and may be a predictor of outcome for infants exposed *in utero* to alcohol.

Mattson *et al.*[11] studied two children previously diagnosed as having FAS. Neuropsychological evaluations were carried out, as well as magnetic resonance imaging (MCI) and electrophysiology. The electrophysiological analysis indicated moderately abnormal EEGs for both subjects, with theta activity dominating the records, and occasional delta activity recorded from posterior head regions. In both subjects, MRI analysis showed abnormalities in the corpus callosum as well as reduced volumes of several brain structures. Similarly, neuropsychological evaluation showed both to have deficits in a variety of memory functions, including tests of verbal memory and memory for motor sequences. Considered together, these results indicate a constellation of effects associated with FAS, and suggest that the cognitive deficits are a reflection of the underlying abnormal brain morphology and electrophysiology. Importantly, these results were obtained in individuals diagnosed with FAS and examined as adolescents, demonstrating persisting deficits after prenatal alcohol exposure, at least in those children with a diagnosis of FAS.

B.   EVOKED-POTENTIAL DATA

The functional integrity of the auditory system has also been examined in FAS using brainstem auditory-evoked potentials. Because the procedures are non-invasive, they are particularly useful in assessing neural transmission of sensory input within the brain. Pettigrew and Hutchinson[12] measured auditory-evoked potentials in full- and pre-term infants born to mothers who were heavy alcohol users during pregnancy. In normal birth weight, full-term infants, the auditory-evoked potentials were generally normal, while variability in the evoked response, including occasional absences of peak V, was observed in the pre-term, alcohol-exposed infants. In addition, brainstem conduction time (BCT), a measure of the speed of conduction of sensory input through auditory relays, was reduced in these pre-term infants compared to full-term infants. Because BCTs generally decrease with age, it was suggested that alcohol exposure delayed neuronal maturation of the auditory system. In a more recent study, Rintelmann et al.[13] studied auditory brainstem responses (ABRs) in a group of full-term neonates who were exposed prenatally to alcohol, but did not have the dysmorphologies associated with the diagnosis of FAS. They found abnormal ABRs suggestive of a developmental delay due to alcohol exposure. Such findings in humans are supported by similar findings in rats exposed prenatally to alcohol.[14]

C.   CONCLUSIONS

In conclusion, EEG abnormalities are associated with prenatal alcohol exposure in humans. One effect of prenatal alcohol exposure appears to be a disruption of sleep/wake cycles. This was suggested by studies demonstrating that sleep states and sleep EEGs were abnormal in infants of mothers who consumed large amounts of alcohol during pregnancy. These effects were evident as early as 30 weeks gestational age, and could still be detected out to eight or nine years of age in some children. Prenatal alcohol exposure also affected sensory systems. Both visual- and auditory-evoked potentials have been reported to be abnormal in infants exposed prenatally to alcohol. The general findings suggest that alcohol exposure delays development of sensory neural systems. The results in humans appear to be generally consistent, although relatively few such studies have been carried out. Additional human research in this area would appear to be warranted and, as suggested by Yellin,[15] such research could result in the development of electrophysiological techniques as useful tools in the diagnosis of FAS and in the prediction of risk for future developmental problems.

III. ANIMAL STUDIES

Animals exposed prenatally to alcohol display behavioral and cognitive deficits similar to those found in human FAS cases. Rats that are exposed to alcohol during gestation demonstrate impairments in radial-arm maze,[16-18] inhibitory avoidance,[19-21] and T-maze[22] performance. Using these animal models, researchers are able to directly examine the effects of various exposure parameters on behavior and the corresponding neurophysiology in a manner that is not possible in human studies.

A.   *IN VIVO* ELECTROPHYSIOLOGICAL DATA
1. Theta Activity

In vivo recordings from many species, including the rat, cat, and rabbit, reveal that the hippocampus often displays a slow rhythmic activity with a principal frequency that lies in the theta (4–12 Hz) range (see Bland,[23] for a complete review). Based on pharmacological and behavioral evidence, two different types of theta activity can be discerned. Type I theta is most evident during voluntary movements, such as walking, running, swimming, rearing, jumping, and digging.[24] Type II theta occurs in the absence of movement, and may be related to attention and cognition. In contrast to type I theta, type II is abolished by the administration of cholinergic antagonists, such as atropine.[25]

We have recently completed the only study that we are aware of which examines the effects of prenatal alcohol exposure on hippocampal theta activity in animals.[26] Using rats that were either untreated, exposed prenatally to 4 or 6 g/kg/day, or pair-fed to the 6 g/kg group, we collected theta while the animals were moving and while still, then took a ratio of the relative power of the theta range during those periods. A significantly higher ratio of moving-to-still theta activity was observed in the 6 g/kg male group as compared to controls. This was attributed to either an increase in type I (movement-related) or a decrease in type II (immobility-related) theta. Experiments are currently being conducted to further explore these possibilities using cholinergic antagonists.

2. Event-Related Potentials

Event-related potentials (ERPs) are a useful tool for the diagnosis of neurological deficits. Typically, the averaged time-linked EEG response to a sensory stimulus is measured in different brain areas, and the amplitude and latency of the response is then used as an index of brain function. In one such study, pregnant rats were fed a liquid diet consisting of 35% ethanol-derived calories (EDCs) or pair-fed to the alcohol group.[27] At approximately PD 120, a series of auditory tones was presented to the offspring, and the ERPs measured from the cortex, amygdala, and hippocampus. Those rats exposed prenatally to alcohol demonstrated longer latencies of the first positive (P1) and negative (N1) ERPs measured in the hippocampus, while latencies were unaffected in the amygdala and cortex. This suggested that either information processing was impaired in these subjects, or the rates of neurotransmission were slowed.

Church and Holloway[14] used a longitudinal approach to study the effects of prenatal alcohol exposure on ERPs. Using the offspring of pregnant rats fed either a liquid diet of 40% EDCs, allowed free access to food, or pair-fed to the alcohol group, auditorily evoked potentials were obtained at PDs 14–70. Throughout the recording period, ERP latencies of all three groups decreased as a function of age, indicating maturation of the auditory pathways. ERP latencies of the alcohol group, however, were considerably longer than control latencies at all stages of development. This suggests that maturation of the neural pathways responsible for the transmission of auditory information is retarded by prenatal exposure to alcohol.

B.   *IN VITRO* ELECTROPHYSIOLOGICAL DATA

The *in vitro* slice preparation is well-suited for studying the local circuitry and pharmacological responses of the central nervous system. To prepare *in vitro* slices, the animal is usually sacrificed by decapitation, the brain quickly removed, and the area of interest dissected away and sliced using a small tissue chopper. The tissue is kept viable in a well containing artificial cerebral spinal fluid bubbled with oxygen and maintained at a physiologically relevant temperature. After preparation, the slices are transferred to a recording chamber where neurophysiological measures can be obtained. Typically, an electrode is used to stimulate a fiber tract, and the resultant effect on the population of postsynaptic neurons surrounding the recording electrode is obtained. This effect can take several forms. The two which are usually measured are the slope of the population excitatory postsynaptic potential (pEPSP) or the population spike (PS). The pEPSP is an aggregate measure of the graded excitatory and inhibitory potentials elicited in the postsynaptic neurons by neurotransmitter released from the stimulated axons. A greater slope would thereby indicate a greater response by the postsynaptic neurons. The PS, on the other hand, is a summation of action potentials elicited by the stimulation. Since the action potential is an all-or-none phenomenon, the amplitude of the PS is not dependent on the amplitude of the action potentials themselves, but rather, on the number of neurons producing action potentials.

1. Long-Term Potentiation

For more than two decades, researchers have known that synaptic efficacy can be enhanced by patterned electrical stimulation of specific neuronal pathways, a phenomenon predicted by Hebb in 1949.[28] This enhancement, now referred to as *long-term potentiation* (LTP), can be induced in a matter of seconds, but lasts from a few minutes to several days.[29] Because LTP is rapidly expressed, maintained for long periods of time, stimulus-specific, and sensitive to the same types of pharmacological treatments which alter memory consolidation, it is viewed as a possible cellular mechanism of learning and memory.[30-31]

To date, only a few published studies have focused their attention on the effects of prenatal alcohol exposure on LTP, and the results have been mixed. Swartzwelder et al.[32] examined LTP in hippocampal slices obtained from adult (PDs 50–70) rats that were untreated, exposed prenatally to 18.8% EDCs, or pair-fed to the alcohol group. LTP was evoked in the slices by tetanizing the Schaffer collaterals (10-sec, 60-Hz stimulus train) with a current that evoked a PS in the CA1 region that was 20% of maximum. This procedure produced a 140% increase in the PS of the untreated group, a 260% increase in the pair-fed group, but only a 75% increase in the alcohol group, when tested 30 minutes after administration of the stimulus train. While the control groups were not statistically different from one another, LTP produced in the alcohol group was significantly lower than both the untreated and pair-fed groups.

In a more recent study, Tan et al.[21] examined the electrophysiology of hippocampal slices taken from adult (PDs 90–120) rats that were untreated, exposed prenatally to 17.5% or 35% EDCs, or pair-fed to the 35% EDC group. LTP was induced by stimulating the Schaffer collaterals (200-msec, 400-Hz stimulus train at a current that evoked a 1-mV PS). This procedure produced a 210% increase in the PS of the untreated group, a 135% increase in the pair-fed group, and a 170% and 60% increase in the 17.5% and 35% EDC groups, respectively. Although the pattern of results suggested a prenatal alcohol effect on LTP, none of the differences among the groups were statistically significant.

We recently presented data from another study on the effects of prenatal alcohol exposure on the electrophysiological characteristics of young rats (PDs 25–32) in which we also failed to find prenatal alcohol effects on LTP.[33] The rats were either untreated, exposed prenatally to 4 or 6 g/kg/day, or pair-fed to the 6 g/kg group. Again, no significant differences were found in hippocampal CA1 LTP among the four groups immediately, 10, 20, or 30 minutes after tetanizing the Schaffer collateral pathway (200-msec, 400-Hz stimulus train at a half-maximal current intensity). Given this discrepancy in results, it may be premature to state that prenatal alcohol exposure adversely effects LTP.

2. Paired-Pulse Inhibition and Facilitation

A second stimulus pulse which is presented shortly after an initial pulse (on the order of tens of msec) will subsequently elicit a smaller response from the *in vitro* hippocampal slice as compared to the first pulse. This phenomenon, called *paired-pulse inhibition*, is believed to be caused by the activation of recurrent inhibition.[34] At longer intervals, facilitation of the second pulse results, presumably from either feed-forward excitation or a decrease in recurrent inhibition.[35]

As with LTP, the data are sparse concerning the effects of prenatal alcohol exposure on paired-pulse ratios. In one of the earliest studies, Hablitz[36] compared Schaffer collateral paired-pulse responses of pair-fed control rats to those exposed prenatally to 35% alcohol. He observed significantly less paired-pulse inhibition of hippocampal slices in the alcohol group than in controls when the interpulse interval was shorter than 20 msec, but found significantly greater facilitation between 40–100 msec.

Similar results have been obtained in our laboratory.[21] Using the same preparation described above, rats that were exposed prenatally to 35% alcohol had significantly less hippocampal paired-pulse inhibition at 10 msec as compared to the control groups, and demonstrated enhanced facilitation between 20–160 msec. In a follow-up study using a 4 and 6 g/kg/day prenatal-exposure protocol, however, we were unable to find differences in paired-pulse inhibition or facilitation.[33] Again, given the paucity of data, it may be too early to draw definitive conclusions about the effects of prenatal alcohol exposure on paired-pulse inhibition and facilitation.

3. Input/Output Curves

In an input/output (I/O) curve, the electrophysiological response (e.g., PS amplitude) of the *in vitro* slice is plotted against the intensity of the stimulus, and typically follows a sigmoidal function. This sigmoidal function can be altered by changes in either the slope, which signifies the strength of the slice's response at a given stimulus intensity, or the asymptote, which indicates the maximum response that the slice can produce. Such I/O curves have been used for years to assess the stability and responsiveness of *in vitro* slices, but the data are usually reported anecdotally, and have rarely been used to examine prenatal alcohol effects.

While Hablitz[36] did not report significant differences in the I/O curve between hippocampal slices taken from prenatally exposed rats and pair-fed controls, an interesting pattern was evident. He reported that the mean stimulus intensity required to elicit a threshold response was 55 μA in the controls and 61 μA in slices taken from ethanol-exposed subjects, while the maximum responses obtained from these slices were 150 and 145 μA, respectively, possibly indicating a trend towards less responsiveness in slices taken from prenatally exposed animals.

Our lab has recently studied the relationship between prenatal alcohol exposure and I/O curves in the hippocampal slice.[33] Using untreated and pair-fed controls, and rats exposed prenatally to 4 and 6 g/kg/day alcohol, we found a significant decrease in the maximum response (asymptote) that could be elicited by slices taken from the 6 g/kg group as compared to controls. This decrease could theoretically be caused by a number of different factors. Since the amplitude of the PS is dependent on the number of neurons producing action potentials, any treatment which would reduce this number (e.g., a reduction in cell count, action potential threshold, transmitter release, postsynaptic receptor number, etc.) would also affect PS amplitude. The effects of prenatal alcohol exposure on these different measures are discussed in the next section.

C.   ANATOMICAL AND PHARMACOLOGICAL CORRELATES

To understand the data presented above, it is helpful to review the anatomical and pharmacological changes which underlie these electrophysiological results. The purpose of this section is to aid in the understanding of the electrophysiological data presented above, therefore, the literature presented here is not meant to be complete.   Since the electrophysiological studies focused mainly on the hippocampus, the anatomical and pharmacological data in this review will be similarly weighted. For the same reason, much of the anatomical and pharmacological data pertaining to the cerebellum, while relevant to many of the behavioral effects of prenatal alcohol exposure, have been purposely omitted, since electrophysiological data for that structure are completely lacking.

1. Anatomy

Gross anatomical measurements have demonstrated that the effects of prenatal alcohol exposure can have widespread effects on the developing brain. Viirre et al.[37] exposed rats prenatally to 49% EDCs, then measured brain height, width, and area. Adult rats exposed prenatally to alcohol had a significantly smaller total brain area than controls, while the size of the ventricles was more than double that of controls. Lopez-Tejero et al.[38] found significant decreases in gross brain weight, as well, as a result of prenatal exposure to 25% alcohol. This difference was apparent on PDs 0, 1, and 4, but disappeared by PD 15, indicating that, for some measurements, the effects of prenatal alcohol exposure may not be permanent.

Alterations in neuronal morphology, spine density, and receptor function and density have all been noted following exposure to alcohol prenatally. A few studies examining hippocampal morphology following prenatal alcohol exposure report a selective loss of neurons. Barnes and Walker,[39] for instance, observed a 20% decrease in the number of pyramidal neurons in the hippocampal formation of the adult (PD 60) rat following 35% prenatal alcohol exposure. This decrease was seen mainly in area CA1; while there did appear to be a reduction in area CA3, it did not reach significant proportions. No effects were observed on granule cells in the dentate gyrus (DG). Abdollah et al.[40] saw a similar effect in adult (PDs 90–100) guinea pigs that were exposed prenatally to 4 g/kg/day of alcohol. Pyramidal neurons were reduced by 25% in area CA1, but no significant reductions were obtained in area CA3. The DG was not examined.

The preferential loss of pyramidal cells in the hippocampus following prenatal alcohol exposure may be due to the relatively early acquisition and differentiation of those neurons. In mice and rats, precursor pyramidal cells begin to proliferate around gestational day (GD) 16 and stop around GD 19, whereas the majority of precursor granule cells do not begin to divide until the postnatal period.[41-42] This would reduce the exposure of granule cells in the DG to prenatal alcohol, thus limiting the damage in the hippocampus to pyramidal cells. Experiments on neonatal rats appear to support this conclusion. West et al.[43] observed a 10% decrease in the number of granule cells in the DG following postnatal (PDs 4–10) alcohol exposure in rats, while pyramidal cells in areas CA1 and CA3 were not significantly affected.

The number of dendritic spines on surviving pyramidal cells also appear to be reduced following prenatal alcohol exposure. Abel et al.[44] found a 30% decrease in spine density on the apical and basilar dendrites of pyramidal CA1 neurons of adult (PD 90) rats. There was also a shift from type I (long, thin-necked, with small end bulbs) to type II (short, thin-necked, with large end bulbs) spines. Even greater spine density reductions have been reported by others. Ferrer et al.[45] noted over a 50% reduction in CA1 spine densities in young (PD 15) rats. Kuge et al.[46] saw similar reductions in 2-, 14-, 21-, and 70-day-old rats. However, it should be noted that the magnitude of difference between prenatally exposed animals and controls appears to be reduced in adult animals,[45-46] suggesting that the aberrant effects of prenatal alcohol exposure may be reduced with time. As was also seen above, alcohol given prenatally appeared to have no significant effect on the synaptic density within the DG.[47]

West and colleagues[48-50] have been able to show that, while the number and synaptic densities of neurons in the DG are little affected by prenatal alcohol exposure, the distribution of their axon projections is significantly altered. After a diet of 35% EDCs throughout gestation, offspring show an aberrant distribution of mossy fiber terminals in the infra-pyramidal region of the hippocampus. Since most granule cells are not present during prenatal alcohol exposure, alterations in mossy fiber projections are probably related to changes in the target cells, namely, the pyramidal neurons of area CA3.

In the cerebral cortex, prenatal alcohol exposure may delay the proliferation and distribution of neurons. Miller[51] exposed rats to a 6.7% alcohol solution on GD 6 to birth, resulting in a delay in the generation of new cortical neurons, as measured by the uptake of ^{3}H-thymidine, and interference with the migration of those neurons generated. Dendritic arborization and spine densities of cortical neurons may also be affected by prenatal alcohol exposure, albeit, to a lesser extent than that observed in the hippocampus. Hammer and Scheibel[52] observed a substantial decrease in the number of dendritic branches in pyramidal neurons in the sensory-motor cortex of newborn rats exposed prenatally to a 5% alcohol solution. They also reported dendritic varicosities and putative growth cones, indicating abnormal development of these cells. Delayed maturation of these cells has also been demonstrated following prenatal exposure to 25% alcohol.[38] In this study, a significant reduction in the number of basilar dendritic branches in young, alcohol-exposed rats was observed, along with a 10% decrease in the number of dendritic spines. Both of these differences were gone, however, by PD 30. Stoltenburg-Didinger and Spohr [53] examined the types of spines present on cortical pyramidal neurons and found that prenatal exposure to 35% EDCs in rats produces a substantial increase in the number of abnormal, long spines with prominent terminal heads, while the number of normal, stubby, mushroom-shaped spines decreases.

2. Pharmacology

Pharmacological studies of animal models of FAS have tended to focus on excitatory amino acids. The excitatory amino acids are believed to play a major role in a number of physiological and pathological processes, ranging from synaptic plasticity (as demonstrated by LTP) to mechanisms of cell death.

In a study of ^{3}H-glutamate binding, Farr et al.[54] used the offspring of pregnant rats given a liquid diet of either 3.35% or 6.70% EDCs. They found a significant and substantial reduction in the density of specific glutamate binding in the dorsal and ventral hippocampus, and in the posterior neocortex as compared to controls at PD 45. Significant binding differences in the anterior neocortex, entorhinal cortex, caudate nucleus, lateral septal nucleus, and pars anterior hippocampus were not observed. In a later study, this same group reported that the glutamate binding sites found to be reduced by prenatal alcohol exposure in the hippocampus were predominantly N-methyl-D-aspartate (NMDA)-sensitive,[55] and were only affected by exposure to alcohol during the third trimester of gestation in the rat.[56] Several electrophysiological studies have also demonstrated a reduction in the sensitivity of hippocampal neurons to NMDA following prenatal alcohol exposure, possibly through an alteration of the MK-801 and Mg^{++} modulatory site found inside the ion channel.[57-59]

It is unclear whether kainate receptors are affected by prenatal alcohol exposure. Farr et al.[60] measured ^{3}H-vinylidene kainic acid binding in PD 45 rats that had been exposed prenatally to 3.35% or 6.70% alcohol, and found that the number of these binding sites was significantly reduced in the hippocampus, entorhinal cortex, and cerebellum as compared to controls. However, a later study did not observe significant kainate binding differences in these groups, nor did they demonstrate significant changes in binding to (RS)-α-amino-3-hydroxy-5-methyl-4-isoxazolepropionate (AMPA)-sensitive sites.[61]

D.   CONCLUSIONS

Prenatal exposure to alcohol in animals can lead to a variety of potential postnatal physiological effects, including an alteration of theta activity and delayed maturation of ERPs, as well as decreased LTP, paired-pulse inhibition, and neuronal responsiveness. Concomitant reductions in neuronal counts, dendritic arborization, dendritic spine densities, and NMDA-sensitive glutamate binding densities may help to explain some of these effects. Many of these findings, however, have yet to be replicated, indicating that much work is still needed in this field in order to fully understand the mechanisms and manifestations of FAS.

REFERENCES

1. **Jones, K.L. and Smith, D.W.**, Recognition of the fetal alcohol syndrome in early infancy, *Lancet*, 2, 999, 1973.
2. **Havlicek, V. and Childiaeva, R.**, EEG component of fetal alcohol syndrome, *Lancet*, 2, 477, 1976.
3. **Havlicek, V., Childiaeva, R., and Chernick, V.**, EEG frequency spectrum characteristics of sleep states in infants of alcoholic mothers, *Neuropadiatrie*, 8, 360, 1977.
4. **Chernick, V., Childiaeva, R., and Ioffe, S.**, Effects of maternal alcohol intake and smoking on neonatal electroencephalogram and anthropometric measurements, *Am. J. Obstet. Gynecol.*, 146, 41, 1983.
5. **Ioffe, S., Childiaeva, R., and Chernick, V.**, Prolonged effects of maternal alcohol ingestion on the neonatal electroencephalogram, *Pediatrics*, 74, 330, 1984.
6. **Majewski, F.**, Alcohol embryopathy: Some facts and speculations about pathogenesis, *Neurobehav. Toxicol. Teratol.*, 3, 129, 1981.
7. **Spohr, H.L. and Steinhausen, H.**, Follow-up studies of children with fetal alcohol syndrome, *Neuropediatrics*, 18, 13, 1987.
8. **Scher, M.S., Richardson, G.A., Coble, P.A., Day, N.L., and Stoffer, D.S.**, The effects of prenatal alcohol and marijuana exposure: Disturbances in neonatal sleep cycling and arousal, *Pediatr. Res.*, 24, 101, 1988.
9. **Ioffe, S. and Chernick, V.**, Development of the EEG between 30 and 40 weeks gestation in normal and alcohol-exposed infants, *Dev. Med. Child Neurol.*, 30, 797, 1988.
10. **Ioffe, S. and Chernick, V.**, Prediction of subsequent motor and mental retardation in newborn infants exposed to alcohol *in utero* by computerized EEG analysis, *Neuropediatrics*, 21, 11, 1990.
11. **Mattson, S.N., Riley, E.P., Jernigan, T.L., Ehlers, C.L., Delis, D.C., Jones, K.L., Stern, C., Johnson, K.A., Hesselink, J.R., and Bellugi, U.**, Fetal alcohol syndrome: A case report of neuropsychological, MRI, and EEG assessment of two children, *Alc. Clin. Exp. Res.*, 16, 1001, 1992.

12. **Pettigrew, A.G. and Hutchinson, I.,** Effects of alcohol on functional development of the auditory pathway in the brainstem of infants and chick embryos, in *Mechanisms of Alcohol Damage In Utero*, West, J.R., Ed., Oxford University Press, New York, 1986, chap. 10.

13. **Rintelmann, W.R., Simpson, T.H., Church, M.W., and Root, L.E.,** Effects of Maternal Alcohol And/or Cocaine on Neonatal ABRs, presented at the American Speech and Hearing Association, October 1994, 85.

14. **Church, M.W. and Holloway, J.A.,** Effects of prenatal ethanol exposure on the postnatal development of the brainstem auditory evoked potential in the rat, *Alc. Clin. Exp. Res.*, 8, 258, 1984.

15. **Yellin, S.M.,** The study of brain function impairment in fetal alcohol syndrome: Some fruitful directions for research, *Neurosci. Biobehav. Rev.*, 8, 1, 1984.

16. **Hall, J.L., Church, M.W., and Berman, R.F.,** Radial arm maze deficits in rats exposed to alcohol during midgestation, *Psychobiology*, 22, 181, 1994.

17. **Reyes, E., Wolfe, J., and Savage, D.D.,** The effects of prenatal alcohol exposure on radial-arm maze performance in adult rats, *Physiol. Behav.*, 46, 45, 1989.

18. **Zimmerberg, B., Sukel, H.L., and Stekler, J.D.,** Spatial learning of adult rats with fetal alcohol exposure: Deficits are sex-dependent, *Behav. Brain Res.*, 42, 49, 1991.

19. **Abel, E.L.,** *In utero* alcohol exposure and developmental delay of response inhibition, *Alc. Clini. Exp. Res.*, 6, 369, 1982.

20. **Lochry, E.A. and Riley, E.P.,** Retention of passive avoidance and T-maze escape in rats exposed to alcohol prenatally, *Neurobehav. Toxicol. Teratol.*, 2, 107, 1980.

21. **Tan, S.E., Berman, R.F., Abel, E.L., and Zajac, C.S.,** Prenatal alcohol exposure alters hippocampal slice electrophysiology, *Alcohol*, 7, 507, 1990.

22. **Riley, E.P., Lochry, E.A., Shapiro, N.R., and Baldwin, J.,** Response preservation in rats exposed to alcohol prenatally, *Pharmacol. Biochem. Behav.*, 10, 255, 1979.

23. **Bland, B.H.,** The physiology and pharmacology of hippocampal formation theta rhythms, *Prog. Neurobiol.*, 26, 1, 1986.

24. **Vanderwolf, C.H.,** Hippocampal electrical activity and voluntary movement in the rat, *Electroencephalogr. Clin. Neurophysiol.*, 26, 407, 1969.

25. **Kramis, R.C., Vanderwolf, C.H., and Bland, B.H.,** Two types of hippocampal rhythmical slow activity in both the rabbit and the rat: Relations to behavior and effects of atropine, diethyl ether, urethane and pentobarbital, *Exp. Neurol.*, 49, 58, 1975.

26. **Cortese, B.M., Krahl, S.E., Berman, R.F., and Hannigan, J.H.,** Effects of prenatal alcohol exposure on hippocampal theta activity in the rat, *Alcohol*, in press.

27. **Kaneko, W.M., Riley, E.P., and Ehlers, C.L.,** Electrophysiological and behavioral findings in rats prenatally exposed to alcohol, *Alcohol*, 10, 169, 1993.

28. **Hebb, D.O.,** *The Organization of Behavior*, Wiley Press, New York, 1949.

29. **Bliss, T.V.P. and Collingridge, G.L.,** A synaptic model of memory: Long-term potentiation in the hippocampus, *Nature*, 361, 31, 1993.

30. **Izquierdo, I.,** Pharmacological evidence for a role of long-term potentiation in memory, *FASEB J.*, 8, 1139, 1994.

31. **Izquierdo, I. and Medina, J.H.,** Correlation between the pharmacology of long-term potentiation and the pharmacology of memory, *Neurobiology of Learning and Memory*, 63, 19, 1995.

32. **Swartzwelder, H.S., Farr, K.L., Wilson, W.A., and Savage, D.D.,** Prenatal exposure to ethanol decreases physiological plasticity in the hippocampus of the adult rat, *Alcohol*, 5, 121, 1988.

33. **Krahl, S.E., Berman, R.F., and Hannigan, J.H.,** Effects of prenatal ethanol exposure on the electrophysiological characteristics of CA1 neurons in hippocampal slices, *Alc. Clin. Exp. Res.* 19(Suppl.), 50A, 1995.

34. **Andersen, P.,** Interhippocampal impulses: II. Apical dendritic activation of CA1 neurons, *Acta Physiologica Scandinavica*, 48, 178, 1960.

35. **Dunwiddie, T.V., Mueller, A., Palmer, M., Stewart, J., and Hoffer, B.,** Electrophysiological interactions of enkephalins with neuronal circuitry in the rat hippocampus. I. Effects on pyramidal cell activity, *Brain Res.*, 184, 311, 1980.

36. **Hablitz, J.J.,** Prenatal exposure to alcohol alters short-term plasticity in the hippocampus, *Exp. Neurol.*, 93, 423, 1986.

37. **Viirre, E., Cain, D.P., and Ossenkopp, K.-P.,** Prenatal ethanol exposure alters rat brain morphology but does not affect amygdaloid kindling, *Neurobehav. Toxicol. Teratol.*, 8, 615, 1986.

38. **Lopez-Tejero, D., Ferrer, I., Llobera, M., and Herrera, E.,** Effects of prenatal ethanol exposure on physical growth, sensory reflex maturation and brain development in the rat, *Neuropathol. Appl. Neurobiol.*, 12, 251, 1986.

39. **Barnes, D.E. and Walker, D.N.,** Prenatal ethanol exposure permanently reduces the number of pyramidal neurons in rat hippocampus, *Dev. Brain Res.*, 1, 333, 1981.

40. **Abdollah, S., Catlin, M.C., and Brien, J.F.,** Ethanol neurobehavioural teratogenesis in the guinea pig: Behavioural dysfunction and hippocampal morphologic change, *Can. J. Physiol. Pharmacol.,* 71, 776, 1993.

41. **Altman, J. and Bayer, S.,** Postnatal development of the hippocampal dentate gyrus under normal and experimental conditions, in *The Hippocampus,* Vol. 1, Isaacson, R.L. and Pribram, K.H., Eds., Plenum Press, New York, 1975, 95.

42. **Schlessinger, A.R., Cowan, W.M., and Gottlieb, D.I.,** An autoradiographic study of the time of origin and the pattern of granule cell migration in the dentate gyrus of the rat, *J. Comp. Neurol.,* 159, 149, 1975.

43. **West, J.R., Hamre, K.M., and Cassell, M.D.,** Effects of ethanol exposure during the third trimester equivalent on neuron number in rat hippocampus and dentate gyrus, *Alc. Clin. Exp. Res.,* 9, 190, 1986.

44. **Abel, E.L., Jacobson, S., and Sherwin, B.T.,** *In utero* alcohol exposure: Functional and structural brain damage, *Neurobehav. Toxicol. Teratol.,* 5, 363, 1983

45. **Ferrer, I., Galofré, F., López-Tejero, D., and Llobera, M.,** Morphological recovery of hippocampal pyramidal neurons in the adult rat exposed *in utero* to ethanol, *Toxicology,* 48, 191, 1988.

46. **Kuge, T., Asayama, T., Kakuta, S., Murakami, K., Ishikawa, Y., Kuroda, M., Imai, T., Seki, K., Omoto, M., and Kishi, K.,** Effect of ethanol on the development and maturation of synapses in the rat hippocampus: A quantitative electron-microscopic study, *Environ. Res.,* 62, 99, 1993.

47. **Hoff, S.F.,** Synaptogenesis in the hippocampal dentate gyrus: Effects of *in utero* ethanol exposure, *Brain Res. Bull.,* 21, 47, 1988.

48. **West, J.R., Hodges, C.A., and Black, A.C., Jr.,** Prenatal exposure to ethanol alters the organization of hippocampal mossy fibers in rats, *Science,* 211, 957, 1981.

49. **West, J.R. and Hodges-Savola, C.A.,** Permanent hippocampal mossy fiber hyperdevelopment following prenatal ethanol exposure, *Neurobehav. Toxicol. Teratol.,* 5, 139, 1983.

50. **West, J.R. and Pierce, D.R.,** The effect of *in utero* ethanol exposure on hippocampal mossy fibers: An HRP study, *Dev. Brain Res.,* 15, 275, 1984.

51. **Miller, M.W.,** Effects of alcohol on the generation and migration of cerebral cortical neurons, *Science,* 233, 1308, 1986.

52. **Hammer, R.P., Jr. and Scheibel, A.B.,** Morphological evidence for a delay of neuronal maturation in fetal alcohol exposure, *Exp. Neurol.,* 74, 587, 1981.

53.   **Stoltenburg-Didinger, G. and Spohr, H.L.,** Fetal alcohol syndrome and mental retardation: Spine distribution of pyramidal cells in prenatal alcohol-exposed rat cerebral cortex; a Golgi study, *Dev. Brain Res.,* 11, 119, 1983.

54.   **Farr, K.L., Montano, C.Y., Paxton, L.L., and Savage, D.D.,** Prenatal ethanol exposure decreases hippocampal ^{3}H-glutamate binding in 45-day-old rats, *Alcohol,* 5, 125, 1988.

55.   **Savage, D.D., Montano, C.Y., Otero, M.A., and Paxton, L.L.,** Prenatal ethanol exposure decreases hippocampal NMDA-sensitive [3H]-glutamate binding site density in 45-day-old rats, *Alcohol,* 8, 193, 1991.

56.   **Savage, D.D., Queen, S.A., Sanchez, C.F., Paxton, L.L., Mahoney, J.C., Goodlett, C.R., and West, J.R.,** Prenatal ethanol exposure during the last third of gestation in rat reduces hippocampal NMDA agonist binding site density in 45-day-old offspring, *Alcohol,* 9, 37, 1991.

57.   **Lee, Y.-H., Spuhler-Phillips, K., Randall, P.K., and Leslie, S.W.,** Effects of prenatal ethanol exposure on N-methyl-D-aspartate-mediated calcium entry into dissociated neurons, *J. Pharmacol. Exp. Ther.,* 271, 1291, 1994.

58.   **Morrisett, R.A., Martin, D., Wilson, W.A., Savage, D.D., and Swartzwelder, H.S.,** Prenatal exposure to ethanol decreases the sensitivity of the adult rat hippocampus to *N*-methyl-D-aspartate, *Alcohol,* 6, 415, 1989.

59.   **Nadler, J.V., Martin, D., Bowe, M.A., Morrisett, R.A., and McNamara, J.O.,** Kindling, prenatal exposure to ethanol and postnatal development selectively alter responses of hippocampal pyramidal cells to NMDA, in *Excitatory Amino Acids and Neuronal Plasticity,* Ben-Ari, Y., Ed., Plenum Press, New York, 1990, 407.

60.   **Farr, K.L., Montano, C.Y., Paxton, L.L., and Savage, D.D.,** Prenatal ethanol exposure decreases hippocampal ^{3}H-vinylidene kainic acid binding in 45-day-old rats, *Neurotoxicol. Teratol.,* 10, 563, 1989.

61.   **Martin, D., Savage, D.D., and Swartzwelder, H.S.,** Effects of prenatal ethanol exposure on hippocampal ionotropic-quisqualate and kainate receptors, *Alc. Clin. Exp. Res.,* 16, 816, 1992.

Chapter 5

THE EFFECTS OF PRENATAL ALCOHOL EXPOSURE
ON HEARING AND VESTIBULAR FUNCTION

Michael W. Church

I. INTRODUCTION

The pattern of defects associated with the Fetal Alcohol Syndrome (FAS) include: (1) prenatal and/or postnatal growth retardation, (2) craniofacial anomalies, (3) nervous system defects, and (4) malformations of the skeletal system and internal organs.[1-2]

Perhaps the most devastating consequences of prenatal alcohol exposure are its effects on the nervous system. These can include deficient[3] and developmentally delayed myelination of nerve fibers,[4] delayed and altered dendritic growth,[5-8] fewer dendritic spines,[9] abnormal synaptogenesis,[10-11] abnormalities in neuronal ultrastructure,[12-13] retarded neural development,[10,14] fewer neurons,[15] altered cerebral metabolism,[16] abnormal neurochemistry,[17-18] abnormal neural cell migration,[19-20] enhanced cell death,[21-22] microencephaly and heterotopia,[19] incomplete cerebral cortex, and agenesis of the corpus callosum.[19]

These nervous system effects underlie the sensory and neurobehavioral problems that can occur in children born to alcohol-abusing women. The neurobehavioral effects can include mental impairment ranging from minor learning disabilities to mental retardation, hyperactivity, distractibility, short attention span,[23-24] poor judgement, impulsivity, poor social skills,[23] poor visual and auditory memory,[25] and hyper-responsivity to stress.[23,26-28] The sensory problems include ocular,[29-30] somatosensory,[15] auditory,[31-36] and possibly vestibular problems.[35-36]

When considering the intellectual development of a child, it is important to appreciate the adverse influences of sensory impairment. There is no doubt that normal postnatal development of higher central nervous system (CNS) structures is critically dependent on normal sensory function. For example, the now classical research on the developing visual system found that sensory deprivation during a critical period of postnatal maturation interfered with the normal development of visual perception, neural synapses, dendritic arbors and spines, myelination, cell sizes, cell numbers and organization.[37-39] Similar observations have been made concerning sensory deprivation in the developing auditory system of laboratory animals[38,40] and humans.[41-43] The principle of critical periods for sensory systems states that there are specific developmental stages wherein an animal or human is programmed to utilize sensory stimulation optimally and that subsequent stimulation has gradually diminishing influence on the organism's development. In humans, the critical period of hearing and language development occurs during the first 2 or 3 years of life.[44] A hearing impairment at this age, even in an otherwise normal child, is a form of sensory deprivation which can lead to permanent speech, language and intellectual deficits; cause distractibility, hyperactivity, and developmental delays; and impair academic performance.[44-47] These facts should be kept in mind when considering the adverse effects of prenatal alcohol exposure on the auditory system.

This chapter focuses primarily on prenatal alcohol exposure and the auditory system. The vestibular system is also reviewed because it is embryologically, anatomically and functionally similar to the auditory system and because the inner ear and eighth cranial nerve contain the peripheral nervous systems of both these senses.

A.   EMBRYOLOGY OF THE INNER EAR

Before discussing the nature of the congenital hearing disorders caused by prenatal alcohol exposure, it may be helpful to review some auditory embryology.

The mammalian embryo has three primitive tissue (germ) layers from which all the organs are formed. These are the ectoderm, endoderm and mesoderm. The ectoderm is the external surface layer. It becomes the skin and related structures such as hair, teeth, nails and sweat glands. It also invaginates to form the neural groove which is the precursor of the central nervous system, including the optic cup which forms the eye and the otic pit which forms the endolymphatic portion of the ear. The endoderm is the internal surface area of the embryo. It forms the pharynx and related structures such as the Eustachian tube, middle ear and mastoid cavities, the thyroid gland, the larynx, trachea, bronchi, lungs and the intestinal tract. The mesoderm lies between the ectoderm and endoderm and forms bone, muscle, cartilage, vasculature, and such internal organs as the heart, kidney and reproductive organs.

The first stage of inner ear development begins with the formation of the otic anlage which is comprised of neuroepithelial cells from the surface ectoderm. The otic anlage forms the otic placode (plate) which appears as a thickening on the ectoderm surface. This occurs about the middle of the third week of gestation in humans. The otic placode then invaginates about the 23rd day to make a cuplike structure known as the otic pit or otic cup. The otic pit closes about the 30th day to form the otic vesicle or otocyst. This is accompanied by penetration of the eighth cranial nerve into the otic vesicle wall and by an encapsulation of mesoderm which will form the otic capsule. The otic vesicle then differentiates into the pars inferior and the pars superior which mature respectively into the auditory and vestibular end organs.

Both the auditory and vestibular end organs are innervated by the eighth cranial nerve. This nerve's embryonic origin is still controversial. Many embryologists believe that the eighth nerve ganglion is of neural crest origin. Other studies indicate that the cells of this ganglion are of placode origin and that the contribution of the neural crest to this ganglion is minimal. The majority of the eighth nerve's supporting cells (i.e., glia and Schwann cells) are formed by neural crest cells.[48-49]

Another important aspect of embryonic development is the formation of the five branchial arches on the embryo's head about the 4th week of gestation. These arches are separated by external grooves. Parts of the lower head and neck are formed from the first two branchial arches and grooves. The inner ear, mandible, malleus, incus, tensor tympani and tensor veli palatini are derived from the first (mandibular) arch. The hyoid bone and stapes, are derived from the second (hyoid) arch. Together, the malleus, incus and stapes comprise the inner ear ossicles. The ossicles are located in the middle ear cavity and are the smallest bones in the body. Their function is to help amplify and transduce sound between the outer and inner ears.

The external ear is formed by hillocks derived from both the first and second branchial arches. The external auditory canal is formed by the first branchial groove (pouch) and becomes a passageway to the middle ear cavity and Eustachian tube. The eardrum (tympanic membrane), derived from ectodermal tissue of the first branchial groove, forms a barrier between these external and internal portions of the passageway. The middle ear cavity and Eustachian tube are derived from the first, second and third branchial arches and the intervening endodermal pouches. The first branchial arch is penetrated by the trigeminal (fifth cranial) nerve, while the second branchial arch is penetrated by the facial (seventh cranial) and by the auditory (eighth cranial) nerves.

One principle of embryonic development is that a congenital abnormality whose origin is derived from one particular primitive tissue layer will usually be accompanied by congenital abnormalities in other organs derived from the same primitive layer. For example, a congenital eye anomaly involves a structure whose origin is ectodermal. This is an origin shared by portions of the inner ear. Therefore, the presence of a congenital eye anomaly traditionally suggests that the infant might also have a congenital inner ear anomaly. In fact, there are many congenital disorders characterized in part by both eye and ear anomalies such as Usher's syndrome, Eldridge's syndrome, Mobius syndrome, and Waardenburg's syndrome.[44,50]

Another embryonic principle concerns timing. During the first 6 to 12 weeks of embryonic life, organs are being formed. Alcohol (or any other teratogen) may cause malformations of organs that are developing during that period. For example, maternal rubella, if contracted during the first 3 months of pregnancy, can cause low birth weight, cardiac and ocular defects, microcephaly, mental retardation, dental abnormalities and behavior problems as well as congenital hearing loss. These teratogenic effects do not occur if maternal rubella is contracted later in pregnancy.

Another clinical correlation concerns multiple congenital anomalies related to the first and second branchial arches. For example, patients with Möbius syndrome can have sixth and seventh cranial nerve aplasia, malformations of the external ear, submucous cleft palate, dental malocclusions, mastoid dysplasia, anomalies of the middle ear ossicles and sensorineural hearing loss. Some other familiar syndromes that show an association between craniofacial anomalies and hearing loss are the otopalatodigital syndrome, orofacial syndrome II of Mohr, Alpert's syndrome, Treacher Collin's syndrome, Klippel-Feil syndrome, Crouzon's syndrome, Pierre Robin's syndrome and Down's syndrome. There is also a general association between hearing loss and cleft palate[44,51] as well as between hearing loss and mental impairment.[44,52]

B.   STRUCTURE AND FUNCTION OF THE INNER EAR

To understand the nature of hearing and vestibular disorders, it may be helpful to review the structure and function of the auditory and vestibular systems. The bony labyrinth of the inner ear consists of two components: the cochlea (which contains the auditory receptor system) and the vestibular labyrinth (which contains the vestibular receptor system).

1. The Auditory System

Humans and many other animals use sounds as sources of information. They can signal the presence of predator or prey. They can be used for social communication among and between species. Sounds reach their most complex and communicative form in human language. Without proper hearing, language can become unintelligible, making the learning of and the communication through language very difficult, if not impossible.

Sounds consist of pressure waves that are transmitted through the air and which are characterized by frequency (pitch) and amplitude (loudness). Sound reception requires transduction of pressure waves to the auditory sensory receptor cells and then the sequential transmission of neural signals from the receptor cells to the auditory nerve, the brainstem auditory pathway and certain cortical structures of the brain. The transduction process requires sound to pass down the external auditory canal. The sound pressure waves strike the tympanic membrane. Vibrations then flow across the ossicles (the malleus, incus and stapes bones) of the middle ear to vibrate. Ossicular vibration exerts an amplifying lever action on the oval window of the cochlea.

The cochlea (from the Greek word for "snail shell") is spiral shaped and has three internal chambers (scala vestibuli, scala tympani, cochlear duct), which run the length of the cochlea and are separated by membraneous tissue. The scala vestibuli and scala tympani are filled with perilymphatic fluid. The cochlear duct is filled with endolymphatic fluid. Both fluids are rather similar to the aqueous humor of the eye and to cerebral spinal fluid (CSF). The endolymph is secreted by the stria vascularis which is a choroidal vascular bed similar to the ciliary bodies of the eye (which produce the aqueous humor) and the choroid plexus of the brain's ventricular system (which produces the CSF). The cochlear duct also contains the sensory organ for hearing, the organ of

Corti, which lies on the basilar membrane. The organ of Corti, consists of the sensory receptor cells, supporting cells, and the tectorial membrane. The sensory receptor cells are called "hair cells" because of the hairlike stereocilia that protrude from the cell's cuticular surface. The organ of Corti has one row of inner hair cells (IHC) and three rows of outer hair cells (OHC) that are innervated by afferent fibers from the auditory branch of the eighth cranial nerve whose cell bodies are located in the spiral ganglion. The tectorial membrane projects over the hair cells like a shelf. The ends of the OHC stereocilia make contact with the under surface of the tectorial membrane.

Movements of the oval window create waves in the endolymphatic fluid, causing the basilar membrane and the organ of Corti to move relative to the tectorial membrane. This causes a shearing motion on the hair cell stereocilia, resulting in a mechanical stimulation of the hair cells. This initiates neural impulses as neurotransmitters are released by the hair cells to stimulate the auditory nerve. There is a tonotopic arrangement to the cochlea such that low frequency sounds cause maximal displacement at the apex (upper end) of the basilar membrane while high frequency sounds cause maximal displacement at the base (lower end). The stereocilia of the hair cells recall their embryonic origin as ciliated neuroepithelial cells like those that form the sensory receptor cells of the eye (rods, cones) and like the ciliated neuroepithelial cells that line the brain's ventricles.

The auditory nerve fibers enter the brainstem at the cochlear nucleus located in the medulla. The brainstem auditory pathway is complex. Simplistically, neural information passes from the cochlear nucleus to the superior olivary complex, lateral lemniscus, inferior colliculus, medial geniculate body, the thalamocortical radiations and then to the auditory cortex in the brain's temporal lobe.

The Eustachian tube connects the middle ear cavity to the back of the throat. Collapsed most of the time, it opens when one swallows or blows one's nose. When open, it lets air pass between the throat and middle ear cavity, allowing air pressure within the cavity to equalize with that on the outer side of the eardrum. The Eustachian tube's opening in the throat is controlled by the tensor veli palatini muscles.

2. The Vestibular System

The vestibular system provides us with our sense of balance and is used for the control of various muscles. Without a properly functioning vestibular system, we would not be able to stand, walk or run without constantly staggering and falling over.

The vestibular organ is comprised of the vestibular sacs and the semicircular canals. Both are filled with endolymphatic fluid. The sensory organs of the semicircular canals respond maximally to angular acceleration and deceleration of the head. The ampulla, an enlargement in the canal, contains the crista or sensory organ. The crista contains hair cells whose stereocilia are embedded in an overlying gelatinous mass called the cupula. As one's head accelerates or decelerates, the endolymphatic fluid pushes against the cupula which causes a shearing force on the hair cell stereocilia.

The vestibular sacs (utricle and saccule) have patches of receptive tissue called maculae. The maculae have hair cells whose stereocilia are embedded in an overlying gelatinous mass that contains small calcium carbonate crystals called otoconia. The weight of the otoconia causes a shearing force on the stereocilia as one's head changes position.

The hair cells of the semicircular canals and vestibular sacs are innervated by afferent fibers from the vestibular branch of the eighth cranial nerve. The cell bodies of this branch are contained in the vestibular ganglion. Messages from the vestibular nerve enter the brainstem at the vestibular nuclei or enter the cerebellum. Neural messages are subsequently sent to nuclei controlling eye muscles, head and neck muscles, and to motor neurons of the limbs.

C.   HEARING DISORDERS

As mentioned earlier, there are common embryologic mechanisms that underlie craniofacial, central nervous system, ocular, vestibular and hearing anomalies. Ocular anomalies associated with FAS in humans include strabismus (cross-eyed, cock-eyed), hypertelorism (widely spaced eyes), hypotelorism (closely spaced eyes), abnormal slanting of the palpebral fissures, ptosis, epicanthal folds, microphthalmia, anomalies of the cornea and lens, coloboma (holes) of the iris and retina, tortuous retinal vessels, hypoplastic optic disc and nerve.[29-30,36,53-54] Craniofacial anomalies associated with FAS include microtia or otherwise misshapened external ears, stenosis of the ear canal, lowset and/or posteriorly rotated ears, maxillary hypoplasia, micrognathia, retrognathia, dental malocclusions, missing and rotated teeth, crooked and crowded teeth, cleft lip, cleft palate, short or anteverted nose, flat nasal bridge, thin upper lip, flat philtrum, high arched or narrow or banded palate.[19,32,35-36,55-56] Animal models of FAS have exhibited similar ocular [29-30,57-64] and craniofacial anomalies.[57,60,65-69]

Since FAS is characterized by a litany of congenital craniofacial, CNS and ocular anomalies and since such anomalies are traditionally associated with childhood hearing disorders,[44] a high prevalence of hearing disorders in FAS children should be anticipated. Recent human and animal research support this conjecture. There are at least four types of hearing disorders that can result from prenatal alcohol exposure. These include developmental delays in the maturation of the auditory system, sensorineural hearing loss, intermittent conductive hearing loss secondary to recurrent serous otitis media, and central hearing loss. Each is described below.

1. Developmental Delay

Developmental delay refers to a retardation of growth and maturation. One of the hallmarks of prenatal alcohol exposure is delayed maturation of the nervous system.[9] Consequently, we used the <u>auditory brainstem response</u> (ABR) to assess otoneurological maturation in an animal model of FAS. Specifically, we examined laboratory rats that were prenatally exposed to alcohol by administering alcohol-containing diets to their mothers during pregnancy. The offspring were examined from the ages of 2 to 10 weeks. This time period encompassed the beginning of hearing perception in the rat to when its nervous system fully matures.

The ABR is commonly used to evaluate otoneurological functioning in laboratory animals and humans who cannot be easily tested by more conventional tests, such as infants and mentally impaired children. The ABR is a short-latency far-field sensory evoked potential elicited by a series of clicks or tone pips. ABRs are recorded with surface electrodes and extracted from background brain electrical activity by a computer averaging technique. In the rat and many other laboratory rodents, the ABR is comprised of at least four vertex-positive waves labeled P1 through P4, occurring within 6 msec post stimulus.[31,70-72] Although each wave may reflect activity from several anatomical sites, the chief neural generators in the laboratory rodent are believed to be the auditory nerve (P1), the cochlear nucleus (P2), the superior olivary complex (P3) and the inferior colliculus (P4).[72] The reader should be aware that the human ABR can have seven waveforms and its neural generators are more complex than the rodent's.[73] But in general, the ABR's waves reflect sequential action along the brainstem auditory pathway with wave P1 latency and the P1-P4 interpeak latency used, respectively, as measures of peripheral and brainstem transmission times. Clinically, ABRs are widely used to evaluate peripheral and retrocochlear hearing loss, demyelinating diseases, and the effects of toxic agents.[71,74] In terms of postnatal development, ABR latencies decrease monotonically with increasing age in concert with the brain's maturation.[70,75] Thus, ABRs can provide a useful, noninvasive measure of peripheral and brainstem auditory pathway maturation.

Figure 1 compares the ABRs of control animals and animals prenatally exposed to alcohol that were gathered early (day 17) and late (day 70) in the developmental period. As this figure illustrates, some alcohol exposed animals had prolonged ABR latencies and decreased ABR amplitudes in comparison with controls. Figure 2 compares the maturational changes in the ABR latencies for control and alcohol exposed offspring. The control data came from both untreated and pair-fed nutritional control groups. As this figure indicates, the ABR latencies of the alcohol group were prolonged at each stage of development. The differences between the two groups were greatest during the early stages of development, while a "catch-up" trend was seen in the alcohol group during the later stages of development. It is notable that even at maturity (day 70) there were still statistically significant prolongations in the ABR waves of the prenatally exposed offspring,[33] suggesting some permanent auditory defect. It was also noteworthy that the prenatally undernourished control group showed normal postnatal ABR development, indicating that undernutrition was not the cause of the ABR abnormalities in the alcohol group.

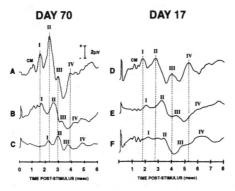

Figure 1. ABRs from control and alcohol-exposed offspring. Traces A-C were collected at 70 days of age. Trace A was collected from a typical control animal, while traces B and C were from animals prenatally exposed to alcohol. Traces D-F were collected at 17 days of age. Trace D was collected from a typical control animal, while traces E and F were from animals prenatally exposed to alcohol. Animals prenatally exposed to alcohol had lower ABR amplitudes and prolonged latencies compared to control cohorts at both the pup and young adult ages. All six traces were from different animals. (Modified from Church & Holloway, 1984.[33] With permission.)

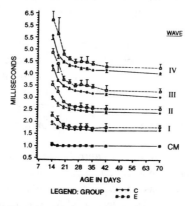

Figure 2. Mean (± SD) ABR and cochlear microphonic (CM) latencies as a function of postnatal maturation in control (C) and ethanol (E) treated rats. ABR latencies for the E group were prolonged in comparison to the C group throughout postantal development. Latency differences were greatest early in development and narrowed somewhat between postnatal days 17 and 23, suggesting a "catch up" trend. (Modified from Church & Holloway, 1984.[33] With permission.)

Maturation of the auditory pathway in an animal model of FAS has also been studied by Pettigrew.[36] Using field potential and extracellular spike potential recordings of the auditory nerve and several brainstem auditory nuclei of developing chicken embryos, he observed a maturational delay in the calcium-dependent mechanisms of neural transmission. In addition, several animal studies have reported a maturational delay in pinna (external ear) development[33,76-77] and a general retardation of physical development.[1]

Despite these animal studies, only a few human studies have evaluated the hearing maturation in infants prenatally exposed to alcohol. In one study, the ABR recordings of such infants revealed delayed development of normal auditory thresholds in 3 of 7 preterm infants. This condition persisted past term equivalent in 2 of the infants.[36] We have also evaluated neonates who were prenatally exposed to alcohol and/or cocaine and occasionally observed that such infants have abnormal ABRs.[78] In some cases, the abnormal ABRs might reflect permanent hearing disorder; but in most cases, the abnormal ABRs were probably due to delayed maturation of the auditory system.

While the term "developmental delay" implies that the child eventually "catches up," it does not mean that the child is entirely normal. For example, a study of high risk infants with developmentally delayed ABRs found that half of the children later experienced serious academic problems (e.g., dyslexia, attention deficits) in elementary school.[79] Consequently, a developmental delay in the ABR caused by prenatal alcohol exposure is clinically important because it may reflect a permanent, global central nervous system insult that later results in learning disabilities. This also points out the value of neonatal ABR screening of drug-exposed and other high-risk infants. Namely, such ABR screening can result in the early identification and early intervention of the adversely affected child. This, in turn, should result in a better patient outcome.

2. Sensorineural Hearing Loss

Both animal and human studies indicate that prenatal exposure to high levels of alcohol can sometimes result in permanent hearing impairment in the form of congenital sensorineural hearing loss (SNHL). SNHL results from damage to the sensory end organs (i.e., the cochlear hair cells) and/or auditory nerve. Traditionally, damage to the sensory end organ and the auditory nerve are not easily differentiated, so the resulting hearing loss is combined as "sensorineural." Some causes of SNHL include ototoxic drugs, noise trauma, presbycusis, certain genetic disorders, prenatal exposure to teratogens and viruses (especially maternal rubella, thalidomide, meningitis, syphilis, cytomegalovirus), cretinism, irradiation, perinatal anoxia, and perinatal hyperbilirubinemia.[52]

Our previously mentioned study on prenatal alcohol exposure not only observed delayed maturation of the auditory system, but also provided evidence of a permanent abnormality.[33] That is, prolonged ABR latencies were still present in some of the mature animals. In a follow-up study, we investigated the exact nature of this permanent abnormality. We found that 6 (19%) of the 32 rats in the prenatal alcohol group had significantly elevated ABR thresholds when tested as adults, indicating that these particular animals had significant, permanent hearing losses. By employing a technique called

ABR latency-intensity (L-I) profiles, we were able to determine that the hearing losses experienced by these animals were in the form of SNHL.[31] These ABR findings have since been replicated by two other animal studies using laboratory rats[34,80] and an unpublished study using mice.

To provide anatomical verification of possible hair cell damage, we histologically examined the cochleas of several animals with ABR evidence of SNHL. This included animals from two different studies using laboratory rats [34] as well as one unpublished study using laboratory mice. These animals showed punctate damage to the auditory sensory epithelium in the form of missing hair cells and hair cells with malformed stereocilia. This damage was confined mostly to the three rows of outer hair cells, but damaged inner hair cells were occasionally observed. This damage, as it occurred in a rat model, is illustrated in Figure 3.

This hair cell damage, while reproducible across several animal studies, did not seem extensive enough to fully account for the amount of hearing loss as indicated by the ABR data. That is, the ABR data indicated dramatic losses in auditory acuity but the same animals had only punctate hair cell damage. Consequently, other damage to the peripheral auditory system must have occurred. Specifically, there may have been damage to the auditory nerve, perhaps in the form of fewer synaptic connections with the hair cells, fewer auditory nerve fibers, and/or less myelination of the auditory nerve fibers.

Support for this conjecture comes from several recent embryology studies. Using mouse embryos exposed to alcohol, Kotch and Sulik[22] observed excessive cell death in the otic placode. This cell death affected the neural progenitor cells which develop into the auditory nerve, as well as the hair cells. Similarly, Cartwright and Smith[81] using chick embryos exposed to alcohol, observed enhanced cell death in the neural crest cells that later differentiate into the cranial ganglia (such as the spiral ganglia), as well as enhanced cell death in the otic vesicle. Apparently, alcohol causes excessive production of reactive oxygenated free radicals (e.g., superoxide anion, hydrogen peroxide) which damage the highly vulnerable neural crest cells.[21,82] Earlier studies using fish embryos[62] and chicken embryos [83] similarly observed alcohol-induced abnormalities in the developing otic vesicles. These effects provide a basis for the SNHL seen in FAS children and animal models of FAS.

After initially observing SNHL in an animal model of FAS,[31] we wanted to know if such a hearing disorder also occurred in children with FAS. Several publications had reported isolated cases of SNHL in FAS children,[84-86] but no systematic study of SNHL in this population had been conducted and the authors did not draw a connection between the prenatal alcohol exposure and the SNHL. Consequently, we evaluated one group of FAS children who were patients of the Craniofacial Clinic, University of Colorado Health Sciences Center in Denver, CO and a second group of FAS children who were patients of the Communications Disorder Clinic, Children's Hospital in Detroit, MI. Congenital SNHL was observed in 29% (4 of 14) of the FAS children in

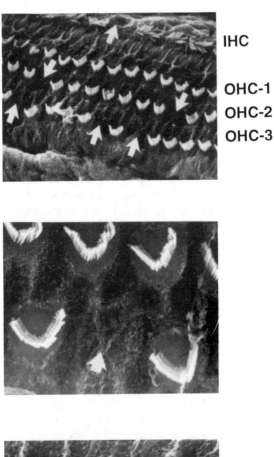

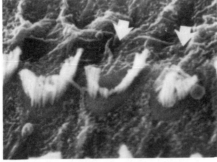

Figure 3. Scanning electron micrographs (SEMs) of the auditory sensory epithelium from a rat prenatally exposed to alcohol (17.5% EDC group). Upper panel: punctate loss of hair cells in the 2nd and 3rd OHC rows and one in the IHC row (arrow heads). Middle panel: a close-up of a missing OHC (arrow-head). Lower panel: OHCs with malformed stereocilia (arrow-heads). (From Church *et al.*, in press.[34] With permission)

Denver[32] and in 27% (6 of 22) of the FAS children in Detroit.[35] These rates for SNHL are similar to those rates seen in other children with craniofacial anomalies such as a 24% rate in Down Syndrome,[87] and a 26% rate in submucous left palate,[88] and greatly exceed the 1% rate seen in the general pediatric population.[44,89]

Pure tone audiograms (PTA) indicated that about half the FAS children with SNHL had predominantly high frequency hearing loss. That is, their hearing was within normal limits (WNL) for tonal frequencies of 2000 Hertz (Hz) and below, but showed a clinically significant hearing loss of 15 dB or more for frequencies above 2000 Hz. This hearing loss was progressively greater for successively higher frequencies, but rarely exceeded 40 decibels (dB) at the highest frequencies tested (8,000 to 10,000 Hz). These would be classified as mild to moderate hearing losses, according to ANSI standards (1969), and would necessitate the use of hearing aid devices. But while a high frequency hearing loss was the most common audiometric profile, some FAS children had hearing losses that were clinically significant only at the low frequencies (i.e., a low frequency hearing loss) while still others had hearing losses that were fairly equivalent at low, middle and high frequencies.[32,35] Our more recent animal studies which used tone pip-evoked ABRs, produced similar results. That is, while a high frequency hearing loss was the most common audiometric profile, hearing loss could nonetheless occur at any frequency.[34,80] The predominance of a high frequency hearing loss is not surprising. Ototoxic agents typically cause high frequency hearing losses.[52,71]

3. Conductive Hearing Loss and Recurrent Serous Otitis Media

Conductive hearing loss (CHL) refers to a hearing loss caused by an interference of sound transmission through the external or middle ear mechanisms. Some common causes of CHL include blockage of the external auditory canal (e.g., ear wax, atresia, foreign objects), damage to the eardrum (e.g., tympanosclerosis, perforation), damage to the middle ear ossicles (e.g., arthritis, fixation, discontinuity), or the impairment of eardrum and ossicular movement by the presence of middle ear fluids (e.g., blood from trauma, puss or serous fluids from infections).

Otitis media (OM) refers to an inflammation of the middle ear. Serous otitis media (SOM) is caused by a middle ear infection and is characterized by the build-up of serous fluid in the middle ear cavity. Recurrent SOM (RSOM) refers to a clinical condition wherein the patient experiences repeated episodes of SOM within a short time span.[44]

For our studies, a hearing loss due to otitis media was considered to be significantly handicapping in young children if (1) the otitis media continued constantly during a 3-month period, (2) the otitis media recurred three or more times despite antibiotic treatment or myringotomy with ventilation tubes in a 6-month period, or (3) a hearing loss of 15 dB or greater occurred constantly for 3 months or half the time during a 6-month period.[32,87] A hearing loss of

15 dB or more is considered to be clinically significant in young children because it can significantly and adversely affect speech and language acquisition, behavior, and academic performance.[44,90]

Intermittent CHL caused by RSOM is common in children with congenital craniofacial anomalies.[91] So, it was not surprising when we observed a high rate of RSOM in FAS children. In our Denver study, 93% (13 out of 14) of the FAS children had clinically significant CHL due to RSOM while 77% (17 out of 22) of the FAS children in the Detroit study had this disorder.[35] The FAS children in our two studies had RSOM rates that were similar to (or exceeded) those of other craniofacial children. For example, Down syndrome has an otitis-proness rate of 62%,[87] overt cleft palate has a rate of 50% to 90%,[51,92-93] submucous cleft palate has a rate of 39%.[88] These rates greatly exceed the 12% to 20% otitis-proneness rates reported for the general pediatric population.[45,47,94-95]

Both of our human studies observed that episodes of RSOM started early in infancy and occurred repeatedly throughout childhood. All the children who were in adolescence or young adulthood continued to be otitis prone. This is in contrast to cleft palate children who show a decrease in the incidence and severity of RSOM as they grow older.[93] It also suggests that otitis proneness is a life-long problem for FAS patients and that they will require life-long management for this condition.

Clinicians have long been aware of an association between craniofacial anomalies and otitis proneness. Eustachian tube dysfunction is regarded as a significant factor for the otitis proneness of such patients. This dysfunction is probably due in part to Eustachian tube tortuosity, stenosis or deficiencies in the muscles (the veli palatini) surrounding the proximal opening of the Eustachian tube.[51] Such malformations impair proper aeration and drainage of the middle ear cavity, leading to any increased risk for middle ear disease. In addition to Eustachian tube dysfunction, immunodeficiency and a subsequent increased risk for upper respiratory tract infections have been suggested as an etiologic factor in the otitis proneness of FAS children.[32,35,96] The high incidences of otitis media, pneumonia and allergies in FAS children certainly suggest that they can have immune deficiency problems.[32,35,96]

Because cleft palate is traditionally associated with otitis proneness,[51,94] and since there was a high incidence of cleft palate in our FAS patients, one question is whether the otitis proneness was concentrated in the patients with cleft palate. In combing the Denver and Detroit study, we found that the incidence of otitis proneness in FAS patients with (14 out of 16 = 87.5%) and without cleft palate (16 out of 20 = 80%) were highly similar. So the FAS patient without a cleft palate is just as likely to be otitis prone as the one with a cleft palate. Perhaps this is not too surprising because several craniofacial syndromes that are not strongly associated with cleft palate can be accompanied by increased incidences of RSOM. These include Down's, Crouzon's, Apert's and Turner's syndromes and patients with dentofacial abnormalities.[91] Thus, clinicians need to be mindful that even the non-cleft palate FAS patient is at high risk for RSOM and the associated CHL.

In addition to our two human studies, there have been a few case studies commenting on the tendency for otitis proneness in FAS patients. For example, Streissguth *et al.*[97] observed RSOM in 5 out of 9 (56%) FAS patients, S. Johnson *et al.*[96] observed this condition in 7 out of 13 (54%) such children, and Becker *et al.*[98] identified 3 out of 8 (38%) FAS children with positive histories for RSOM. K.G. Johnson[99] reported on a single FAS child who suffered form RSOM. These findings were based on incidental rather than systematic observations and with no stated criteria for determining RSOM. Thus, these studies may have overlooked some cases of clinically significant otitis-proneness. Nonetheless, the incidences of otitis proneness in the Streissguth, S. Johnson, and Becker studies were clearly high by any standard.

4. Central Hearing Loss

The central auditory nervous system (CANS) is comprised of the brainstem auditory nuclei and tracts (e.g., the cochlear nuclei, acoustic stria, superior olivary complexes, lateral lemnisci, inferior colliculi, medial geniculate bodies) and cortical structures such as the thalamocortical radiations, primary and secondary auditory cortices. Damage to any one of these regions can result in a central hearing loss. A central hearing loss can range from an impaired ability to understand speech sounds (despite a normal pure tone audiogram) to complete deafness. Both human and animal FAS studies have provided electrophysiological and behavioral evidence of central hearing loss. These observations are summarized below.

Because the P1 and P4 components of the rodent auditory brainstem response are generated by the auditory nerve and superior colliculus, respectively, the P1-P4 interpeak latency (IPL) of the ABR provides a measure of neural transmission time along the brainstem portion of the auditory pathway. Such IPL measures have been useful in detecting the presence of central auditory dysfunction due to demyelinating disease like Korsakoff's syndrome (a condition caused by chronic alcoholism),[100-101] and multiple sclerosis,[102] as well as brainstem lesions caused by toxic agents.[71,103]

Consequently, we examined the P1-P4 IPL in rats that were prenatally exposed to alcohol. These animals were the offspring of dams who received liquid diets containing 17.5% or 35% ethanol-derived calories (EDC). The offspring were evaluated at the adult ages of 6, 12 and 18 months with ABRs evoked by 2000, 4000 and 8000 Hz tone pips. Regardless of age or tone frequencies, the two alcohol-exposed groups had significantly longer IPLs than untreated and pair-fed (nutritional) control groups.[34] This prolongation of the IPL indicated a slowing of neural transmission time along the brainstem portion of the auditory pathway. This could be due to deficient myelination or impaired synaptic efficency caused by the prenatal alcohol exposure.

Auditory evoked potentials generated primarily by the auditory cortex and other higher order CNS structures can be abnormal in rats prenatally exposed to alcohol[31,104] as well as in FAS children.[105-106] These findings suggest that central auditory disorders might extend beyond the brainstem region to include the diencephalon, auditory cortex and related structures. Such effects would be consistent with anatomical studies that found structural abnormalities in the brain's cortex. These abnormalities included heterotopia and dysgenesis of the cortical gyri in FAS children[19,107] and animal models of FAS.[108] Dysgenesis and agensis of the corpus callosum (CC) have also been observed in animal[109-110] and human FAS studies.[19] The CC is important in various aspects of central auditory information processing and is frequently abnormal in children with learning disabilities.[111] Thus, this region is another likely source of central auditory dysfunction in FAS patients and animal models.

We recently had the opportunity to evaluate 12 FAS children for central hearing disorders using the Competing Sentence Test (CST) and the Word Recognition with Ipsilateral Noise (WRIN) Test. The CST is a dichotic listening task that requires the subject to attend to and report back different, but phonemically balanced sentences presented simultaneously with one sentence in one ear and the other sentence in the opposite ear. The WRIN is a figure-ground test that assesses the subject's ability to identify a word in the presence of background noise. All 12 (100%) of our FAS subjects were clinically impaired on these tests, indicating significant central auditory processing disorders.[35] These disorders could be due to either brainstem or cortical dysfunction.

D.   VESTIBULAR FUNCTION

Since the auditory system can be adversely affected by prenatal alcohol exposure, it seems logical to anticipate that vestibular function may be affected as well.

Observations from a number of behavioral studies in animal models of FAS are suggestive of abnormal vestibular function. These studies have evaluated behaviors that are dependent in part on balance, such as the righting reflex (time to regain the normal prone position after being placed on the back), negative geotaxis (reversal to a climbing position after being placed head downwards on an inclined surface), free-fall righting (ability to land on a surface in a prone position after being dropped a certain height from a supine position), ability to retain balance on a balance beam or rotary drum, as well as walking or running gait. While the abnormalities of these behaviors can reflect motor (muscle movement) or cerebellar problems, they can also be due to vestibular problems.

Delayed maturation of the righting reflex has been observed by some researchers.[112-114] but not by others.[77,115-116] Delayed maturation of negative geotaxis has been reported by some[113,117] but not by others.[77,116] Similarly, delayed maturation of the righting reflex has been seen by some[116] but not by others.[77,117] The inconsistencies in these results may reflect differences in the amount and timing of prenatal alcohol exposure.

Abnormal balance, coordination and ataxia problems have been observed in FAS children.[107,118] Similarly, studies using a laboratory rat model of FAS have observed abnormal balance and walking gait.[119-121] Histological evaluations of such human[107] and animal brain tissue[119] as well as recent brain imaging studies of FAS children[122-123] have implicated cerebellar dysfunction in these disorders. The possible influence of a vestibular disorder was never investigated.

Several anatomical studies have provided more direct evidence that prenatal alcohol exposure can damage the vestibular system. As mentioned earlier, several studies have shown that alcohol can damage the embryonic precursors of the inner ear and eighth cranial nerve, both of which serve the vestibular as well as the auditory system. More specific to the vestibular system, Nordemar[124] found that exposing explants of the mouse's embryonic inner ear caused various abnormalities to the sensory epithelium of the crista ampullaris. This included the hair cells, supporting cells, basal lamina and the innervation. The pathology was most extensive to the hair cells which showed vacuolizations, edema, disintegration of cytoplasm and cell organelles, and even complete cell destruction. Nerve endings were sometimes absent. In an earlier study which exposed fish embryos to alcohol, Stockard[62] observed malformed ampullae and semicircular canals.

Despite these observations, vestibular function in FAS children had not been investigated until recently when we evaluated six FAS patients (aged 6 to 26 years) who were a part of a larger study on auditory and language disorders.[35] The caloric <u>electronystagmogram (ENG)</u> results were normal for all subjects except one who showed a mild but clinically significant unilateral weakness. <u>Rotary chair</u> results were normal for all subjects. The caloric and rotary chair tests should have been consistent with each other, however. Thus, we concluded that there was no compelling evidence of abnormal vestibular function in our patients. While there may still have been subtle abnormalities present, our data were strong enough to rule out any major loss of vestibular nerve or hair cells. In addition, three of the six patients had mild sensorineural hearing loss, but the one case with the possible vestibular abnormality did not have sensorineural hearing loss. Thus, we saw no evidence of a relation between damage to the auditory and vestibular systems. All of the subjects had full-blown FAS, including central hearing disorders, multiple craniofacial anomalies, and significant mental impairments. Thus, the lack of significant vestibular dysfunction was not due to a lack of severe prenatal insult. In view of these considerations, it is our general opinion that the abnormal balance and gait exhibited by FAS children and animal models are more likely due to a cerebellar dysfunction than vestibular dysfunction. We cannot, however, rule out the possibility that vestibular dysfunction can occur in some FAS cases.

II. SUMMARY

In conclusion, FAS children are at high risk for a variety of hearing disorders. These include a developmental delay in the maturation of the auditory system, congenital sensorineural hearing loss, intermittent conductive hearing loss secondary to recurrent serous otitis media, and central hearing disorders. These conclusions are supported by converging evidence from both animal and human studies. These results are also consistent with a vast literature showing strong associations between such hearing disorders and craniofacial anomalies, mental impairment and ocular defects.

Adequate hearing is necessary for proper speech and language acquisition as well as for a child to attain his or her full intellectual potential. A child with a hearing loss, who is otherwise normal, will tend to exhibit hyperactivity, distractibility and learning disabilities if intervention for the hearing loss is delayed beyond the critical period of speech and language development.[44] Problems with speech, language, hyperactivity, distractibility and learning disabilities are characteristic of the typical FAS child.[1,23,32,35,97,125] While the hearing disorders of the FAS child are certainly not the sole cause of these behavioral problems, hearing impairment will significantly worsen them. Early identification and intervention for hearing disorders should help the FAS child achieve his or her full potential and ameliorate behavioral problems.

Early identification of hearing disorders should begin as soon as the first few days of life with ABR screening in the newborn nursery.[78] Intervention should start within the first few months of life with good nutrition and a language stimulation program for the developmentally delayed as well as the hearing-impaired infant. Conductive hearing loss due to RSOM should be treated with antibiotics and myringotomies. The child with sensorineural hearing loss should be habilitated with hearing aids.

The association between FAS and vestibular disorders is less clear. While animal studies have demonstrated that embryonic alcohol exposure can damage the vestibular system, we were unable to find clear evidence of vestibular disorders in a small group of FAS children. The problems of balance and gait shown by FAS children and animal models of FAS are most likely cerebellar, than vestibular, in origin. These conclusions are quite tentative, however, and more research on vestibular problems in FAS children need to be conducted.

Women who abuse alcohol are also frequent abusers of other drugs such as nicotine (cigarette smoking), cocaine and opiates. All of these drugs have been implicated in causing childhood hearing disorders through prenatal exposure.[126-130] Because of this, a question is raised about how much of the hearing disorders in FAS children is due to alcohol and how much is due to other drugs. The animal studies on prenatal alcohol exposure have controlled for these factors and clearly show that prenatal alcohol exposure is sufficient to cause hearing loss. Moreover, prenatal alcohol exposure is strongly implicated in the creation of the craniofacial and ocular anomalies associated with childhood hearing disorders while prenatal exposure to cigarette smoking, cocaine and opiates have very weak associations with craniofacial and ocular anomalies.[128,131-132]

Related questions concern the amount of prenatal alcohol exposure needed to cause childhood hearing disorders and whether children with partial expression of FAS (i.e., fetal alcohol effects or FAE) have hearing disorders. Our original premise was that FAS children have hearing disorders because they have the craniofacial, ocular and CNS disorders traditionally associated with hearing loss.[32-33,35] Based on this premise, children who are prenatally exposed to alcohol but have no craniofacial anomalies should have fewer hearing problems. This hypothesis has yet to be tested, however. Further, FAS children are usually born to the most severely alcoholic women. Thus, very high levels of prenatal alcohol exposure are probably needed to cause hearing disorders. Despite these restrictive conditions of high prenatal alcohol exposure and craniofacial anomalies, FAS is still one of the most common birth defects syndromes and probably one of the more common causes of childhood hearing, speech and language disorders. Consequently, all FAS children should be evaluated thoroughly for hearing, speech and language disorders. Conversely, children with craniofacial, hearing, speech and/or language disorders should be evaluated for a possible FAS diagnosis. Such evaluations will insure proper intervention and a better patient outcome.

ACKNOWLEDGMENTS

This work was supported in part by NIH grants P50 AA07606 from the National Institute on Alcohol Abuse and Alcoholism and R01 DA05536 from the National Institute on Drug Abuse.

REFERENCES

1. **Abel, E.L.,** *Fetal Alcohol Syndrome and Fetal Alcohol Effects,* Plenum Press, New York, 1984.
2. **Rosett, H.,** A clinical perspective of the fetal alcohol syndrome, editorial, *Alc. Clin. Exp. Res.,* 4, 119-122, 1980.
3. **Majedcki, T., Beskid, M., Skladzinski, J., and Marciniak, M.,** Effect of ethanol application during pregnancy on the electron microscopic image of a newborn brain, *Materia. Medica. Polona.,* 8, 365-370, 1976.
4. **Rosman, N.P. and Malone, M.J.,** Reversal of delayed myelinogenesis in the fetal alcohol syndrome, *Neurology,* 27, 369, 1977.

5. **Hammer, J.W. and Scheibel, A.B.,** Morphologic evidence for a delay of neuronal maturation in fetal alcohol exposure, *Exp. Neurol.,* 74, 587-596, 1981.

6. **Miller, M.W., Chiaia, N.L., and Rhoades, R.W.,** Intracellular recording and injection study of corticospinal neurons in the rat somatosensory cortex: Effect of prenatal exposure to ethanol, *J. Comp. Neurol.,* 297, 91-105, 1990.

7. **Shetty, A.K., Burrows, R.C., and Phillips, D.E.,** Alterations in neuronal development in the substantia nigra pars compacta following in utero ethanol exposure: Immunohistochemical and Golgi studies, *Neuroscience,* 52, 311-322, 1993.

8. **Smith, D.E., Foundas, A., and Canale, J.,** Effect of perinatally administered ethanol on the development of the cerebellar granule cell, *Exp. Neurol.,* 92, 491-501, 1986.

9. **Sherwin, B.T., Jacobson, S., Troxell, S.L., Rogers, A.E., and Pelham, R.W.,** A rat model (using a semipurified liquid diet) of the fetal alcohol syndrome, in *Currents in Alcoholism,* Vol. 2, Grune and Stratton, New York, 1980, 15-30.

10. **Miller, M.W.,** Effects of alcohol on the generation and migration of cerebral cortical neurons, *Science,* 233, 1308-1310, 1986.

11. **Miller, M.W.,** Effects of prenatal exposure to ethanol on neocortical development: I. Cell proliferation in the ventricular and subventricular zones of the rat, *J. Comp. Neurol.,* 287, 326-338, 1989.

12. **Al-Rabai, S. and Miller, M.W.,** Effect of prenatal exposure to ethanol on the ultrastructure of layer V of mature rat somatosensory cortex, *J. Neurocytol.,* 18, 711-729, 1989.

13. **Mohamed, S.A., Nathaniel, E.J.H., Nathaniel, D.R., and Snell, L.,** Altered Purkinje cell maturation in rats exposed prenatally to ethanol, *J. Cytol. Exp. Neurol.,* 97, 35-52, 1987.

14. **Miller, M.W. and Robertson, S.,** Prenatal exposure to ethanol alters the postnatal development and transformation of radial glia to astrocytes in rat cortex, *J. Comp. Neurol.,* 337, 253-266, 1993.

15. **Miller, M.W. and Muller, S.J.,** Structure and histogenesis of the principal sensory nucleus of the trigeminal nerve: Effects of prenatal alcohol exposure, *J. Comp. Neurol.,* 282, 570-580, 1989.

16. **Vingan, R.D., Dow-Edwards, D.L., and Riley, E.P.,** Cerebral metabolic alterations in rats following prenatal alcohol exposure: A deoxyglucose study, *Alc. Clin. Exp. Res.,* 10, 22-26, 1986.

17. **Light, K.E., Serbus, D.C., and Santiago, M.,** Exposure of rats to ethanol from postnatal days 4 to 8: Alterations of cholinergic neurochemistry in the cerebral cortex and corpus striatum at day 20, *Alc. Clin. Exp. Res.,* 13, 29-35, 1989.

18. **Rawat, A.K.,** Nucleic acid and protein synthesis inhibition in developing brain by ethanol in the absence of hypothermia, *Neurobehav. Toxicol. Teratol.,* 7, 161-166, 1985.

19. **Jones, K.L. and Smith, D.W.,** Recognition of the fetal alcohol syndrome in early infancy, *Lancet,* 1, 999-1001, 1973.

20. **West, J.R., Hodges, C.A., and Black, A.C., Jr.,** Prenatal exposure to ethanol alters the organization of hippocampal mossy fibers, *Science,* 211, 957-959, 1981.

21. **Chen, S.Y. and Sulik, K.K.,** The role of free radicals in ethanol-induced neural crest cell death, *Teratology,* 51, 181, 1995.

22. **Kotch, L.E. and Sulik, K.K.,** Patterns of ethanol-induced cell death in the developing nervous system of mice; neural fold states through the time of anterior neural tube closure, *Int. J. Dev. Neurosci., 10, 273-279, 1992.*

23. **Streissguth, A.P., Aase, J.M., Clarren, S.K., Randels, S.P., LaDue, R.A., and Smith, D.F.,** Fetal alcohol syndrome in adolescents and adults, *J. Am. Med. Assoc.,* 265, 1961-1967.

24. **Riley, E.P. and Vorhees, C.V.,** Eds., in *Handbook of Behavioral Teratology,* Plenum Press, New York, 1986.

25   **Olson, H.C., Feldman, J., and Streissguth, A.P.,** Neuropsychological deficits and life adjustment in adolescents and adults with fetal alcohol syndrome, *Alc. Clin. Exp. Res.,* 16, 380, 1992.

26. **Bilitzke, P. and Church, M.W.,** Prenatal cocaine and alcohol exposures affect rat behavior in a stress test (the Porsolt swim test), *Neurobehav. Teratol.,* 14, 359-364, 1992.

27. **Taylor, A.N., Branch, B.J., Liu, S.H., and Kokka, N.,** Long-term effects of fetal ethanol exposure on pituitary-adrenal responses to stress, *Pharmacol. Biochem. Behav.,* 16, 585-589, 1982.

28. **Weinberg, J.,** Hyperresponsiveness to stress: Differential effects on prenatal ethanol on males and females, *Alc. Clin. Exp. Res.,* 12, 647-652, 1988.

29. **Stromland, K.,** Ocular abnormalities in the fetal alcohol syndrome, *Acta. Ophthalmol.,* 63 (Suppl. 171), 1-50, 1985.

30. **Stromland, K. and Pinazo-Duran, M.D.,** Optic nerve hypoplasia: Comparative effects in children and rats exposed to alcohol during pregnancy, *Teratol.,* 50, 100-111, 1994.

31. **Church, M.W.,** Chronic *in utero* alcohol exposure affects auditory function in rats and in humans, *Alcohol.,* 4, 231-239, 1987.

32. **Church, M.W. and Gerkin, K.P.,** Hearing disorders in children with Fetal Alcohol Syndrome: Findings from case reports, *Pediatrics,* 82, 147-154, 1988.

33. **Church, M.W. and Holloway, J.A.,** The effects of prenatal alcohol exposure on postnatal development of the brainstem auditory evoked potential in the rat, *Alc. Clin. Exp. Res.,* 8, 258-263, 1984.

34. **Church, M.W., Abel, E.L., Kaltenbach, J.A., and Overbeck, G.W.,** Effects of prenatal alcohol exposure and aging on hearing function in the rat: Preliminary observations, *Alc. Clin. Exp. Res.,* (in press).

35. **Church, M.W., Eldis, F., Blakley, B.W., and Bawle, E.V.,** Disorders of hearing, speech, language, vestibular function and orthodontia in children with fetal alcohol syndrome (FAS), (in preparation).

36. **Pettigrew, A.G.,** Prenatal alcohol exposure and development of sensory systems, in *Alcohol and Brain Development,* West, J.R., Ed., Oxford University Press, New York, 1986.

37. **Globus, A. and Scheibel, A.B.,** The effect of visual deprivation on cortical neurons: A Golgi study, *Exp. Neurol.,* 19, 331-345, 1967.

38. **Risen, A.H.,** Effects of stimulus deprivation on the development and atrophy of the visual sensory system, *Am. J. Orthopsychiat.,* 30, 23-36, 1960.

39. **Wiesel, T.N.,** Postnatal development of the visual cortex and the influence of environment, *Nature,* 299, 583-592, 1982.

40. **Webster, D.B. and Webster, M.,** Neonatal sound deprivation affects brainstem auditory nuclei, *Arch. Otolaryngol.,* 103, 392-396, 1977.

41. **Dennis, W.,** Children of the Creche, in *Century Psychology Series,* Prentice-Hall, New York, 1973.

42. **Downs, M.,** The familiar sounds test and other tests for hearing screening in children, *J. Sch. Health,* 26, 77-87, 1956.

43. **McKay, H., Sinisterra, L., McKay, A., Gomez, J., and Lloreda, P.,** Improving cognitive ability in chronically deprived children, *Science,* 200, 270-278, 1978.

44. **Northern, J.L. and Downs, M.,** *Hearing in Children,* 3rd Edition, Williams & Wilkins, Baltimore, 1984.

45. **Holm, V.A. and Kunze, L.H.,** Effects of chronic otitis media on language and speech development, *Pediatrics,* 43, 833-839, 1969.

46. **Lewis, N.,** Otitis media and linguistic incompetence, *Arch. Otolaryngol.,* 102, 387-390, 1976.

47. **Teele, D.W., Klein, J.O., and Rosner, B.A.,** Epidemiology of otitis media in children, *Ann. Otol. Rhinol. Laryngol.,* 68 (Suppl. 89), 5-6, 1980.

48. **Anniko, M.,** Embryonic development of vestibular sense organs and their innervation, in *Development of Auditory and Vestibular Systems,* Romand, R., Ed., Academic Press, New York, 1983.

49. **Van de Water, T.R.,** Embryogenesis of the inner ear: "*In vitro* studies," in *Development of Auditory and Vestibular Systems,* Romand, R., Academic Press, New York, 1983.

50. **Bergstrom, L.,** Congenital deafness, in *Hearing Disorders,* Northern, J.L., Ed., Little, Brown & Co., Boston, 1976.

51. **Holborow, C.A.,** Deafness associated with cleft palate, *J. Laryngoscop.,* 76, 762-773, 1966.

52. **Paparella, M.M. and Schachern, P.A.,** Sensorineural hearing loss in children--nongenetic, in *Otolaryngology,* 3rd Edition, Paparella, M.M., Shumrick, D.A., Gluckman, J.L., and Meyer, W.L., Eds., WB Saunders Co., Philadelphia, 1991, 1561-1578, chap. 40.

53. **Garber, J.M.,** Steep corneal curvature: A fetal alcohol syndrome landmark, *J. Am. Optometric. Assoc.,* 55, 595-598, 1984.

54. **Miller, M.T., Epstein, R.J., Sugar, J., Pinchoff, B.S., Sugar, A., Gammon, J.A., Mittelman, D., Dennis, R.F., and Ksreal, J.,** Anterior segment anomalies associated with the fetal alcohol syndrome, *J. Ped. Ophthalmol. Strabismus,* 21, 8-18, 1984.

55. **Jones, K.L., Smith, D., Howie, W., Ulleland, C.N., and Streissguth, A.P.,** Pattern of malformation in offspring of chronic alcoholic mothers, *Lancet,* 1, 1267-1271, 1973.

56. **Vitez, M., Koranyi, G., Gonczy, E., Rudas, T., and Czeizel, A.,** A semi-quantitative score system for epidemiologic studies of fetal alcohol syndrome, *Am. J. Epidemiol.,* 119, 301-308, 1984.

57. **Padmanabhan, R., Hameed, M.S., and Sugathan, T.W.,** Effects of acute doses of ethanol on pre- and postnatal development in the mouse, *Drug Alcohol Depend.,* 14, 197-208, 1984.

58. **Pinazo-Duran, M.D., Renau-Pigueres, J., and Guerri, C.,** Developmental changes in the optic nerve related to ethanol consumption in pregnant rats: Analysis of the ethanol-exposed optic nerve, *Teratology,* 48, 305-322, 1993.

59. **Zajac, C.S., Bunger, P.C., and Moore, J.C.,** Neuron development in the superior colliculus of the fetal mouse following maternal alcohol exposure, *Teratol.,* 38, 37-43, 1988.

60. **Gikins, M.L.A., Damjanov, I., and Rubin, E.,** The differential transplacental effects of ethanol in four mouse strains, *Neurobehav. Toxicol. Teratol.,* 2, 235-237, 1980.

61. **Kronick, J.B.,** Teratogenic effects of ethyl alcohol administered to pregnant mice, *Am. J. Obstet Gynecol.,* 124, 676-680, 1976.

62. **Stockard, C.R.,** The influence of alcohol and other anaesthetics on embryonic development, *Am. J. Anat.,* 10, 369-392, 1910.

63. **Stockard, C.R.,** The artificial production of eye abnormalities in the chick embryo, *Anat. Rec.,* 8, 33-41, 1914.

64. **Laale, H.W.,** Ethanol induced notochord and spinal cord duplications in the embryo of the Zebrafish, Brachydanio rerio, *J. Exp. Zool.,* 177, 51-64, 1971.

65. **Webster, W.S., Walsh, D.A., Lipson, A.H., and McEwen, S.E.,** Teratogenesis after acute alcohol exposure in inbred and outbred mice: Implications for the study of the fetal alcohol syndrome, *Teratology,* 2, 227-234, 1980.

66. **Webster, W.S., Walsh, D.A., McEwen, S.E., and Lipson, A.H.,** Some teratogenic properties of ethanol and acetaldehyde in C57BL/6J mice: Implications for the study of the fetal alcohol syndrome, *Teratology,* 27, 231-243, 1983.

67. **Sulik, K.K. and Johnston, M.C.,** Sequence of developmental alterations following acute ethanol exposure in mice: Craniofacial features of the fetal alcohol syndrome, *Am. J. Anat.,* 166, 257-269, 1983.

68. **Randall, C.L. and Taylor, W.J.,** Prenatal ethanol exposure in mice: Teratogenic effects, *Teratology,* 19, 305-312, 1979.

69. **Padmanabhan, R. and Muawad, W.M.R.A.,** Exencephaly and axial skeletal dysmorphogenesis induced by acute doses of ethanol in mouse fetuses, *Drug Alcohol Depend.,* 16, 215-227, 1985.

70. **Church, M.W., Williams, H.L., and Hollway, J.A.,** Postnatal development of the brainstem auditory evoked potential and far field cochlear microphonic in non-sedated rat pups, *Dev. Brain Res.,* 14, 23-31, 1984.

71. **Church, M.W., Kaltenbach, J.A., Blakley, B.A., and Burgio, D.L.,** The comparative effects of sodium thiosulfate, diethyldithiocarbamate, fosfomycin and WR-2721 on ameliorating cisplatin-induced ototoxicity, *Hearing Res.,* 86, 195-286, 1995.

72. **Henry, K.R.,** Auditory brainstem volume-conducted responses: Origins in the laboratory mouse, *J. Am. Audit. Soc.,* 4, 173-178, 1979.

73. **Moller, A.R.,** Neural generators of auditory evoked potentials, in *Principles & Application in Auditory Evoked Potentials,* Jacobson, J.T., Ed., Allyn and Bacon, Boston, 1993.

74. **Jacobson, J.T.,** *Principles & Application in Auditory Evoked Potentials,* Allyn and Bacon, Boston, 1993.

75. **Salamy, A., Eggermont, J., and Eldredge, L.,** Neurodevelopment and auditory function in preterm infants, in *Principles & Applications in Auditory Evoked Potentials,* Jacobson, J.T., Ed., Allyn and Bacon, Boston, 1993.

76. **Anandam, N., Felegi, W., and Stern, J.M.,** *In utero* alcohol heightens juvenile reactivity, *Pharmacol. Biochem. Behav.,* 13, 531-535, 1980.

77. **Gallo, P.V. and Weinberg, J.,** Neuromotor development and response inhibition following prenatal ethanol exposure, *Neurobehav. Toxicol. Teratol.,* 4, 505-513, 1982.

78. **Rintelmann, W.F., Church, M.W., Simpson, T.H., and Root, L.E.,** Effects of maternal alcohol and/or cocaine on neonatal ABRs, *Am. Speech & Hearing Assoc.,* October issue, 85, 1994.

79. **Murray, A., Javel, E., and Watson, C.S.,** Prognostic validity of auditory brainstem evoked response screening in newborn infants, *Am. J. Otolaryngol.,* 6, 120-131, 1985.

80. **Berman, R.F., Beare, D.J., Church, M.W., and Abel, E.L.,** Audiogenic seizure susceptibility and auditory brainstem response in rats prenatally exposed to alcohol, *Alc. Clin. Exp. Res.,* 16, 490-498, 1992.

81. **Cartwright, M.M. and Smith, S.M.,** Increased cell death and reduced neural crest cell numbers in ethanol-exposed embryos: Partial basis for the fetal alcohol syndrome phenotype, *Alc. Clin. Exp. Res.,* 19, 378-386, 1995.

82. **Davis, W.L., Crawford, L.A., Cooper, O.J., Farmer, G.R., Thomas, D.L., and Freeman, B.L.,** Ethanol induces the generation of reactive free radicals by neural crest cells *in vitro, J. Craniofac. Genet. Devel. Biol.,* 10, 277-293, 1990.

83. **Sandor, S.,** The influence of ethyl alcohol on the developing chick embryo, II. *Rev. Roum. Embryol. Cytol. Ser. Embryol.,* 5, 167-171, 1968.

84. **Grundfast, K.M.,** The role of the audiologist and otologist in the identification of the dysmorphic child, *Ear Hear.,* 4, 24-30, 1983.

85. **Stein, L., Ozdamar, O., Kraus, N., and Paton, J.,** Follow-up of infants screened by auditory brainstem response in the neonatal intensive care unit, *J. Pediatr.,* 103, 447-453, 1983.

86. **Thiringer, K., Kankkunen, A., Liden, G., and Kiklasson, A.,** Perinatal risk factors in the aetiology of hearing loss in preschool children, *Devel. Med. Child. Neurol.,* 26, 799-807, 1984.

87. **Downs, M.P.,** The hearing of Down's individuals, *Sem. Speech Lang. Hear.,* 1, 25-38, 1980.

88. **Bergstrom, L. and Hemenway, W.G.,** Otologic problems in submucous cleft palate, *South Med. J.,* 64, 1172-1177, 1971.

89. **Kilney, P. and Robertson, C.M.T.,** Neurological aspects of infant hearing assessment, *J. Otolaryngol.,* 14 (Suppl. 14), 34-39, 1984.

90. **Kessner, D.M., Snow, C.A., and Singer, J.,** *Assessment of Medical Care in Children, Contrast in Health Status,* Vol. 3, Washington, D.C., Institute of Medicine, National Academy of Sciences, 1973.

91. **Bluestone, C.D.,** Diseases and disorders of the Eustachian tube-middle ear, in *Otolaryngology,* Vol. 2, Paparella, M.N., Shumrick, D.A., Gluckman, J.L., and Meyer, W.L., Eds. W.B. Saunders, Co., Philadelphia, 1991, 1289-1315, chap. 26.

92. **Downs, M.P., Jafek, B., and Wood, R.P.,** Comprehensive treatment of children with recurrent serous otitis media, *Otolaryngol. Head Neck Surg.,* 89, 658-665, 1981.

93. **Graham, M.D.,** A longitudinal study of ear disease and hearing loss in patients with cleft lips and palates, *Trans. Am. Acad. Ophthalmol. Otolaryngol.,* 67, 213-222, 1963.

94. **Howie, V.M., Ploussard, J.H., and Slyer, J.,** The "otitis-prone" condition, *J. Dis. Child.,* 129, 676-678, 1975.

95. **Shurin, P.A., Pelton, S.I., and Finkelstein, B.A.,** Tympanometry in the diagnosis of middle ear effusion, *N. Engl. J. Med.,* 296, 412-417, 1977.

96. **Johnson, S., Knight, R., Marmer, D.J., and Steele, R.W.,** Immune deficiency in Fetal Alcohol Syndrome, *Pediatr. Res.,* 15, 908-911, 1981.

97. **Streissguth, A.P., Aase, J.M., Clarren, S.K., Randels, S.P., LaDue, R.A., and Smith, D.F.,** Fetal alcohol syndrome in adolescents and adults, *J. Am. Med. Assoc.,* 265, 1961-1967, 1991.

98. **Becker, M., Warr-Leeper, G.A., and Leeper, H.A.,** Fetal alcohol syndrome: A description of oral motor, articulatory, short-term memory, grammatical, and semantic disabilities, *J. Commun. Disor.,* 23, 97-124, 1990.

99. **Johnson, K.G.,** Fetal alcohol syndrome: Rhinorrhea, persistent otitis media, choanal stenosis, hypoplastic sphenoids and ethmoid, *Rocky Mt. Med.,* 76, 64-65, 1979.

100. **Rosenhammer, J.H. and Silverskiold, B.P.,** Slow tremor and delayed brainstem auditory evoked responses in alcoholics, *Arch. Neurol.,* 37, 293-296, 1980.

101. **Stockard, J.J., Rossiter, V.S., Widerhold, W.C., and Kobayashi, R.M.,** Brainstem auditory-evoked responses in suspected central pontine myelinolysis, *Arch. Neurol.,* 33, 726-728, 1976.

102. **Stockard, J.J. and Rossiter, V.S.,** Clinical and pathologic correlates of brainstem auditory response abnormalities, *Neurology,* 27, 316-325, 1977.

103. **Rebert, C.S., Houghton, P.W., Howard, P.A., and Pryor, G.T.,** Effects of hexane on the brainstem auditory response and caudal nerve action potential, *Neurobehav. Toxicol. Teratol.,* 4, 79-85, 1982.

104. **Kaneko, W.M., Riley, E.P., and Ehlers, C.L.,** Electrophysiological and behavioral findings in rats prenatally exposed to alcohol, *Alcohol,* 10, 169-178, 1993.

105. **Hrbek, A., Iversen, K., and Olsson, T.,** Evaluation of cerebral function in newborn infants with fetal growth retardation, in *Clinical Applications of Evoked Potentials in Neurology,* Courjon, J. *et. al.,* Eds., Raven Press, New York, 1982, 89-95.

106. **Olegard, R., Sabel, K.G., Aronson, M., Sandin, B., Johansson, P.R., Carlsson, C., Kyllerman, M., Iversen, K., and Hrbek, A.,** Effects on the child of alcohol abuse during pregnancy: Retrospective and prospective studies, *Acta Paediatr. Scans. Suppl.,* 275, 112-121, 1979.

107. **Clarren, S.K.,** Recognition of fetal alcohol syndrome, *JAMA,* 245, 2436-2439, 1981.

108. **Miller, M.W. and Potempa, G.,** Numbers of neurons and glia in mature rat somatosensory cortex: Effects of prenatal exposure to ethanol, *J. Comp. Neurol.,* 293, 92-102, 1990.

109. **Zimmerberg, B. and Mickus L.A.,** Sex differences in corpus callosum: Influence on prenatal alcohol exposure and maternal undernutrition, *Brain Res.,* 537, 115-122, 1990.

110. **Zimmerberg, B. and Scalzi, L.V.,** Commissural size in neonatal rats: Effects of sex and prenatal alcohol exposure, *Int. J. Dev. Neurosci.,* 7, 81-86, 1989.

111. **Musiek, F.E. and Lamb, L.,** Central auditory assessment: An overview, in *Handbook of Clinical Audiology,* 4th ed., Katz, J., Ed., Williams & Wilkins Co., Baltimore, MD, 1994.

112. **Himwich, W.A., Hall, J.S., and MacArthur, W.F.,** Maternal alcohol and neonatal health, *Biol. Psychiatry,* 12, 495-505, 1979.

113. **Lee, M.H., Haddad, R., and Rabe, A.,** Developmental impairments in the progeny of rats consuming ethanol during pregnancy, *Neurobehav. Toxicol. Teratol.,* 2, 198-198, 1980.

114. **Shaywitz, B.A., Klopper, J.H., and Gordon, J.W.,** A syndrome resembling minimal brain dysfunction (MBD) in rat pups born to alcoholic mothers, *Pediatr. Res.,* 10, 451, 1976.

115. **Cogan, D.C., Cohen, L.E., and Sparkman, G.,** Effects of gestational alcohol on the development of neonatal reflexes in the rat, *Neurobehav. Toxicol. Teratol.,* 5, 517-522, 1983.

116. **Shaywitz, B.A., Griffith, G.G. and Warshaw, J.B.,** Hyperactivity and cognitive deficits in developing rat pups born to alcoholic mothers: An experimental model of the expanded fetal alcohol syndrome (EFAS), *Neurobehav. Toxicol., Teratol.,*1, 113-122, 1979.

117. **Demers, M. And Kirouac, G.,** Prenatal effects of ethanol on the behavioral development of the rat, *Physiol., Psychol.,* 6, 517-520, 1978.

118. **Marcus, J.C.,** Neurological findings in the fetal alcohol syndrome, *Neuropediatrics.,* 18, 158-160, 1987.

119. **Hannigan, J.H. and Riley, E.P.,** Prenatal ethanol alters gait in rats, *Alcohol,* 5, 451-454, 1989.

120. **Meyer, L.S., Kotch, L.E., and Riley, E.P.,** Alterations in gait following ethanol exposure during the brain growth spurt in rats, *Alc. Clin. Exp. Res.,* 14, 23-27, 1990.

121. **Meyer, L.S., Kotch, L.E., and Riley, E.P.,** Neonatal ethanol exposure: Functional alterations associated with cerebellar growth retardation, *Neurotoxicol. Teratol.,* 12, 15-22, 1990.

122. **Hannigan, J.H., Martier, S.S., Chugani, H.T., and Sokol, R.J.,** Brain metabolism in children with fetal alcohol syndrome (FAS): A positive emission tomography study, *Alc. Clin. Exp. Res.,* 19, 53A, 1995.

123. **Sowell, E.R., Mattson, S.N., Riley, E.P., and Jernigan, T.L.,** A reduction in the area of the anterior cerebellar vermis in children exposed to alcohol prenatally, *Alc. Clin. Exp. Res.,* 19, 53A, 1995.

124. **Nordemar, H.,** Alcohol and ultrastructural changes in the developing inner ear, *Acta. Otolaryngol.,* 105, 75-81, 1988.

125. **Shaywitz, S.E., Caparulo, B.K., and Hodgson, E.S.,** Developmental language disability as a consequence of prenatal exposure to ethanol, *Pediatrics,* 68, 850-855, 1981.

126. **Church, M.W. and Overbeck, G.W.,** Prenatal cocaine exposure in the Long-Evans rats: III. Developmental effects on the brainstem auditory evoked potential, *Neurotoxicol. Teratol.,* 14, 335-343, 1990.

127. **Church, M.W. and Overbeck, G.W.,** Sensorineural hearing loss as evidenced by the auditory brainstem response following prenatal cocaine exposure in the Long-Evans rat, *Teratol.,* 43, 561-570, 1991.

128. **Church, M.W., Kaufmann, R.A., Keenan, J.A., Martier, S.S., Savoy-Moore, R.T., Ostrea, E.M., Subramanian, M.G.,Welch, R.A., and Zajac, C.S.,** *Effects of prenatal cocaine exposure,* Vol. 3, Watson, R.R., Ed., CRC Press, Boca Raton, 1991, chap. 8.

129. **McCartney, J.S., Fried, P.K., and Watkinson, B.,** Central auditory processing in school-age children prenatally exposed to cigarette smoke, *Neurotoxicol. Teratol.,* 16, 269-276, 1994.

130. **Rosen, T.S. and Johnson, H.L.,** Children of methadone-maintained mothers: Follow-up to 18 months of age, *J. Pediat.,* 101, 192-196, 1982.

131. **Abel, E.L.,** Smoking and pregnancy, *J. Psychoactive Drugs,* 16, 327-338, 1984.

132. **Ostrea, E.M. and Chavez, C.J.,** Perinatal problems (excluding neonatal withdrawal) in maternal drug addiction: A study of 830 cases, *J. Pediatr.,* 94, 292-295.

Chapter 6

FETAL ALCOHOL EXPOSURE
AND FUNCTIONAL IMPLICATIONS OF THE
NEUROIMMUNE-ENDOCRINE NETWORKS

Zehava Gottesfeld

I. MAINTAINING HOMEOSTASIS

Homeostasis is a condition in which the body's internal environment remains constant within certain physiological limits. For the body's cells to survive, the composition of the surrounding fluids must be precisely maintained at all times, including an optimal ("set-point") temperature, steady concentrations of gases, nutrients, ions, water, neurotransmitters and hormones, as well as a well-regulated immune response to antigens. Clearly, challenging the constancy of the internal environment by stressors, poisons, drugs or antigens may compromise the survival of the host.

The immune system normally maintains homeostasis by employing a variety of cells and signalling agents in response to antigenic challenges. Once the defense mechanisms are activated to overcome the challenge, other compensatory mechanisms may be mobilized to ensure a fine-tuning of the immune response, as well as the return to basal conditions thereafter. An increasing body of evidence has indicated that the central nervous system (CNS) plays an important role in immune homeostasis by regulating neural and humoral compensatory mechanisms to restore the internal balance. Thus, the central regulation of immune responsiveness does not differ from that of any other homeostatic system in the body. As illustrated in Figure 1, stimulated lymphoid cells secrete proteinaceous agents ("cytokines"), which play a key role in the regulation and promotion of various immune responses to challenges. In addition, the cytokines mediate immune signals from the activated lymphocytes to the CNS, especially the hypothalamus. The latter, in turn, modulates the immune response by regulating the secretion of hormones from the pituitary-endocrine axis, as well as the autonomic neural output from the spinal cord. In addition, communications among the hypothalamus, neocortex and the limbic system play a role in the regulation of emotions and motivated behavior that are influential in modulating immune functions. Collectively, the maintenance of immune homeostasis represents a major component of an organism's defensive response to stimuli that threaten homeostasis and, therefore, is precisely controlled by the complex compensatory neural and humoral networks (see Ader *et al.,*[1] for further information). Clearly, the functional disruption of the autonomic neural and/or endocrine system by alcohol intake during pregnancy, may compromise the wellness of both the mother and her progeny. The purpose of this chapter is to review the evidence and speculate on the mechanisms which may underlie the immune incompetence associated with exposure to alcohol during early development. Several reviews pertaining to various aspects of this topic were published previously.[2-6]

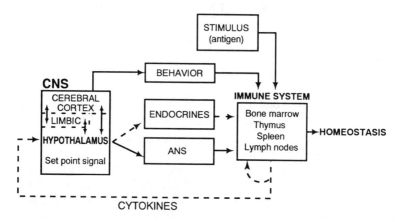

Figure 1. A schematic illustration of the neuroimmune-endocrine networks: maintaining homeostasis following antigenic challenges (details in the text). Solid lines indicate neural pathways, and interrupted lines represent humoral output. ANS, autonomic nervous system.

II. FAE AND IMMUNOCOMPETENCE

A. CELL-MEDIATED IMMUNE RESPONSES
1. *In Vitro* and *In Vivo* Studies

Clinical and experimental evidence has shown that fetal alcohol exposure (FAE) is associated with varied immunocompetence, including suppressed, augmented or unaltered response to challenges as compared with the control subjects. The decreased response has been primarily observed in the cellular immunity of humans and animals. Children diagnosed with fetal alcohol syndrome (FAS) displayed decreased mitogen-induced T-cell proliferation[7-9] and, in a few cases, a blunted T-cell-mediated delayed hypersensitivity response.[7] The suppressed cell-mediated immune reaction is also consistent with the clinical observations in children with FAS. This may help explain the predisposition of these children to viral and fungal infections, as well as to pneumonia caused by *Mycobacterium tuberculosis*,[7] or increased susceptibility to other kind of infections.[8-11] The clinical data have been largely supported by experimental studies. FAE has been associated with a suppressed splenic T-cell proliferative response to the mitogenic lectin Concanavalin-A (Con-A) in weanling pups[12] and adult male,[12-18] but not female rats[16-17] or female CD-1 mice.[19] An impaired Con-A-induced splenic T-cell response to interleukin-2 was also observed in adult FAE rats.[15-16] The effect was, however, age-dependent as demonstrated by a marked suppression between 1.5 and 3 months of age, but not thereafter.[20] FAE was also associated with a reduced Con-A-induced proliferation of thymocytes from near-term fetal mice,[21-22] as well as from 3-week-old male rats.[12] In contrast, however, an increase in thymocytes' proliferative response to Con-A was observed in FAE male rats 30 to 44-days old, and that returned to normal levels by 72 days of age.[23] More recently, Wolcott et al.,[24] reported that FAE in C57Bl/6 mice had no significant effects on the lytic activity of mature natural killer cells. On the other hand, the proliferative response of splenocytes to T-cell mitogens was suppressed during the first 21-days of age, but recovered to control levels by the 4th to 5th week of life. Other investigators observed a decrease in the number of T-helper, T-cytotoxic and T-suppressor cells in fetal as well as weanling mice.[25] Finally, preliminary studies have been reported on cellular immune functions in progeny of nonhuman primates (*Macaca nemestrina*).[26] Males and females, 1 to 3 years of age, were exposed *in utero* to a single weekly dose of ethanol (1.8 g/kg) administered to the mothers for the first 3, 6 or the entire 24-weeks of pregnancy. Peripheral T-cell proliferative response to tetanus toxoid, but not *staphylococcus* enterotoxin B, was significantly decreased in all ethanol-exposed animals compared with the controls. Other parameters, including white blood cell counts, leukocyte subsets and monocyte phagocytic activity were not significantly different from the control values.

There have been only few *in vivo* experiments which test the cell-mediated immune response of FAE animals. Young adult FAE C57Bl/6 mice displayed a marked suppression of the contact hypersensitivity response to the contact allergen trinitrochlorobenzene.[27] In contrast, the response to the contact allergen picryl chloride was enhanced in FAE mice of the same species.[28] In CD-1 mice, however, FAE males and females were not significantly different from their control cohorts in displaying a delayed type hypersensitivity response to subcutaneous injections of Keyhole Limpet Hemocyanin.[19] Another *in vivo* study demonstrated that graft *versus* host responses, a measure of cell-mediated immunity, were markedly suppressed in FAE male and female C57Bl/6 mice compared with the appropriate controls.[27]

Taken together, most studies have demonstrated that FAE is associated with impaired cell-mediated immune responses. The inconsistency may be attributable to the variance reported in the amount, route and duration of alcohol intake during the gestational period; the species, gender and age of the animal model; the type and dose of allergen or mitogen used in the experimental design, as well as the immune test under investigation.

2. FAE and Malignancy

The association of FAE with impaired cellular immunity may be responsible for the increased incidence of malignancies in progeny of mothers which consume alcohol during pregnancy. Most of the tumors reported in these children were of embryonic origin, including neuroblastoma,[29-32] ganglioneuroblastoma,[33] and medulloblastoma;[34] few other types of malignancies have also been reported (Table 2 in Gottesfeld and Abel[2]). In contrast, tumors in humans which consume excessive amounts of alcohol are characteristically found in the oral cavity, esophagus or larynx.[35] This suggests differential mechanistic possibilities which underlie the oncogenic effects of alcohol during prenatal development or adulthood. Few experimental studies have examined the effects of FAE on the susceptibility to tumor induction. In one study, weanling mice which were exposed to prenatal and lactational alcohol displayed increased susceptibility to the induction of primary Rous sarcoma.[36] In another study, FAE further potentiated the estrogen-induced prolactin-secreting pituitary tumor in the adult rat.[37] It remains to be determined as to whether alcohol or its metabolites act as carcinogens *in utero,* co-carcinogens predisposing the offspring to other carcinogens, or as teratogens promoting malignancy indirectly by suppressing the immune system.

B.   HUMORAL-MEDIATED IMMUNE RESPONSES

B-cell function is one of the important defense mechanisms against extracellular antigens, including microbes and their secreted toxins. There has been a paucity of knowledge, however, regarding FAE effects on B-cell-mediated humoral immune response. Johnson *et al.,*[7] reported that children with FAS displayed a marked decrease in the number of circulating B-cells, as well as low *basal* concentrations of immunoglobulins, including IgA, IgG and IgM, in nine out of 13 *unimmunized* individuals with FAS compared with age-matched controls; the data to support this report, however, were not provided by the authors. In contrast, Grossmann *et al.,*[26] were unable to find decreased serum immunoglobulin levels in 1 to 3-year-old nonhuman primates (*Macaca nemestrina*) exposed to once-weekly alcohol *in utero* for gestational periods ranging from 3 to 24 weeks. *In vitro* studies using rats also failed to demonstrate fetal alcohol effects on the humoral immune response, including the proliferative response of splenic B-cells to the mitogen lipopolysaccharide (LPS),[14,16,38] or plaque-forming cell response to a T-dependent antigen sheep red blood cell (SRBC) in CD-1 mice.[19] The effect of FAE on the LPS-induced proliferative response of B-cells in C57Bl/6 mice is apparently age-dependent, because a significantly reduced response at 3-weeks of age recovered to control values by postnatal week 4.[24]

A series of *in vivo* experiments were carried out to study the ability of FAE rats to mount specific humoral immune responses to various T-cell-dependent antigens.[38] The studies demonstrated that in response to immunization with sheep erythrocytes (SRBC) or bovine serum albumin (BSA) coupled with trinitrophenyl (TNP-SRBC or TNP-BSA), serum levels of the immunoglobulins IgM and IgG in FAE male and female rats were not significantly different from those in the pair-fed cohorts. It is noteworthy, however, that there was a higher overall serum IgM level in the female compared to the male rat following primary immunization to TNP-SRBC.

This sexual dimorphic effect is consistent with previous reports showing an augmented immune response in the female,[39-40] and may have been attributable to sex steroids. In contrast, adult rats consuming alcohol displayed a marked impairment of the humoral immune response.[41-42] This suggests differential mechanism associated with alcohol effects on the nascent as compared with mature humoral immune functions.

Rodents sired by alcohol-consuming males are also more susceptible to infection. It was demonstrated that paternal alcoholism contributed to the severity of the ocular infection to *Pseudomonas aeruginosa* in rats. The higher the paternal alcohol consumption, the earlier and the more frequent the cornea of the offspring perforated. The increased susceptibility was species-specific, i.e. it was observed only in Long-Evans and not in Sprague-Dawley rats. Furthermore, there was no effect of the progeny's gender nor interaction between maternal and paternal factors.[43] In mice, the increased susceptibility to *Pseudomonas aeruginosa* infection occurred despite the presence of high titers of antibody specific to the bacterium.[44] This suggests that the differential susceptibility is not due to humoral-mediated immunity, but likely involves a cellular defect.

Taken together, it appears that FAE has a selective effect predominantly on cellular not humoral immune responsiveness.

III. LACTATIONAL ALCOHOL AND IMMUNOCOMPETENCE

Compared with immune effects of exposure to alcohol *in utero,* there is a paucity of information on effects of ethanol in breast milk on the suckling infant. This may have been attributable, at least in part, to the reports that the amount of alcohol ingested by the breast-fed infant is very small relative to the amount consumed by the mother [3,45-46] and, thus, has not been perceived as a risk to the infant. Furthermore, the medical community has strongly advocated breast-feeding during early infancy, primarily because of the milk's protective effect against infection,[47-48] and that may have led to a resurgence of breast-feeding. On the other hand, although it has been documented that the human brain is vulnerable to alcohol during the third trimester, a period of cellular proliferation, migration and maturation ("brain growth spurt," a period equivalent to early postnatal life in the rodent), the brain continues to be vulnerable to alcohol during lactation, when most of the organs, including the endocrine and immune systems, are continuing to develop. Thus, knowledge of the potential adverse effects of lactational alcohol on the infant is of considerable clinical importance.

The limited studies on alcohol and lactation have demonstrated that alcohol has pluripotent effects that contribute to a pattern of behavioral, neurologic, endocrinologic and immunological anomalies in the suckling infant. Nursing mothers who drink may pass on enough alcohol in the milk to retard their children's development of nervous system functions, as shown by an impaired motor function at one-year of age.[49] The authors postulated two mechanisms that could explain the observed motor impairments: one, the developing brain is very sensitive to small quantities of alcohol and/or two, that decreased metabolism of alcohol[50] could have resulted in its accumulation in the suckling infant and, thus, impair the functional development of the brain. In experimental animals, administration of alcohol through breast milk or by other methods during early postnatal life has been associated with extensive brain damage,[51-52] reduced brain development,[53-54] neurochemical changes[55-56] and postnatal growth deficits.[54] The latter anomaly may have been associated with a compromised infantile nutrition that is possibly caused by alterations such as suckling behavior,[57] structure and function of maternal mammary gland,[58-59] anomalous feeding patterns due to alcohol-induced specific flavors and odors in the milk[60] and reduced suckling-induced prolactin which leads to reduced maternal milk production and, consequently, to reduced infantile milk intake.[61]

Alcohol in breast milk may also have a direct pharmacological effect on the neuroendocrine system of the infant. One clinical study reported a case of pseudo-Cushing syndrome associated with an increased level of circulating cortisol in a 4-month-old infant exposed to alcohol by breast-feeding.[62] These observations are reminiscent of clinical patterns caused by alcoholism in adults.[63-65] The clinical manifestations in the infant were rapidly reversed when alcohol was withheld.[62]

It has been well documented that breast-feeding has a protective effect on the infant against various infections (for review see Goldman and Goldblum;[66] Walker;[67] Chandra;[68] Butler;[69] Machtinger;[70] Wilson[71]). Milk has been shown to contain numerous cellular and humoral immune components, including T-cells, B-cells, macrophages, antibodies, lymphokines and interleukins,[72-75] which appear to protect the neonate against environmental antigens before its own immune system is completely developed. Since the defense mechanisms of the nascent immune system is immature, it could be increasingly vulnerable to challenges, including various stressors, infections, drugs and alcohol.

Several lines of evidence have shown that the intake of alcohol through breast milk can compromise immune functions in the suckling infant. Seelig and his coworkers observed that maternal alcohol consumption can adversely influence the transmission of T-cell-mediated immunity to the intestinal parasite Trichinella spiralis (TS) during lactation; that could compromise the ability of the neonate to fight infection.[76-77] In subsequent studies of alcohol-consuming TS-infected lactating rats, the authors suggested that several factors, including a decrease in natural killer cells and specific antibody levels in the milk,[78] a suppressed production of the cytokines tumor necrosis factor and interleukin-6 by milk and blood cells,[79] as well as a marked decrease in the number and distribution of T- and B-cells, may have attributed to the depressed lactational immune transfer to the pups.

Other investigators utilized CD-1 mice in a paradigm of ethanol exposure during pregnancy, pregnancy and lactation, or lactation alone.[80-81] The data show that while all of the ethanol-exposure paradigms were associated with altered phenotypic development of splenic lymphocytes in the 21-day-old offspring, the greatest effect was on differentiation antigen expression that occurred in mice exposed to lactational alcohol during the suckling period.[81] The authors suggested that the marked decrease in specific splenic lymphocyte population, especially the Thy 1.2^+, is attributable to the direct effect of alcohol in the milk. In another study, Giberson and Blakley[80] demonstrated that mice exposed to lactational alcohol displayed an increased susceptibility to a retrovirus-induced lymphocytic leukemia.

Gottesfeld and LeGrue[46] carried out *in vivo* studies to examine cell-mediated immune responses in adult C57Bl/6 mice exposed to lactational alcohol during the first 21 postnatal days. The authors observed persistent deficits in contact hypersensitivity to the allergen TNCB as well as in graft versus host responses. While these data are consistent with the suppression observed in similar cell-mediated immune responses of mice exposed to alcohol *in utero*,[82] the blood alcohol level in the suckling pups was about one third of that in the maternal or fetal blood during the prenatal alcohol exposure. The minimal level of alcohol at which such deficits may occur is not known, nor have the underlying mechanisms been determined. Based on available evidence, however, one can speculate that (1) the nervous and immune system are highly susceptible to small amounts of alcohol during the critical period of early postnatal development, in accord with the observed lactational alcohol-induced brain damage during the rapid brain growth spurt;[52] (2) alcohol may accumulate in the infant;[49] (3) acetaldehyde in milk of the nursing dam may be more deleterious than alcohol *per se* during early postnatal life; (4) effects of early postnatal alcohol may be exacerbated during the withdrawal period, and finally, anomalies such as altered synaptic transmission across the sympatho-lymphoid axis,[46] increased circulating levels of glucocorticoids[62] and, perhaps, other factors yet to be determined, may account for the immune deficits associated with lactational alcohol consumption.

IV. MECHANISTIC POSSIBILITIES FOR THE IMMUNE INCOMPETENCE ASSOCIATED WITH FAE

As indicated above, the brain regulates the responsiveness of lymphoid organs to environmental stimuli via two major controlling elements: (1) neuroendocrine axes, and (2) autonomic neural pathways. Altered immune modulation by the neural and humoral elements, possibly underlies the cellular immune deficit associated with FAE.

A. NEUROENDOCRINE MODULATION OF IMMUNE RESPONSIVENESS

There is a large body of evidence indicating that hormones secreted from the hypothalamo-pituitary-endocrine axis can modulate immune responsiveness by interacting with specific lymphocytic receptors.[1,83-84] Of all neuroendocrine axes, however, that of the hypothalamo-pituitary-adrenal (HPA) outflow has been best studied, presumably because of the important clinical implications of glucocorticoids as potent anti-inflammatory hormones.[85] Exposure to alcohol *in utero* also alters the secretion of hormones from most, if not all neuroendocrine axes, as well as the responsiveness of endocrine glands to stimuli well into adulthood (reviewed by Rudeen and Taylor;[86] Weinberg[87]). In the present review, attention will be focused on the HPA axis, because it influences brain development as well as the ability of the host to cope with and adapt to challenges, including resistance to infections and malignancy.

1. The Hypothalamo-Pituitary-Adrenal Axis

a. Feedback Regulation

Activation of the HPA axis represents a major component of an organism's defensive response to stimuli which threaten homeostasis. Corticotropin releasing hormone (CRH), the major driving force of the HPA axis, is found in neurosecretory cells in the paraventricular nucleus (PVN) of the hypothalamus[88-89] and is influenced by various stimuli, including emotional stress, trauma, diurnal rhythms, cytokine-mediated inflammation, and neurotransmitters such as catecholamines, various peptides, acetylcholine and GABA (Figure 2). The CRH-containing neurons project into the median eminence of the hypothalamus where they terminate on capillaries of the hypophysial-portal vessels. There, CRH is released and transported to the anterior pituitary gland where the hormone stimulates pituitary corticotrophs to synthesize and secrete adrenocorticotropic releasing hormone (ACTH). The latter, a 39-amino acid peptide, is formed from the prohormone pro-opiomelanocortin (POMC) along with β-lipotropin, a 92-amino acid peptide. β-lipotropin is further broken into other smaller active fragments, including β-endorphin. While CRH is the most potent stimulator of ACTH/β-endorphin secretion from the anterior pituitary corticotrophs, the release of ACTH in response to stress is also regulated by other peptides, including arginine-vasopressin and oxytocin as well as by several neurotransmitters, including serotonin, epinephrine and norepinephrine.[90-92] ACTH is transported via the general circulation to the adrenal cortex where it stimulates the synthesis and secretion of glucocorticoids, aldosterone and adrenal androgens. Glucocorticoids (cortisol in human as well as in non-human primates; corticosterone in rodents) are released from the adrenal cortex into the general circulation, where a high proportion of the hormone is bound to an α-globulin ("transcortin" or "corticosteroid-binding globulin") and considered physiologically inactive. The small free-fraction of the glucocorticoid in plasma represents the active fraction of the hormone.[93] As illustrated in Figure 2, the secretion of adrenal glucocorticoids is regulated by several closed negative feedback mechanisms, including a major feedback loop mediated by glucocorticoids to the hypothalamus to suppress the release of CRH, and to the pituitary to inhibit ACTH secretion. Additional feedback loops include the inhibitory effects of ACTH (not shown), β-endorphin as well as CRH *per se* on the CRH neuron.[94] This feedback mechanism enables the organism

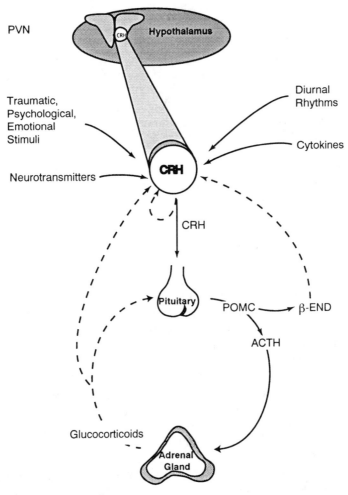

Figure 2. Feedback loops of the hypothalamo-pituitary-adrenal axis (details in the text). Solid lines indicate stimulation, and interrupted lines indicate inhibitory effects. ACTH, adrenocorticotropin hormone; CRH, corticotropin releasing hormone; β-END, β-endorphin; POMC, pro-opiomelanocortin; PVN, paraventricular nucleus of the hypothalamus.

to maintain stable blood levels of glucocorticoids at all times, while simultaneously counteracting environmental stimuli which may be threatening to the body's homeostasis.

b. Immune System - HPA Axis Interactions

Glucocorticoids exert a wide variety of effects on bodily functions, including the modulation of immune responsiveness. It has been well documented that glucocorticoids have potent immunosuppressive as well as anti inflammatory actions.[95-96] Previous studies demonstrated that chronic elevation of circulating glucocorticoids, whether by exogenous administration or induced by stress, was associated with lymphocytopenia, thymic involution and loss of splenic as well as lymph node tissue mass.[97-98] In addition, glucocorticoids have been found to suppress T cell-mediated immunity,[99-101] possibly by acting directly on lymphocytic receptors for corticosteroids, ACTH, POMC-derived peptides and CRH.[102] Another possibility suggests that glucocorticoids inhibit the secretion of cytokines,[96,101,103] which play an important role in the stimulation and promotion of a variety of immune responses. This is based on studies showing increased circulating levels of glucocorticoids during the course of the immune response to antigenic challenges.[104-105] Subsequent studies proposed that the increased secretion of glucocorticoids following immunization is mediated by cytokines.[106]

Interleukin-1 (IL-1) is the cytokine most studied for its effect on the HPA axis. Activation of the immune system results in the release of IL-1 from activated macrophages and monocytes. It stimulates T-cell proliferation, antibody production, release of neutrophils from bone marrow and causes fever. In addition, IL-1 stimulates CRH release from the PVN[107-110] and induces the increase in plasma ACTH, POMC-derived peptides and corticosterone.[106,108,111-113] These effects were blocked by deafferentation of the medial basal hypothalamus[114] and by immunoneutralization of endogenous CRH.[107-108] While these observations strongly suggest a central effect of IL-1 action, the exact site is still controversial. Several investigators suggested that IL-1 in the circulation can stimulate CRH-containing axon terminals in the median eminence and/or CRH cell bodies in the PVN of the hypothalamus.[108,115] Other investigators proposed that the neural connections between brainstem catecholaminergic nuclei and the PVN,[116] play a role in the mediation of IL-1 effects on the release of CRH.[117-119] Subsequent studies utilizing the immediate early gene c-fos, considered an early marker of neuronal activation,[120-121] lend support to this view.[122] The latter authors demonstrated a temporally dynamic response to IL-1-induced activation of the HPA axis, which was preceded by the activation of the area postrema and nucleus of the solitary tract. These brainstem regions contain the cell bodies of ascending catecholaminergic pathways to the PVN[116] and, thus, may initiate the response of the HPA axis to the cytokine.

While there is strong evidence for the central effect of IL-1, its effect on pituitary corticotrophs and/or the adrenal cortex cannot be ruled out. In fact, it has been suggested that the POMC-derived peptides ACTH and β-endorphin may also act as immunomodulators and are involved, perhaps, in the fine-tuning of the inflammatory response[96] by inhibiting splenocyte production of the cytokine interferon and its responsiveness to antigenic challenges.[95,123-124] Other cytokines, including IL-2, IL-6, IL-8 and tumor necrosis factor, can not be ruled out as active mediators in the interaction between the immune and the HPA and, possibly, other neuroendocrine axes (reviewed in Jones and Kennedy[125]).

Taken together, a feedback loop appears to exist between the HPA axis and the immune system. Cytokines released from stimulated lymphocytes activate the HPA axis to release glucocoticoids in order to counter the overly active immune system, while a negative feedback mechanism of glucocorticoids regulates the HPA axis at the hypothalamic and pituitary levels. Clearly, an immune response to antigenic challenges, if left unchecked by defective glucocorticoid secretion, will produce adverse immune effects that may lead to diseases and pathogenesis.[126]

c. Influence of FAE on Immune - HPA Axis Interactions

A growing body of evidence indicates that alcohol consumption during pregnancy can elicit profound effects on both maternal and fetal HPA axes (for recent reviews see Rudeen and Taylor,[86] and Weinberg[87]). Exposure to alcohol *in utero* may influence, directly or indirectly, the HPA axis during early development as well as after maturity. Studies with neonatal rats have demonstrated that levels of glucocorticoids in plasma, brain and adrenal gland, as well as of CRH and ACTH in the hypothalamus and pituitary gland, respectively, are significantly higher compared with the control cohorts.[12,127] In contrast, adult rats exposed to prenatal alcohol display normal basal levels of plasma corticosterone and β-endorphin. The anomalies in HPA axis activity become apparent, however, when the FAE adult rat is challenged.[128-130] These studies have shown that the animals exhibit a heightened stress response, which is expressed by increased plasma levels of corticosteroid and β-endorphin, as well as retarded recovery from the stress response. Furthermore, the anomalies are sexually dimorphic depending on several experimental variables, including the test parameters, the nature and intensity of the stressor, and the time course of the challenge.[131] In order to dissociate between effects of increased corticosteroid levels in pregnant rats consuming alcohol and effects of the alcohol *per se* on the HPA axis of the progeny, Redei et al.,[17] used adrenalectomized dams. They observed that FAE markedly increased POMC gene expression in the anterior pituitary of adult male, but not female rats. The increase was reversed by maternal adrenalectomy. Furthermore, the hypothalamic levels of CRH mRNA were increased in FAE male, while maternal adrenalectomy had no effect on the CRH synthesis. These results were at variance, however, with those of Lee et al.,[132] which showed that adrenalectomy of the pregnant dam reversed the increased hypothalamic CRH expression in the FAE offspring. These differences are difficult to interpret, since in the latter study the adrenalectomized dams were supplemented with corticosterone. In addition, the alcohol exposure in the study by Lee et al.,[132] was confined to the second gestational week and no gender-related distinctions were made.

Clearly, the functional disturbances in the HPA and/or β-endorphin axes could account for the persistent cellular immune deficits associated with FAE. Only a few studies have attempted to show a direct relationship between an altered activity of the HPA axis and the immune incompetence associated with exposure to prenatal alcohol. Redei et al.,[17] demonstrated that maternal adrenalectomy reversed the deficit in cellular immunity (shown by a suppressed proliferative response of splenocytes to Con-A stimulation) in male rats exposed to alcohol in utero. In the same study, the authors also showed that maternal adrenalectomy during gestation had a reversal effect on the FAE-induced increase in POMC in the anterior pituitary. Gottesfeld and Ullrich[38] used in vivo studies to examine effects of FAE on circulating corticosterone levels during the course of the immune response to sheep erythrocytes (humoral immunity). The data showed that there were no significant differences in the immune response to SRBC nor in the activation of the HPA axis between peripubertal FAE male rats and their control cohorts. Taken together, this suggests a selective relationship between functional anomalies of the HPA axis and cellular, not humoral, immune incompetence associated with FAE.

Effects of IL-1 on activation of the HPA axis was also studied in FAE young weanling (22 to 24-day-old) rats and their pair-fed controls.[133] The investigators demonstrated that following a systemic administration of IL-1, the release of ACTH and β-endorphin, but not corticosterone, was markedly decreased in the FAE pups and also, although to a lesser extent, in the pair-fed compared with the control cohorts. There were no significant differences, however, in the CRH-induced ACTH release among the three groups. The possible relationship among alcohol, nitric oxide and neurotoxicity[134] led Lee and Rivier[135] to test the hypothesis that the blunted pituitary response to IL-1 in FAE young rats is associated with increased nitric oxide production in the fetal brain. This hypothesis was based on previous studies showing similar effects of IL-1 and nitric oxide on the HPA axis of adult rats.[136] The study showed that inhibiting the formation of nitric oxide by an arginine derivative augmented ACTH secretion, and reversed the blunted pituitary response to IL-1 caused by FAE.[135] The authors suggested that exposure to alcohol in utero increases endogenous levels of nitric oxide and that may alter the response of the HPA axis to IL-1.[133,135] The altered responsiveness of the HPA axis to the cytokine appears to be consistent with observations of a decreased fever induction by lipopolysaccharide (LPS) in FAE rats.[137] Normally, the systemic administration of the endotoxin LPS activates peripheral macrophages to produce and release cytokines (e.g., IL-1, IL-6) that may induce fever by activating, at least in part, CRH neurons.[138] In the study by Yirmiya et al.,[137] FAE appeared to have impaired the LPS-induced release of endogenous cytokines and/or the response of the HPA axis to IL-1. Fever is an important factor which normally enables the host to cope with bacterial infections by enhancing immunological responses. Thus, the functional impairments of the HPA axis may account, at least in part, for the cellular immune deficits associated with FAE.

While this review has focused on the HPA axis as one possible neuroendocrine mechanism to account for the cellular immune deficit associated with FAE, other neuroendocrine axes should not be overlooked as possible factors. For example, the hypothalamo-pituitary-thyroid axis and the hypothalamo-pituitary-gonadal axis, have both been implicated in immune modulation,[84] and other functional anomalies associated with FAE.[139-142] However, more studies are needed to demonstrate a direct relationship between the alcohol-related cellular immune incompetence and the dysfunction of the indicated neuroendocrine axes.

B.   AUTONOMIC NEURAL MODULATION OF IMMUNE RESPONSIVENESS

The autonomic nervous system (ANS) innervates all of the tissues of the immune system, including the primary lymphoid organs (bone marrow and thymus) and secondary lymphoid organs (spleen, lymph nodes and gut-associated lymphoid tissue/GALT). Both the sympathetic (noradrenergic) and the parasympathetic (cholinergic) branches of the ANS innervate immune tissues.[143-144] It is noteworthy, however, that while there have been reports on the presence of cholinergic projections to lymphoid organs[145] as well as of muscarinic cholinergic receptors on lymphocytes,[146] the role of the parasympathetic system in immune modulation remains controversial.[147] In contrast, there is a great deal of evidence indicating that the sympathetic nervous system plays an important role in immune modulation.[148-149] This review will focus, therefore, on dynamic metabolic changes in the sympathetic innervation of lymphoid organs ("sympatho-lymphoid axis"), as an additional mechanistic possibility for the immune anomalies associated with FAE.

1. The Sympatho-Lymphoid Axis

It has been well documented that the sympatho-lymphoid axis provides the anatomical link between the brain and the immune system. Both the primary and secondary lymphoid organs are extensively innervated by noradrenergic (NA) postganglionic sympathetic nerve fibers.[144,148] The thymus receives NA innervation from the superior cervical ganglion and the upper sympathetic chain. These fibers enter the thymus with the vasculature, which displays its highest density at the junction between the thymic cortex and medulla. Some NA fibers branch off the vasculature into the parenchyma and end among thymocytes. The spleen receives NA sympathetic innervation mainly from the superior mesenteric/coeliac ganglionic complex. The postganglionic NA fibers enter the spleen at the hilar region along with the vasculature and then arborize into the parenchyma forming synapse-like contacts with T lymphocytes.[150]

Development of the sympathetic noradrenergic innervation of lymphoid organs has been studied extensively in the rat spleen.[151-152] In the spleen of the neonate rat, sympathetic axon terminals are relatively sparse but increase in number during early postnatal life. Ackerman et al.,[151-152] observed that maturation of the splenic noradrenergic innervation is temporally linked to the development of lymphoid compartmentation,[153-155] consistent with the hypothesis that sympathetic innervation of the immune system facilitates the ontogeny of lymphoid organs and the development of immunocompetence.[152]

Adrenoceptors, both α- and to a greater extent β-subtype, have been identified and characterized on human and rodent lymphocytes.[156-158] Thus, alterations in levels of norepinephrine may influence lymphocyte adrenoceptors and their mediation of immune capacity. This is supported by studies in which sympathetic neurons were manipulated by surgical or chemical means. Thus, it has been reported that following sympathectomy there was an enhancement of antibody formation (plaque-forming cells) against a T-dependent antigen,[159] as well as an increased activity of natural killer cells,[160] characterized as a defense mechanism against certain tumor cells or viral-infected normal cells. The enhanced immune response following sympathectomy suggests that this is attributable to the loss of noradrenergic inhibitory influences on certain aspects of immune responsiveness.[161] This is supported by reports of a transient decline in norepinephrine (NE) concentration in spleen during the course of the immune response[159] suggesting that the decrease in levels of NE may be necessary for optimal lymphocytic proliferation. On the other hand, it may be argued that the decreased tissue levels of NE may be associated with increased release, or turnover of the amine that is necessary for the suppression of any further expansion of the lymphocytic population following immunization. This is supported by observations of increased amounts of splenic catecholaminergic metabolites correlated with decreased density of β-adrenoceptors on splenic lymphocytes following antigenic exposure.[162-163]

The mechanism by which sympathetic neural modulation of immunity occurs is not completely understood. It has been shown, however, that the amine-adrenoceptor interaction is linked to second messenger systems, including cyclic AMP formation,[164-166] increased cyclic AMP concentrations blocks IL-2-stimulated proliferation of T-lymphocytes.[167]

While the evidence for a direct communication between cells of the immune system and sympathetic axon terminals is well documented, other studies have suggested an additional, indirect sympathetic immunomodulation via central regulation of autonomic outflow. This suggestion is supported by observations of changes in firing rates as well as in NE parameters (decreased levels, increased turnover) in discrete hypothalamic nuclei following antigenic challenges or IL-1 administration.[117,168-169] The IL-1-induced release of splenic NE was shown to be associated with activation of CRH-containing neurons in the hypothalamus.[170] This confirms previous observations of suppressed splenic natural killer cell activity mediated by CRH-induced activation of sympathetic neurons.[171-172] Similarly, a transient suppression of peripheral immune cell reactivity was mediated by CRH through activation of the HPA axis as well as the sympathetic nervous system following intracerebroventricular administration of IL-1 or lipopolysaccharide.[173-175]

Finally, it is noteworthy that along with the catecholamines, the sympatho-lymphoid axis co-releases a number of neuropeptides, including vasoactive intestinal peptide, cholecystokinine, neuropeptide Y, somatostatin, substance P, opioid peptides and others.[144] Their source has not been determined, although some peptides in lymphoid organs may be released from lymphocytes.[176] The peptidergic immunomodulation is probably mediated by receptors which have been identified on lymphoid cells.[144,177-179]

Taken together, the sympatho-lymphoid axis clearly plays an important role in immunomodulation. While the underlying mechanisms remain to be determined, it has been suggested that the regulation of the sympathetic outflow occurs at two levels: (1) locally, at the level of lymphoid organs, that would allow rapid responsiveness of sympathetic axon terminals to activation or perturbations of immune functions, and (2) through the CNS, possibly CRH neurons, that would permit long-term regulation and coordination of the neuroendocrine, autonomic and immune systems.[149]

2. FAE and Sympathetic-Immune System Interactions

As indicated above, the sympatho-lymphoid axis plays an important role in the regulation of immune responses. Thus, Gottesfeld et al.[27,82] conducted a series of studies, utilizing neurochemical and histochemical methods, to look for a peripheral neurotransmitter correlate of immune anomalies characteristic of FAE. Mice exposed to prenatal alcohol displayed persistent deficits of cell-mediated immune responsiveness and selective neurochemical changes, indicative of altered transmission across the sympatho-lymphoid synapse. The anomalies included low concentrations of NE in the spleen and thymus, but not the heart of the young-adult FAE mice. The amine deficits were observed as early as postnatal day one, and became progressively larger as the animal grew older. This may have been caused by the thymic and splenic weight-gain restriction in the FAE mice.[82] Normally, NE levels undergo relatively little changes despite fluctuation in neuronal activity, mainly because the rate of synthesis and release of the amine are at equilibrium.[180] Thus, the reduced levels of splenic and thymic NE in FAE mice suggests that the synthesis of the amine does not keep up with the enhanced release. This was demonstrated by the increased turnover rate of NE selectively in lymphoid organs.[27] The possibility that the decrease in NE levels may also reflect alcohol-related neuronal damage and/or paucity of sympathetic projections onto lymphoid organs is unlikely, as indicated by the histofluorescence data.[27] Both the distribution of noradrenergic varicosities and their density in the splenic white pulp were unaffected by the FAE. The results, thus, suggest that the noradrenergic defect in the FAE mice is metabolic, not structural. Furthermore, the enhanced release of the amine produced a selective reduction in the number of binding sites, not affinity, of β-adrenoceptors in the spleen and thymus of the FAE mice. Similar to the pattern of amine deficits, the decrease in the density of β-adrenoceptors in lymphoid organs was noted as early as postnatal day one, and became more pronounced with age compared with the pair-fed cohorts.[82] Taken together, the fact that the alcohol-related changes occurred in spleen and thymus but not the heart tissue suggests that the neurochemical changes were organ-specific and not related to a generalized effect on the sympathetic nervous system. The site of alcohol action remains speculative: One possibility is that it acts at a local level, on sympathetic axon terminals in lymphoid tissues. Alternatively, or an additional possibility is that alcohol regulates the sympatho-lymphoid axis indirectly, by activating CRH neurons in the CNS. As indicated above, alcohol induces the central release of CRH, and this neuropeptide activates the pituitary-adrenal axis as well as the sympathetic neural outflow[171-172] that may account for the cellular immune deficits characteristic of FAE.

Sympathetic neurons require nerve growth factor (NGF) for their development and maintenance,[181-182] as indicated by cell survival, neurite elongation and induction of neurotransmitter biosynthetic enzymes in response to NGF.[182-183] In addition, NGF may have a role in modulating immune responses[184] including enhanced proliferative response of rat splenic lymphocytes to lectins[185] and expression of NGF receptors on lymphocyte subpopulations in humans and rodents.[186] Because the first obligatory step in NGF action is binding to NGF receptors on sympathetic axon terminals,[187] a study was carried out to characterize the expression of NGF receptors in lymphoid organs and heart of FAE infant mice.[82] It was observed that FAE mice displayed a selective enhancement of NGF binding in lymphoid organs, particularly in the thymus. The data suggest that FAE may disrupt the immunomodulatory effects of NGF. While the mechanism by which exposure to alcohol *in utero* may disrupt NGF modulation of immune function are not known, several possibilities come to mind: (1) FAE associated with hypo-thyroidism during early infancy[139-140,188] may disrupt sympathetic neural devel-opment[189] that may be mediated by NGF; [190-192] (2) increased glucocorticoid levels in pregnant mothers consuming alcohol[193] may influence the development of noradrenergic neural expression[194-195] as well as NGF activity[196-197] in the offspring. This may partly account for the adverse effects of maternal glucocorticoids on the immune system of the FAE offspring;[17] and (3) FAE may interfere with the biosynthesis of NGF.[198-200] This is consistent with recent studies showing that administration of exogenous NGF to infant rats exposed to prenatal alcohol reversed the deficits in splenic NE levels.[201]

Taken together, the developmental changes in the sympatho-lymphoid axis along with altered NGF function may account, at least in part, for the cellular immune incompetence associated with FAE.

V. SUMMARY

There is probably no single mechanism which can account for such a complex biological phenomenon as immune modulation. Disruption of any of the functional components, whether neural, humoral, or immune-derived factors, can be translated into immune deficiency. Hence, exposure to alcohol during critical developmental periods may impair immune responsiveness to challenges by either acting directly on the nascent lymphoid cells, or indirectly by perturbing neuroendocrine systems or components of the autonomic nervous system that are closely involved in immune modulation.

ACKNOWLEDGMENTS

The author's research cited herein has been supported in part by NIAAA grants AA06158 and AA09131, as well as by a Biomedical Research Support Grant. The author wishes to thank her collaborators, students and technicians who have contributed to various aspects of the studies. A special note of gratitude to Diana Parker for her expert secretarial assistance and to Rama Grenda for the art work.

REFERENCES

1. **Ader, R., Felten, D.L., and Cohen, N.,** Eds., *Psychoneuroimmunology*, 2nd ed. 1991.
2. **Gottesfeld, Z. and Abel, E.L.,** Maternal and paternal alcohol use: Effects on the immune system of the offspring, *Life Sci.*, 48, 1, 1991.
3. **Gottesfeld, Z.,** Neuroimmune effects of prenatal and early postnatal alcohol exposure, in *Alcohol, Immunity and Cancer*, Yirmiya, R. and Taylor, A. N., Eds., CRC Press, Boca Raton, Florida, 1993, chap. 8.
4. **Giberson, P.K. and Weinberg, J.,** Fetal alcohol syndrome and functioning of the immune system, *Alcohol. Health Res. World*, 16, 29, 1992.

5. **Chiappelli, F., Wong, C., Yirmya, R., Norman, D., Chang, M-P., and Taylor, A.,** Fetal alcohol exposure and neuroimmune surveillance, in *Alcohol, Immunity and Cancer*, Yirmiya R. and Taylor A.N., Eds., CRC Press, Boca Raton, 1993, Chap. 9.

6. **Watson, R.R. and Gottesfeld, Z.,** Neuroimmune effects of alcohol and its role in AIDS, *Adv. Neuroimmunol.*, 3, 151, 1993.

7. **Johnson, S., Knight, R., Marmer, D.J., and Steele, R.W.,** Immune deficiency in fetal alcohol syndrome, *Pediatr. Res.*, 15, 908, 1981.

8. **Ammann, A.J., Wara, D.W., Cowan, M.J., Barrett, D.J., and Stiehm, E.R.,** The DiGeorge syndrome and the fetal alcohol syndrome, *Am. J. Dis. Child.*, 136, 906, 1982.

9. **Calvani, M., Ghirelli, D., Fortuna, C., Lalli, F., and Marcolini, P.,** Fetal alcohol syndrome: Clinical, metabolic, and immunologic follow-up in 14 cases, *Minerva Pediatr.*, 37, 77, 1985.

10. **DiGeorge, A.M.,** Congenital absence of the thymus and its immunologic consequences: Concurrence with congenital hypoparathyroidism, *Birth Defects*, 4, 116, 1968.

11. **Church, M. and Gerkin, K.P.,** Hearing disorders in children with fetal alcohol syndrome: Findings from case reports, *J. Pediatr.*, 82, 147, 1988.

12. **Redei, E., Clark, W.R., and McGivern, R.F.,** Alcohol exposure *in utero* results in diminished T-cell function and alterations in brain corticotropin-releasing factor and ACTH content, *Alc. Clin. Exp. Res.*, 13, 439, 1989.

13. **Chang, M.-P., Yamaguchi, D.T., Yeh, M., and Taylor, A.N.,** Mechanism of the impaired T-cell proliferation in adult rats exposed to alcohol *in utero*, *Int. J. Immunopharmacol.*, 16, 345, 1994.

14. **Monjan, A.A. and Mandell, W.,** Fetal alcohol and immunity: Depression of mitogen-induced lymphocyte blastogenesis, *Neurobehav. Toxicol.*, 2, 213, 1980.

15. **Norman, D.C., Chang, M.-P., Castle, S.C., and Van Zuylen, J.E.,** Diminished proliferative response of Con-A blast cells to interleukin 2 in adult rats exposed to ethanol *in utero*, *Alc. Clin. Exp. Res.*, 13, 69, 1989.

16. **Weinberg, J. and Jerrells, T.R.,** Suppression of immune responsiveness: Six differences in prenatal ethanol effects, *Alc.Clin. Exp. Res.*, 15, 525, 1991.

17. **Redei, E., Halasz, I., Li, L.-F., Frystowsky, M.B., and Aird, F.,** Maternal adrenalectomy alters the immune and endocrine functions of fetal alcohol-exposed, *Endocrinology*, 133, 452, 1993.

18. **Tewari, S., Diano, M., Bera, R., Nguyen, Q., and Parekh, H.,** Alterations in brain polyribosomal RNA translation and lymphocyte proliferation in prenatal ethanol-exposed rats, *Alc. Clin. Exp. Res.*, 16, 436, 1992.

19. **Zidell , R.H., Hatoum, N.S., and Thomas, P.T.,** Fetal alcohol effects: Evidence of developmental impairment in the absence of immunotoxicity, *Fund. Appl. Toxicol.*, 10, 189, 1988.

20. **Norman, D.C., Chang, M.-P., Wong, C.M.K., Branch, B.J., Castle, S., and Taylor, A.N.,** Changes with age in the proliferative response of splenic T cells from rats exposed to ethanol *in utero*, *Alc. Clin. Exp. Res.*, 15, 428, 1991.

21. **Ewald, S.J. and Frost, W.W.,** Effect of prenatal exposure to ethanol on development of the thymus, *Thymus*, 9, 211, 1987.

22. **Ewald, S.J. and Walden, S.M.,** Flow cytometric and histological analysis of mouse thymus in fetal alcohol syndrome, *J. Leukocyte Biol.*, 44, 434, 1988.

23. **Wong, C.M.K., Chiappelli, F., Chang, M.-P., Norman, D.C., Cooper, E.L., Branch, B.J., and Taylor, A.N.,** Prenatal exposure to alcohol enhances thymocyte mitogenic responses postnatally, *Int. J. Immunopharmacol.*, 14, 303, 1992.

24. **Wolcott, R.M., Jennings, S.R., and Chervenak, R.,** *In utero* exposure to ethanol affects postnatal development of T- and B-lymphocytes, but not natural killer cells, *Alc. Clin. Exp. Res.*, 19, 170, 1995.

25. **Ewald, S.J. and Huang, C.,** Lymphocyte populations and immune responses in mice prenatally exposed to ethanol, *Alcohol, Immumodulation and AIDS*, 191, 1990.

26. **Grossman, A., Astley, S.J., Liggitt, H.D., Clarren, S.K., Shiota, F., Kennedy, B., Thouless, M.E., and Maggio-Price, L.,** Immune function in offspring of nonhuman primates (*Macaca nemestrina*) exposed weekly to 1.8 g/kg ethanol during pregnancy: Preliminary observations, *Alc. Clin. Exp. Res.*, 17, 822, 1993.

27. **Gottesfeld, Z., Christie, R., Felten, D.L., and LeGrue, S.J.,** Prenatal ethanol exposure alters immune capacity and noradrenergic synaptic transmission in lymphoid organs of the adult mouse, *Neuroscience,* 35, 185, 1990.

28. **Clausing, P., Günther, B., Emmendörfer, A., Lohmann-Matthes, M.-L., Taylor, L.D., Newport, G., and Paule, M.G.,** Neuroimmune effects of prenatal ethanol exposure in CD-1 rats and C57BL/6 mice, *Adv. Biosci.*, 86, 503, 1993.

29. **Kinney, H., Faix, R., and Brazy, J.,** The fetal alcohol syndrome and neuroblastoma, *Pediatrics*, 66, 130, 1980.

30. **Kiess, W., Linderkamp, O., Hadorn, H.-B., and Haas, R.,** Fetal alcohol syndrome and malignant disease, *Eur. J. Pediatr.*, 143, 60, 1984.

31. **Kahn, A., Bader, J.L., Hoy, G.R., and Sinks, L.F.,** Hepatoblastoma in child with fetal alcohol syndrome, *Lancet,* 1, 1403, 1979.

32. **Zaunschirm, A. and Muntean, W.,** Fetal alcohol syndrome and malignant disease, *Eur. J. Pediatr.*, 141, 256, 1984.

33. **Holt, C.P. and Favara, B.,** Eleventh Annual Meeting of the Soc. Pediatr. Onc., Lisbon, Portugal, p. 761, 1979.

34. **Cohen, M.M., Jr.,** Neoplasia and the fetal alcohol and hydantoin syndromes, *Neurobehav. Toxicol. Teratol.,* 3, 161, 1981.

35. **Rothman, K.J.,** Alcohol, in *Persons at High Risk of Cancer; An Approach to Cancer Etiology and Control,* Fraumeni, J.F., Ed., Academic Press, New York, 1975.

36. **Haughton, G. and Ellis, F.,** Increased susceptibility to induction of primary rous sarcoma in C57BL/105ScSn following perinatal exposure to dietary ethanol, *Alc. Clin. Exp. Res.,* 5, 347, 1981.

37. **Gottesfeld, Z., Trippe, K., Wargovich, M.J., and Berkowitz, A.S.,** Fetal alcohol exposure and adult tumorigenesis, *Alcohol,* 9, 465, 1992.

38. **Gottesfeld, Z. and Ullrich, S.E.,** Prenatal alcohol exposure selectively suppresses cell-mediated but not humoral immune responsiveness, *Int. J. Immunopharmac.,* 17, 247, 1995.

39. **Goble, F.C. and Konopka, E.A.,** Sex as a factor in infectious disease, *Trans. N.Y. Acad. Sci.,* 35, 325, 1973.

40. **Krzych, U., Strausser, H.R., Bressler, J.P., and Goldstein, A.L.,** Quantitative differences in immune responses during various stages of estrous cycle in female BALB/mice, *J. Immun.,* 121, 1603, 1979.

41. **Jerrells, T.R., Marietta, C.A., Eckardt, M.J., Majchrowicz, E., and Weight, F.F.,** Effects of ethanol administration on parameters of immunocompetency in rats, *J. Leuk. Biol.,* 39, 499, 1986.

42. **Jerrells, T.R., Perritt, D., Eckardt, M.J., and Marietta, C.,** Alterations in interleukin-2 utilization by T cells from rats treated with ethanol-containing diet, *Alc. Clin Exp. Res.,* 14, 245, 1990.

43. **Hazlett, L.D., Barrett, R.P., Berk, R.S., and Abel, E.L.,** Maternal and paternal alcohol consumption increase offspring susceptibility to *Pseudomonas aeruginosa* ocular infection, *Ophthalmic Res.,* 81, 381, 1989.

44. **Berk, R.S., Montgomery, I.N., Hazlett, L.D., and Abel, E.L.,** Paternal alcohol consumption: Effects on ocular and serum antibody response to *Pseudomonas aeruginosa* infection to offspring, *Alc. Clin. Exp. Res.,* 13, 795, 1989.

45. **Swiatek, K.R., Dombrowski, G.J., Jr., and Chao, K.-L.,** The inefficient transfer of maternally fed alcohol to nursing rats, *Alcohol,* 3, 169, 1986.

46. **Gottesfeld, Z. and LeGrue, S.J.,** Lactational alcohol exposure elicits long-term immune deficits and increased noradrenergic synaptic transmission in lymphoid organs, *Life Sci.,* 47, 457, 1990.

47. **Fomon, S.J.,** Reflections on infant feeding in the 1970s and 1980s, *Am. J. Clin. Nutr.,* 46, 171, 1987.

48. **Martinez, G.A. and Krieger, F.W.,** Milk-feeding patterns in the United States, *Pediatrics,* 76, 1004, 1985.

49. Little, R.E., Anderson, K.W., Ervin, C.H., Worthington-Roberts, B., and Clarren, S.K., Maternal alcohol use during breast-feeding and infant mental and motor development at one year, *N. Engl. J. Med.*, 321, 425, 1989.

50. Zorzano, A. and Herrera, E., Decreased *in vivo* rate of ethanol metabolism in the suckling rat, *Alc. Clin. Exp. Res.*, 13, 527, 1989.

51. Diaz, J. and Samson, H.H., Impaired brain growth in neonatal rats exposed to ethanol, *Science*, 208, 751, 1980.

52. Detering, N., Reed, W.D., Ozand, P.T., and Karahasan, A., The effects of maternal ethanol consumption in the rat on the development of their offspring, *J. Nutr.*, 109, 999, 1979.

53. Pierce, D.R. and West, J.R., Alcohol induced microencephaly during the third trimester equivalent: Relationship to dose and blood alcohol concentration, *Alcohol*, 3, 185, 1987.

54. West, J.R., Fetal alcohol-induced brain damage and the problem of determining temporal vulnerablitity: A review, *Alc. Drug Res.*, 7, 423, 1987.

55. Serbus, D.C., Stull, R.E., and Light, K.E., Neonatal ethanol exposure to rat pups: Resultant alterations of cortical muscarinic and cerebellar H[1]-Histaminergic receptor binding dynamics, *Neurotoxicol.*, 7, 257, 1986.

56. Lancaster, F.E., Selvanayagam, P.F., and Hsu, L.L., Lactational ethanol exposure: Brain enzymes and [3H] spiroperidol binding, *Int. J. Dev. Neurosci.*, 4, 151, 1986.

57. Barron, S., Kelly, S.J., and Riley, E.P., Neonatal alcohol exposure alters suckling behavior in neonatal rat pups, *Pharmacol. Biochem. Behav.*, 39, 423, 1991.

58. Steven, W.M., Bulloch, B., and Seelig, L.L., Jr., A morphometric study of the effects of ethanol consumption on lactating mammary glands of rats, *Alc. Clin. Exp. Res.*, 13, 209, 1989.

59. Viñas, O., Vilaró, Herrera, E., and Remesar, X., Effects of chronic ethanol treatment on amino acid uptake and enzyme activities in the lactating rat mammary gland, *Life Sci.*, 40, 1745, 1987.

60. Mennella, J.A. and Beauchamp, G.K., Maternal diet alters the sensory qualities of human milk and the nursing's behavior, *Pediatrics*, 88, 737, 1991.

61. Subramanian, A.G., Chen, X.G., and Bergeski, B.A., Pattern and duration of the inhibitory effect of alcohol administered acutely on suckling-induced prolactin in lactating rats, *Alc. Clin. Exp. Res.*, 14, 771, 1990.

62. Binkiewicz, A., Robinson, M.J., and Senior, B., Pseudo-Cushing syndrome caused by alcohol in breast milk, *J. Pediatr.*, 93, 965, 1978.

63. **Smals, A.G., Kloppenborg, P.W., Njo, K.T., Knoben, J.M., and Ruland, G.M.,** Alcohol induced Cushingoid syndrome, *Br. Med. J.*, 2, 2198, 1976.

64. **Rees, L.H., Besser, G.M., Jeffcoate, W.F., Goldie, D.J., and Marks, V.,** Alcohol-induced pseudo-Cushing's Syndrome, *Lancet*, 1, 726, 1977.

65. **Paton, A.,** Alcohol induced Cushingoid syndrome, *Br. Med. J.*, 2, 1504, 1976.

66. **Goldman, A.S. and Goldblum, R.M.,** Immunologic system in human milk: Characteristics and effects, in *Textbook of Gastroenterology and Nutrition in Infancy*, Lebenthal, E., Ed., Raven Press, New York, 1989.

67. **Walker, W.A.,** Development of intestinal host defense mechanisms and the passive protective role of human milk, *Mead Johnson Symp. on Perinatal and Dev. Med.*, 11, 39, 1977.

68. **Chandra, R.K.,** Immunological aspects of human milk, *Nutr. Rev.*, 36, 265, 1978.

69. **Butler, J.E.,** Immunologic aspects of breast feeding, antiinfectious activity of breast milk, *Seminars in Perinatol.*, 3, 255, 1979.

70. **Machtinger, S.,** Transfer of antigens via breast milk, in *Food Intolerance in Infancy: Allergology, Immunology and Gastroenterology*, Vol 1, Hamburger, N., Ed., Carnation Nutrition Education Series, The Carnation Co., Raven Press, New York, 1989.

71. **Wilson, C.B.,** Immunologic basis for increased susceptibiity of the neonate to infection, *J. Pediatr.*, 108, 1, 1986.

72. **Head, J.R., Beer, A.E., and Billingham, R.E.,** Significance of the cellular component of the maternal immunologic endowment in milk, *Transplant. Proc.*, 9, 1465, 1977.

73. **Goldman, A.S., Ham Pong, A.J., and Goldblum, R.M.,** Host defenses: Development and maternal contributions, *Adv. Pediatr.*, 32, 71, 1985.

74. **Soder, O.,** Isolation of interleukin-1 from human milk, *Int. Arch. Allergy Appl. Immunol.*, 83, 19, 1987.

75. **McGhee, J.R., Michalek, S.M., and Ghanta, V.K.,** Rat immunoglobulins in serum and secretions: Purification of rat IgM, IgA, and IgG and their quantitation in serum, colostrum, milk and saliva, *Immunochem.*, 12, 817, 1975.

76. **Kumar, S.N., Stewart, G.L., Steven, W.M., and Seelig, L.L.,** Maternal to neonatal transmission of T-cell mediated immunity to *Trichinella spiralis* during lactation, *Immunol.*, 68, 87, 1989.

77. **Steven, W.M., Stewart, G.L., and Seelig, L.L.,** The effects of maternal ethanol consumption on lactational transfer of immunity to *Trichinella spiralis* in rats, *Alc. Clin. Exp. Res.*, 16, 884, 1992.

78. **Na, H.R., Chervenak, R., and Seelig, L.L., Jr.,** Effects of maternal alcohol consumption on milk and blood lymphocytes and IgG antibody levels from *Trichinella spiralis*-infected rats, *Alc. Clin. Exp. Res.*, 17, 532, 1993.

79. **Na, H.R. and Seelig, L.L., Jr.,** Effect of maternal ethanol consumption on *in vitro* tumor necrosis factor, interleukin-6 and interleukin-2 production by rat milk and blood leukocytes, *Alc. Clin. Exp. Res.*, 18, 398, 1994.

80. **Giberson, P.K. and Blakley, B.R.,** Effect of ethanol on leukemia susceptibility in mice, *Alc. Clin. Exp. Res.*, 16, 383, 1992.

81. **Giberson, P.K. and Blakley, B.R.,** Effect of postnatal ethanol exposure on expression of differentiation antigens of murine splenic lymphocytes, *Alc. Clin. Exp. Res.*, 18, 21, 1994.

82. **Gottesfeld, Z. and LeGrue, S.J.,** Lactational alcohol exposure elicits long-term immune deficits and increased noradrenergic synaptic transmission in lymphoid organs, *Life Sci.*, 47, 457, 1990b.

83. **Fabris, N. and Provinciali, M.,** Hormones, in *Natural Immunity*, Nelson, D. S., Ed., Vol. 10, 306, 1989.

84. **Berczi, I.,** The pituitary-thyroid axis, in *Pituitary Function and Immunity*, Berczi, I., Ed., CRC Press, Boca Raton, Florida, 1986.

85. **Cupps, T.R. and Fauci, A.S.,** Corticosteroid-mediated immunoregulation in man, *Immunol. Rev.*, 65, 133, 1982.

86. **Rudeen, P.K., and Taylor, A.N.,** Alcohol and neurobiology: Brain development and hormone regulation, in Watson, R. R., Ed., *Fetal Alcohol Neuroendocrinopathies*, CRC Press, Boca Raton, Florida, 1993, chap. 6.

87. **Weinberg, J.,** Prenatal alcohol exposure: Endocrine function of offspring, in *Alcohol and the Endocrine System*, Zakhari, S., Ed., *Res. Monogr.* 23, 363, 1993, chap. 18.

88. **Olschowka, J.A., O'Donohue, T.L., Mueller, G.P., and Jacobowitz, D.M.,** The distribution of corticotropin releasing factor-like immunoreactive neurons in rat brain, *Peptides*, 3, 995, 1982.

89. **Bloom, R.E., Battenberg, E.L.F., Rivier, J, and Vale, W.,** Corticotropin releasing factor (CRF): Immunoreactive neurones and fibers in rat hypothalamus, *Regul. Peptides*, 4, 43, 1982.

90. **Axelrod, J. and Reisine, T.D.,** Stress hormones: Their interaction and regulation, *Science*, 224, 452, 1984.

91. **Plotsky, P., Bruhn, T., and Otto, S.,** Central modulation of immunoreactive arginine vasopressin and oxytocin secretion into the hypophyseal-portal circulation by CRF, *Endocrinol.*, 116, 1669, 1985.

92. **Rivier, C. and Vale, W.,** Modulation of stress-induced ACTH release by CRF, catecholamines, and vasopressin, *Nature*, 305, 325, 1983.

93. **Siiteri, P.K., Murai, J.T., Hammond, G.L., Nisker, J.A., Raymoure, W.J., and Kuhn, R.W.,** The serum transport of steroid hormones, *Recent. Prog. Horm. Res.,* 38, 457, 1982.

94. **Calogero, A.E., Gallucci, W.T., Gold, P.W., and Chrousos, G.P.,** Multiple feedback regulatory loops upon rat hypothalamic corticotropin-releasing hormone secretion, *J. Clin. Invest.,* 82, 767, 1988.

95. **Munck, A., Guyre, P., and Holbrook, N.,** Physiological function of glucocorticoids during stress and their relation to pharmacological actions, *Endocrinol. Rev.,* 5, 25, 1984.

96. **Bateman, A., Singh, A., Kral, T., and Solomon, S.,** The immune-hypothalamic-pituitary-adrenal axis, *Endocrinol. Rev.,* 10, 92, 1989.

97. **Dougherty, T.F.,** Effects of hormones on lymphatic tissue, *Physiol. Rev.,* 32, 379, 1952.

98. **Marsh, J.T. and Rasmussen, A.F.,** Response of adrenals, thymus, spleen and leukocytes to shuttle box and confinement stress, *Proc. Soc. Exp. Biol. Med.,* 104, 180, 1960.

99. **Haynes, B.F. and Fauci, A.S.,** The differential effect of *in vivo* hydrocortisone on the kinetics of subpopulations of human peripheral blood thymus-derived lymphocytes, *J. Clin. Invest.,* 61, 703, 1978.

100. **Besedovsky, H.O., Del Rey, A., and Sorkin, E.,** Neuroendocrine immunoregulation, in *Immunoregulation,* Fabris, W., Garaci, E., and Hadden, J., Eds., Plenum, London, 1983.

101. **Calabrese, J.R., Kling, M.A., and Gold, P.W.,** Alterations in immunocompetence during stress, bereavement, and depression: Focus on neuroendocrine regulation, *Am. J. Psychiatr.,* 144, 1123, 1987.

102. **Blalock, J.E., Harbour-McMenamin, D., and Smith, E.M.,** Peptide hormones shared by the neuroendocrine and immunologic systems, *J. Immunol.,* 135, 858s, 1985.

103. **Gillis, S., Crabtree, G. R., and Smith, K. A.,** Glucocorticoid induced inhibition of T cell growth factor production I. The effect of mitogen induced lymphocyte proliferation, *J. Immunol.,* 123, 1624, 1979.

104.. **Besedovsky, H. O., Sorkin, E., Keller, M., and Muller, J.,** Changes in blood hormone levels during the immune response, *Proc. Soc. Exp. Med.,* 150, 466, 1975.

105. **Dunn, A. J., Powell, M. L., Meitin, C., and Small, P. A., Jr.,** Virus infection as a stressor: Influenza virus elevates plasma concentrations of corticosterone, and brain concentrations of MHPG and tryptophan, *Physiol. Behav.,* 45, 591, 1989.

106. **Besedovsky, H., Del Rey, A., Sorkin, E., and Dinarello, C. A.,** Immunoregulatory feedback between interleukin-1 and glucocorticoid hormones, *Science,* 233, 652, 1986.

107. Berkenbosch, F., Van Oers, J., Del Rey, A., Tilders, F., and Besedovsky, H., Corticotropin releasing factor-producing neurons in the rat activated by interleukin-1, *Science*, 238, 524, 1987.

108. Sapolsky, R., Rivier, C., Yamamoto, G., Plotsky, P., and Vale, W., Interleukin 1 stimulates the secretion of hypothalamic corticotropin releasing factor, *Science*, 238, 522, 1987.

109. Uehara, A., Gillis, S., and Arimura, A., Effects of interleukin-1 on hormone release from normal rat pituitary cells in primary culture, *Neuroendocrinol.*, 45, 343, 1987.

110. Tsagarakis, S., Gillies, G., Rees, L.H., Besser, M., and Grossman, A., Interleukin-1 directly stimulates the release of corticotropin releasing factor from rat hypothalamus, *Neuroendocrinol.*, 49, 98, 1989.

111. Matta, S.G., Singh, J., Newton, R., and Sharp, B.M., The adrenocorticotropin response to interleukin-1β instilled into the rat median eminence depends on the local release of catecholamines, *Endocrinol.*, 127, 2175, 1990.

112. Harbuz, M.S. and Lightman, S.L., Stress and the hypothalamo-pituitary-adrenal axis: Acute, chronic and immunological activation, *J. Endocrinol.*, 134, 327, 1992.

113. Rivier, C., Vale, W., and Brown, W., In the rat, interleukin-1α and -β stimulate adenocorticotropin and catecholamine release, *Endocrinol.* 125, 3096, 1989.

114. Ovadia, H., Abramsky, O., Barak, V., Conforti, N., Saphier, D., and Weidenfeld, J., Effect of interleukin-1 on adrenocorticoid activity in intact and hypothalamic deafferented male rats, *Exp. Brain Res.*, 76, 246, 1989.

115. Rivest, S., Torres, G., and Rivier, C., Differential effects of central and peripheral injection of interleukin-1β on brain *c-fos* expression and neuroendocrine functions, *Brain Res.*, 587, 13, 1992.

116. Sawchenko, P.E. and Swanson, L.W., The organization of noradrenergic pathways from the brainstem to the paraventricular and supraoptic nuclei in the rat, *Brain Res. Rev.*, 4, 275, 1982.

117. Dunn, A.J., Systemic interleukin-1 administration stimulates hypothalamic norepinephrine metabolism paralleling the increased plasma corticosterone, *Life Sci.*, 43, 429, 1988.

118. Kabiersch, A., Del Rey, A., Honegger, C.G., and Besedovsky, H.O., Interleukin-1 induces changes in norepinephrine metabolism in the rat brain, *Brain Behav. Immunol.*, 2, 267, 1988.

119. Chuluyan, H.E., Saphier, D., Rohn, W.M., and Dunn, A.J., Noradrenergic innervation of the hypothalamus participates in adrenocortical responses to interleukin-1, *Neuroendocrinol.*, 56, 106, 1992.

120. **Sheng, M. and Greenberg, M.E.,** The regulation and function of *c-fos* and other immediate early genes in the central nervous system, *Neuron,* 4, 477, 1990.

121. **Morgan, J.I. and Curran, T.,** Stimulus-transcription coupling in the nervous system: involvement of the inducible proto-oncogenesis *fos* and *jun, Annu. Rev. Neurosci.,* 14, 421, 1991.

122. **Brady, L.S., Lynn, A.B., Herkenham, M., and Gottesfeld, Z.,** Systemic interleukin-1 induces early and late patterns of *c-fos* mRNA expression in brain, *J. Neurosci.,* 14, 4951, 1994.

123. **Johnson, H.M., Smith, E.M., Torres, B.A., and Blalock, J.E.,** Regulation of the *in vitro* antibody response by neuroendocrine hormones, *Proc. Natl. Acad. Sci. USA,* 79, 4171, 1982.

124. **Johnson, H.M., Torres, B.A., Smith, E.M., Dion, D.L., and Blalock, J.E.,** Regulation of lymphokine (γ-interferon) production by corticotropin, *J. Immunol.,* 132, 246, 1984.

125. **Jones, T.H. and Kennedy, R.L.,** Cytokines and hypothalamic-pituitary function, *Cytokine,* 5, 531, 1993.

126. **Sternberg, E.M., Hill, J.M., Chrousos, G.P., Kamilaris, T., Listwack, S.J., Gold, P.W., and Wilder, R.,** Inflammatory mediator-induced hypothalamic-pituitary-adrenal axis activation is defective in streptococcal cell wall arthritis-susceptible Lewis rats, *Proc. Natl. Acad. Sci. USA,* 86, 2374, 1989.

127. **Weinberg, J.,** Prenatal ethanol exposure alters adrenocortical development of offspring, *Alc. Clin. Exp. Res.,* 13, 73, 1989.

128. **Taylor, A.N., Branch, B.J., Nelson, L.R., Lane, L.A., and Poland, R.E.,** Prenatal ethanol and ontogeny of pituitary-adrenal responses to ethanol and morphine, *Alcohol,* 3, 255, 1986.

129. **Weinberg, J.,** Hyperresponsiveness to stress: differential effects of prenatal ethanol on males and females, *Alc. Clin. Exp. Res.,* 12, 647, 1988.

130. **Angelogianni, P. and Gianoulakis, C.,** Prenatal exposure to ethanol alters the ontogeny of the β-endorphin response to stress, *Alc. Clin. Exp. Res.,* 13, 564, 1989.

131. **Weinberg, J. and Gianoulakis, C.,** Fetal ethanol exposure alters glucocorticoid and β-endorphin responses to stress, *Soc. Neurosci. Abstr.,* 17, 1596, 1991.

132. **Lee, S., Imaki, T., Vale, W., and Rivier, C.,** Effect of prenatal exposure to ethanol on the activity of the hypothalamic-pituitary-adrenal axis of the offspring: importance of the time of exposure to ethanol and possible modulating mechanisms, *Molec. Cell. Neurosci.,* 1, 168, 1990.

133. **Lee, S. and Rivier, C.,** Prenatal alcohol exposure blunts interleukin-1-induced ACTH and β-endorphin secretion by immature rats, *Alc. Clin. Exp. Res.,* 17, 940, 1993.

134. Lancaster, F.E., Alcohol, nitric oxide, and neurotoxicity: is there a connection? A review, *Alc. Clin. Exp. Res.*, 16, 539, 1992.

135. Lee, S. and Rivier, C., Prenatal alcohol exposure alters the hypothalamic-pituitary-adrenal axis response of immune offspring to interleukin-1: is nitric oxide involved?, *Alc. Clin. Exp. Res.*, 18, 1242, 1994.

136. Rivier, C. and Shen, G.H., In the rat, endogenous nitric oxide modulates the response of the hypothalamic-pituitary-adrenal axis to interleukin-1β, vasopressin, and oxytocin, *J. Neurosci.*, 14(4), 1985, 1994.

137. Yirmiya, R., Pliati, M.L., Chiappelli, F., and Taylor, A.N., Fetal alcohol exposure attenuates lipopolysaccharide-induced fever in rats, *Alc. Clin. Exp. Res.*, 17, 906, 1993.

138. Tilders, F.J.H., DeRijk, R.H., Van Dam, A.-M., Vincent, V.A.M., Schotanus, K., and Persoons, J.H.A., Activation of the hypothalamus-pituitary-adrenal-axis by bacterial endotoxins: routes and intermediate signals, *Psychoneuroendocrinol.*, 19, 209, 1994.

139. Gottesfeld, Z. and Silverman, P.B., Developmental delays associated with prenatal alcohol exposure are reversed by thyroid hormone treatment, *Neurosci. Lett.*, 109, 42, 1990.

140. Hannigan, J.H., Alcohol exposure and maternal-fetal thyroid function: impact on biobehavioral maturation, in *Alcohol and Endocrine System*, Zakhari, S., Ed., *Res. Monogr.*, 23, 313, 1993, chap. 16.

141. McGivern, R.F., Raum, W.J., Salido, E., and Redei, E., Lack of prenatal testosterone surge in fetal rats exposed to alcohol: alterations in testicular morphology and physiology, *Alc. Clin. Exp. Res.*, 12, 243, 1988.

142. Kelce, W.R., Ganjam, V.K., and Rudeen, P.K., Inhibition of testicular steroidogenesis in the neonatal rat following acute ethanol exposure, *Alcohol*, 71, 75, 1990.

143. Bulloch, K., The innervation of immune system tissues and organs, in *The Neuro-Immune-Endocrine Connection*, Cotman, C.W., Ed., Raven Press, New York, 1987.

144. Felten, D.L., Felten, S.Y., Carlson, S.L., Olschowka, J.A., and Livnat, S., Noradrenergic and peptidergic innervation of lymphoid tissue, *J. Immunol.*, 135, 755s, 1985.

145. Bulloch, K. and Moore, R.Y., Innervation of the thymus gland by brain stem and spinal cord in mouse and rat, *Am. J. Anat.*, 162, 157, 1981.

146. Maslinski, W., Kullberg, M., Nordström, O., and Bartfai, T., Muscarinic receptors and receptor-mediated actions on rat thymocytes, *J. Neuroimmunol.*, 17, 265, 1988.

147. **Felten, S.Y. and Felten, D.L.,** Innervation of lymphoid tissue, in *Psychoneuroimmunology*, Ader, R., Felten, D. L., and Cohen, N., Eds., Academic Press, New York, pp. 27-69, 1991.

148. **Felten, D.L., Felten, S.Y., and Bellinger, D.L.,** Noradrenergic sympathetic neural interactions with the immune system: Structure and function, *Immunol. Rev.*, 100, 225, 1987.

149. **Madden, K.S., Sanders, V.M., and Felten, D.L.,** Catecholamine influences and sympathetic neural modulation of immune responsiveness, *Annu. Rev. Pharmacol. Toxicol.*, 35, 417, 1995.

150. **Felten, D.L. and Olschowka, J.,** Noradrenergic sympathetic innervation of the spleen. II. Tyrosine hydroxylase (TH)-positive nerve terminals from synaptic-like contacts on lymphocytes in the splenic white pulp, *J. Neurosci. Res.*, 18, 37, 1987.

151.. **Ackerman, K.D., Felten, S.Y., Bellinger, D.L., and Felten, D.L.,** Noradrenergic sympathetic innervation of the spleen: III. Development of innervation in the rat spleen, *J. Neurosci. Res.*, 18, 49, 1987.

152. **Ackerman, K.D., Felten, S.Y., Dijkstra, C.D., Livnat, S., and Felten, D.L.,** Parallel development of noradrenergic innervation and cellular compartmentation in the rat spleen, *Exp. Neurol.*, 103, 239, 1989.

153. **Classen, E., Kors, N., Dijkstra, C. D., and van Rooijen, N.,** Marginal zone of the spleen and the development of specific antibody-forming cells against thymus-dependent and thymus-independent type-2 antigens, *Immunology*, 57, 399, 1986.

154. **Kimura, S., Eldridge, J.H., Michalek, S.M., Morisaki, I., Hamada, S., and McGhee, J.R.,** Immunoregulation in the rat: ontogeny of B cell response to types 1, 2, and T-dependent antigens, *J. Immunol.*, 134, 2839, 1985.

155. **Veerman, A.J.P.,** The postnatal development of the white pulp in the rat spleen and the onset of immunocompetence against a thymus-dependent antigen, *Z. Immun. Forsch.*, 150, 45, 1975.

156. **Johnson, D.L. and Gordon, M.A.,** Characteristics of adrenergic binding sites associated with murine lymphocytes isolated from spleen, *J. Immunopharmacol.*, 2, 435, 1980.

157. **Sanders, V.M. and Munson, A.E.,** Norepinephrine and antibody response, *Pharmacol. Rev.*, 37, 229, 1985.

158. **Williams, L.T., Snyderman, R., and Lefkowitz, R.J.,** Identification of beta-adrenergic receptors in human lymphocytes by (-) ^{3}H-alprenolol binding, *J. Clin. Invest.*, 57, 149, 1976.

159. **Besedovsky, H.O., Del Rey, A.E., Sorkin, E., Da Prada, M., and Keller, H.H.,** Immunoregulation mediated by the sympathetic nervous system, *Cell Immunol.*, 48, 346, 1979.

160. Livnat, S., Felten, S.Y., Carlson, S.L., Bellinger, D.L., and Felten, D.L., Involvement of peripheral and central catecholamine systems in neural-immune interactions, *J. Neuroimmun.*, 10, 5, 1985.

161. Madden, K.S. and Livnat, S., Catecholamine action and immunologic reactivity, in *Psychoneuroimmunology*, Ader, R., Felten, D. L. and Cohen, N., Eds., pp. 283-310, 1991.

162. Fuchs, B.A., Albright, J.W., and Albright, J.F., β-adrenergic receptors on murine lymphocytes: Density varies with cell maturity and lymphocyte subtype and is decreased after antigen administration, *Cell. Immunol.*, 114, 231, 1988.

163. Fuchs, B.A., Campbell, K.S., and Munson, A.E., Norepinephrine and serotonin content of the murine spleen: Its relationship between to lymphocyte β-adrenergic receptors density and the humoral immune response *in vivo* and *in vitro*, *Cell. Immunol.*, 117, 339, 1988.

164. Coffey, R.G. and Hadden, J.W., Neurotransmitters, hormones and cyclic nucleotides in lymphocyte regulation, *Fed. Proc.*, 44, 112, 1985.

165. Strom, T.D., Lundin, A.P., and Carpenter, C.B., The role of cyclic nucleotides in lymphocyte activation and function, *Prog. Clin. Immunol.*, 3, 115, 1977.

166. Watson, J., The influence of intracellular levels of cyclic nucleotides on cell proliferation and induction of antibody synthesis, *J. Exp. Med.*, 141, 97, 1975.

167. LeGrue, S. J., Does interleukin-2 stimulus-response coupling result in the generation of intracellular second messenger?, *Lymphokine Res.*, 7, 187, 1988.

168. Besedovsky, H.O., Sorkin, E., Felix, D., and Haas, H., Hypothalamus changes during the immune response, *Eur. J. Immunol.*, 7, 323, 1977.

169. Besedovsky, H.O., Del Rey, A.E., Sorkin, E., Da Prada, M., Burri, R., and Honegger, C., The immune response evokes changes in brain noradrenergic neurons, *Science*, 221, 564, 1983.

170. Shimizu, N., Hori, T. and Nakane, H., An interleukin-1β-induced noradrenaline release in the spleen is mediated by brain corticotropin-releasing factor: An *in vivo* microdialysis study in conscious rats, *Brain Behav. Immunol.*, 7, 14, 1994.

171. Irwin, M., Hauger, R.L., Brown, M., and Britton, K.T., CRF activates autonomic nervous system and reduces natural killer cytotoxicity, *Am. J. Physiol.*, 255, R744, 1988.

172. Irwin, M., Hauger, R.L., Jones, L., Provencio, M., and Britton, K.T., Sympathetic nervous system mediates central corticotropin-releasing factor induced suppression of natural killer cytotoxicity, *J. Pharmacol. Exp. Ther.*, 255, 101, 1990.

173. **Sundar, S.K., Becker, K.J., Cierpial, M.A., Carpenter, D.C., Rankin, L.A., Fleener, S.L., Ritchie, J.C., Simson, P. E., and Weiss, J.M.,** Intracerebroventricular infusion of interleukin 1 rapidly decreases peripheral cellular immune responses, *Proc. Natl. Acad. Sci. USA*, 86, 6398, 1989.

174. **Sundar, S.K., Cierpial, M.A., Kitts, C., Ritchie, J.C., and Weiss, J.M.,** Brain IL-1-induced immunosuppression occurs through activation of both pituitary-adrenal axis and sympathetic nervous system by corticotropin-releasing factor, *J. Neurosci.*, 10(11), 3701, 1990.

175. **Sundar, S., Cierpial, M., Kamaraju, L., Long, S., Hsieh, S., Lorenz, C., Aaron, M., Rithcie, J., and Weiss, J.,** Human immunodeficiency virus glycoprotein (gp 120) infused into rat brain induces interleukin-1 to elevate pituitary adrenal activity and decrease peripheral cellular immune responses, *Proc. Natl. Acad. Sci. USA*, 88, 11246, 1991.

176. **Smith, E.M. and Blalock, J.E.,** A complete regulatory loop between the immune and neuroendocrine systems operates through common signal molecules (hormones) and receptors, in *Enkephalins and Endorphins, Stress and the Immune System*, Plotnikoff, N. P., Faith, R. E., Murgo, A. J., and Good, R. A., Eds., Plenum Press, New York, 1986.

177. **Bellinger, D.L., Lorton, D., Romano, T.D., Olschowka, J.A., Felten, S.Y., and Felten, D.L.,** Neuropeptide innervation of lymphoid organs, *Annals of the New York Acad. of Sci.*, 594, 17, 1990.

178. **Payan, D.G., McGillis, J.P., Renold, F.K., Mitsuhashi, M., and Goetzl, E.J.,** The immunomodulating properties of neuropeptides, in *Hormones and Immunity*, Berczi, C. and Kovacs, K., Eds., MTP Press, Lancaster, PA, 1986.

179. **Goetzl, E.J., Turck, C.W., and Sreedharan, S.P.,** Production and recognition of neuropeptides by cells of the immune system, in *Psychoneuroimmunology*, Ader, R., Felten, D. L. and Cohen, N., Eds., pp. 263-282, 1991

180. **Brodie, B.B., Costa, E., Dlabac, A., Neff, H.H., and Smookler, H.H.,** Application of steady-state kinetics to the estimation of synthesis rate and turnover time of tissue catecholamines, *J. Pharmac. Exp. Ther.*, 154, 493, 1966.

181. **Hendry, I.A.,** Control in the development of the vertebrate sympathetic nervous system, *Rev. Neurosci.*, 2, 149, 1976.

182. **Levi-Montalcini, R. and Angeletti, P.U.,** Immunosympathectomy, *Pharmac. Rev.*, 18, 619, 1966.

183. **Levi-Montalcini, R. and Hamburger, V.,** Selective growth stimulating effects of mouse sarcoma on the sensory and sympathetic nervous system of the chick embryo, *J. Exp. Zool.*, 116, 321, 1951.

184. **Thorpe, L.W., Morgan, B., Beck, C.,Werrbach-Perez, K., and Perez-Polo, J.R.,** Nerve gorwth factor, in *Cellular and Molecular Aspects of Neural Development and Regeneration,* Gorio, A., de Vellis, J., Perez-Polo, J.R., and Haber, B., Eds., Springer-Verlag, Heidelberg, 1988.

185. **Thorpe, L.W. and Perez-Polo, J.R.,** The influence of nerve growth on the *in vitro* proliferative response of rat spleen lymphocytes, *J. Neurosci. Res.,* 18, 134, 1987.

186. **Thorpe, L.W., Stach, R.W., Morgan, B., and Perez-Polo, J.R.,** The biology of nerve growth factor: Its interaction with cells of the immune system, in *Neural Control of Reproductive Function,* Lakoski, J. M., Perez-Polo, J. R., and Rassin, D. K., Eds., Alan R. Liss Inc., New York, 1989.

187. **Springer, J.E.,** Nerve growth factor receptors in the central nervous system, *Exp. Neurol.,* 102, 354, 1988.

188. **Kornguth, D.I., Rutledge, J.J., Sunderland, E., Siegel, F., Carlson, I., Smallens, J., Juhl, U., and Young, D.,** Impeded cerebellar development and reduced serum thyroxine levels associated with fetal alcohol intoxication, *Brain Res.,* 177, 347, 1979.

189. **Slotkin, T.A.,** Thyroid hormone regulation of sympathetic nervous system development, in *Trends in Autonomic Pharnacology,* Vol. 3, Kalsner, S., Ed., Taylor and Francis, Philadelphia, 1985.

190. **Aloe, L. and Levi-Montalcini, R.,** Comparative studies on testosterone and L-thyroxine effects on the synthesis of nerve growth factor in mouse submaxillary salivary glands, *Exp. Cell. Res.,* 125, 15, 1980.

191. **Walker, P., Weischsel, M.E., Jr., Hoatch, S.B., Poland, R.E., and Fisher, D.A.,** Effect of thyroxine testosterone and corticosterone on nerve growth factor (NGF) and epidermal growth factor (EGF) concentrations in adult female mouse submaxillary gland: Dissociation of NGF and EGF responses, *Endocrinol.,* 109, 582, 1981.

192. **Patel, A.J., Hayashi, M., and Hunt, A.,** Role of thyroid hormone and nerve growth factor in the development of choline acetyltransferase and other cell-specific marker enzymes in the basal forebrain of the rat, *J. Neurochem.,* 50, 803, 1988.

193. **Gallo, P.V. and Weinberg, J.,** Prenatal ethanol exposure: Pituitary-adrenal activity in pregnant dams and offspring, *Neurobehav. Toxicol. Teratol.,* 4, 515, 1982.

194. **Jonakait, G.M., Bohn, M.C., and Black, I.B.,** Maternal glucocorticoid hormones influence neurotransmitter phenotypic expression in embryos, *Science,* 210, 551, 1980.

195. **Jonakait, G.M., Bohn, M.C., Goldstein, M., and Black, I.B.,** Elevation of maternal glucocorticoid hormones alters neurotransmitter phenotypic expression in embryos, *Dev. Biol.,* 88, 288, 1981.

196. **Otten, J. and Thoenen, H.,** Modulatory role of glucocorticoids on NGF-mediated enzyme induction in organ cultures of sympathetic ganglia, *Brain Res.*, 111, 438, 1976.

197. **Otten, J., Bauman, J.B., and Girard, J.,** Stimulation of the pituitary-adrenocortical axis by nerve growth factor, *Nature*, 282, 413, 1979.

198. **De Simone, R. and Aloe, L.,** Influence of ethanol consumption on brain nerve growth factor and its target cells in developing and adult rodents, *Ann. Ist. Super. Sanitá*, 29, 179, 1993.

199. **Heaton, M.B., Swanson, D.J., Paiva, M., and Walker, D.W.,** Ethanol exposure affects trophic factor activity and responsiveness in chick embryo, *Alcohol*, 9, 161, 1992.

200. **Walker, D.W., Heaton, M.B., Smothers, C.T., and Hunter, B.E.,** Chronic ethanol ingestion reduces the neurotrophic activity contained in rat hippocampus, *Alc. Clin. Exp. Res.*, 14, 350, 1990.

201. **Gottesfeld, Z., Simpson, S., Yuwiler, A., and Perez-Polo, J.R.,** Effects of nerve growth factor on splenic norepinephrine and pineal N-acetyltransferase in neonate rats exposed to alcohol *in utero*: Neuroimmune correlates. *Int. J. Dev. Neurosci.*, (in press).

Chapter 7

EARLY NEUROBEHAVIORAL ASSESSMENT OF CHILDREN PRENATALLY EXPOSED TO ALCOHOL

Claire D. Coles

I. WHY IS IT IMPORTANT TO IDENTIFY BEHAVIORAL EFFECTS IN EARLY INFANCY?

Fetal alcohol syndrome (FAS) is the most negative end of the continuum of effects of maternal alcohol abuse in pregnancy which can be identified in living offspring. This disorder is defined by three criteria:[1] 1) characteristic facial dysmorphia; 2) growth retardation and 3) damage to the central nervous system (CNS) which is manifested either through frank neurological damage or inferred due to the observation of behavioral deficits or alterations. However, the effects of prenatal exposure to alcohol, like the effects of many other teratogens,[2] appear to be expressed across a broad range. Vorhees [3] has suggested that the CNS may be most sensitive to teratogens so that neurobehavioral alterations may be apparent in individuals who do not show the physical stigmata. Research on longitudinal samples of moderately exposed children supports this suggestion about neurobehavioral effects. Streissguth et al.,[4] in a well controlled, longitudinal study, have found statistical evidence of specific alcohol-related deficits in otherwise "clinically-normal" middle class children. However, in situations in which experimental control cannot be exercised, it is often difficult to identify those behavioral or neurobehavioral effects which are associated with prenatal exposure and those which are associated with cofactors, including exposure to other substances of abuse, postnatal rearing environment and social class. For these reasons, early identification of effects is important.

A.   EARLY IDENTIFICATION
Early identification of alcohol effects in exposed individuals is desirable for many reasons. When the infant is so identified, early medical and educational interventions become possible which may prevent the development of secondary disabilities. Alcohol-exposed infants often have a number of associated physical problems which may include failure to thrive,[5] otitis media and other hearing problems,[6] visual problems,[7] cardiac defects,[8] and delays in motor and cognitive development.[9] Early identification of children at risk for these disorders allows adequate medical treatment. In addition, there are serious concerns about the effect of the postnatal environment on these high risk, children. Although such studies have not been carried out with alcohol-exposed infants, in other contexts,[10] children who are at biological risk have been shown to be particularly vulnerable to the kind of nonoptimal social

0-8493-7685-8/96/$0.00+$.50
© 1996 by CRC Press, Inc.

circumstances which are likely to be present when the child's caregivers are substances abusers. Conversely, children with relatively mild biological compromise are often greatly benefited by early intervention and may avoid more severe negative outcomes.[11]

While there are significant benefits to the child of early identification of alcohol effects, there are also benefits to the mother and to society in general. The woman who has an alcohol-affected child is almost always herself negatively affected by her alcohol abuse or alcoholism. Two common sequelae of giving birth to an alcohol-affected child are the subsequent birth of another, even more affected, child and early maternal death.[12] If identification of the affected child can be associated with recognition of the mother's substance abuse and social/emotional problems, intervention and treatment are possible and many negative outcomes may be avoided. Since such problems usually become the problems of the community as well as the individual, early identification of affected children is both a clinical responsibility to the individuals involved and a potential benefit to the greater society.

B.   SURVEILLANCE AND RESEARCH

Assessment of the neonate can be useful in other contexts as well. Surveillance of alcohol-affected children is necessary to establish the base rate of occurrence of FAS and related disorders and to monitor the effects of prevention efforts on this rate. Since the identification of the physical traits associated with FAS is somewhat difficult without specialized training, identification of behavioral problems can provide additional evidence for health care professionals.

Finally, neurobehavioral effects of alcohol and other substances of abuse have been the focus of research which seeks to identify those environmental agents which have a negative effect on the fetus and young child. In later infancy and early childhood it can be very difficult to discriminate those behaviors associated with, for instance, abuse and neglect, from those associated with teratogenic substances or other factors which can negatively affect the fetus. This is particularly a problem when there is no information about the neonate's behavior. The neonatal period, immediately after birth, provides a convenient "window" to examine the effects of the prenatal environment. It is in this period during which the individual should show the maximal impact of prenatal exposure--because the child is still under the effect of the drug or in "withdrawal" or because there has not yet been time for other experiences to modify the child's behavior. For this reason, it is vital that appropriate methods be used to examine the behavior of the exposed neonate.

II. CHALLENGES FOR THE NEUROBEHAVIORAL ASSESSMENT OF THE NEWBORN

Although occasionally done by developmental pediatricians and similar specialists for clinical reasons, usually neurobehavioral assessment is carried out for the purposes of research. There are a number of reasons why assessment of newborns is not commonplace, ranging from the theoretical to the practical.

A. LIMITED BEHAVIOR RANGE

In the examination of individuals to determine whether they have neurological or behavioral alterations, the focus is usually on areas considered to be of long-term significance, for instance, intelligence, motor skills, and attention. However, newborn infants are capable of a limited set of behaviors . Most of their time is spent in sleep and feeding with occasional periods of alertness during which they appear to attend briefly to various environment stimuli. Due to the pattern of development characteristic of human infants, neonates are capable of little voluntary movement although they respond reflexively to a variety of stimuli. For instance, while they respond with closure of the hand to the stimulation of their palm (grasp reflex), it will be some months before a voluntary grasp develops which will allow them to pick up objects at will. For this reason, many neonatal tests (e.g., Prechtl,[13] Brazelton[14]) include the examination of reflexive behavior ("primitive reflexes") as well as assessment of motor tone and orienting behavior. The assessment of motor tone may include both active movement (observation of the infant's motor behavior, as in, kicking and arm movements) and passive movement or resistance (in which the infant's limbs and torso are manipulated to gauge the "resistance" of the muscles to such manipulation). Finally, "orienting behavior" is usually measured. This is the response of the infant to auditory and visual stimuli. The alert infant when so stimulated will typically turn eyes or head in the direction of the stimulus and will often search with eyes to locate the source. Some young infants are able to "track" objects as well, following a human face or bright object with their eyes. This behavior is described properly as "orienting" behavior rather than as "attention" since it is not clear that the neonate is capable of maintaining "attention" in the same way as older individuals.

This set of behaviors are often described as measuring "neurobehavioral functioning" because it is assumed that competence or "optimality"[13-14] results from the relative intactness of the child's nervous system. Observation of children who were born prematurely, have known neurological injuries or who have been exposed to various toxins has shown that systemic alterations in these neurobehavioral signs can be observed and that there can be a relationship between such observations and both the child's risk status and its later development.[15]

B.   DISCONTINUITY

Measurement during the neonatal period is problematic for another reason. When there is interest in the measurement of ability and/or behavior, the goal is usually to explain current behavior or to predict later abilities. Due to the nature of development in infancy, there can be a limited relationship between what can be observed in the newborn period and what is considered to be of interest in later childhood. For instance, investigators and clinicians are often interested in how a toxin will affect an exposed child's later attention (usually defined as activity level and cooperativeness with adult instructions) and ability level (intelligence or academic potential). However, what can be measured in the neonatal period are orientation behavior and "neurobehavioral" optimality. Sometimes these earlier behaviors will be abnormal or nonoptimal and sometimes they will be related to nontypical behavior which is measured in later childhood. However, due to the nature of early development, it is unlikely that what was measured earlier is genuinely the precursor of what has been measured later. It is more probable that functions at both times were affected by a global deficit or by the conditions that produced the global deficit.[16]

C.   ACUTE AND PERSISTENT EFFECTS

The discrimination of acute and persistent neurobehavioral effects in the neonate can be difficult. In the assessment of individuals of other ages, the goal is typically to identify traits which are persistent and enduring and, for that reason, have meaning for the person's current and future functioning. In the assessment of the newborn, it is usually impossible to discriminate behaviors which are "traits" since there is no behavioral history to evaluate. In addition, because the behavioral repertoire of the neonate is limited, it can be difficult to distinguish what are acute effects of an immediate event and what are the manifestation of more persistent alterations which may have meaning for long-term development. This problem is particularly salient when dealing with the effects of psychoactive substances to which the infant has been exposed prenatally. Psychoactive substances, by definition, affect the nervous system and produce, in both adults and neonates, a variety of worrisome signs. In addition, the infant may have developed a physiological dependence to alcohol or other drugs due to prenatal exposure. (This dependence should be distinguished from "addiction" as seen in adults, which includes a psychological component.[17]) Certain drugs, particularly CNS depressants (see Table 1) are known to be associated with neonatal withdrawal syndrome[18] and, for this reason are associated with a particular set of behaviors. These behaviors and other signs of NWS are discussed below.

However, some of these agitated, aroused behaviors are similar to those which might be shown by an infant who was still under the effects of a CNS stimulant like amphetamine or cocaine, or by an infant with CNS damage leading to behavioral irritability, as is occasionally seen in preterm infants or infants with other kinds of neurological damage. For this reason, in the child being evaluated for the effects of psychoactive substances, it may be inappropriate to interpret such behavior when observed in the first few days of life. Supportive evidence should be obtained, including maternal self report of the use of various psychoactive substances, medical history and urine toxicology reports. The infant should then be observed over time to determine whether observed effects are persistent.

TABLE 1

CNS DEPRESSANTS ASSOCIATED WITH NEONATAL WITHDRAWAL SYNDROME

Opiates/narcotics

Methadone
Heroin
Codeine
Pentazocine (Talwin)
Propoxyphene (Darvon)
Other narcotics

Other drugs

Alcohol
Barbiturates
Bromine
Chlordiazepoxide (Librium)
Diazepam (Valium)
Diphenhydramine (Benadryl)
Ethchlorvynol (Placidyl)

D.   PROFESSIONAL TRAINING

Accurate assessment of infants, like the assessment of older individuals, requires education and training which is not widely available. Such training must be based on a understanding of physiology, medical issues related to pregnancy and infancy, as well as of child development. In addition, the person must understand the requirement of testing and assessment. Since such an educational process is rare and the need for it often overlooked, there is widespread misunderstanding of the usefulness of early infant assessment. When the existing procedures are carried out by poorly trained personnel, the information which is collected can be inaccurate and subject to random error. The frequent result is that the interpretation of findings is inaccurate or biased by the expectations of the observer. Some of the confusion associated with the "crack baby" phenomenon may have resulted from this kind of inaccurate assessment process[19] which led to "over-interpretion." Finally, since assessment of neonates must be carried out by professionals trained to a high level of expertise and because the "window" during which such assessment can occur in the neonatal nursery is brief (and becoming briefer with managed care), carrying out such procedures can be expensive and difficult to arrange.

E.   CONFOUNDING FACTORS

Often, when the assessment is for the purposes of research, the investigators wish to identify the effects of a particular agent (e.g., alcohol) on the infant. However, in human studies it is extraordinarily difficult to separate the effects of such a toxin from the background "noise" provided by the numerous potential confounding factors which may also be affecting the individual child. Most often, when the mother has misused alcohol in pregnancy, she has also smoked cigarettes and frequently has used other drugs as well.[19] In addition, the child may be affected by the quality of maternal nutrition and her health status, by obstetrical medications, and numerous other factors. Interpretation of neonatal behavior should include an understanding of potential confounding factors.

III. METHODS FOR ASSESSMENT OF NEUROBEHAVIORAL FUNCTION IN THE NEONATE

A.   WHAT CAN BE MEASURED?

1. Physical Characteristics

The most obvious things to measure are physical characteristics particularly in a person who is not yet capable of communication and whose social behavior is limited. In the child exposed to toxins or who is suspected of having a genetic or chromosomal disorder, birth defects and dysmorphisms are the most obvious features to be looked for. A second area which is often evaluated is the child's physiological status particularly heart rate and respiration,[20] vagal tone[21] and similar functions which are known to be abnormal in preterm infants and in those with neurological damage. In addition to the basic physiological parameters, heart rate is a useful measure because it varies in response to different kinds of stimuli and can be used as a measure of stress as well as a way to monitor orientation and attention. Sometimes these factors are included in or correlated with the neurobehavioral assessment.

Electroencephographic (EEG) measurement of infant sleep states or of response to environmental stimuli are also used to measure the intactness of the nervous system.[22-24] Physiological measures of stress have also been collected in newborns. These have included both heart rate and respiration[20] and cortisol levels[25] which have been used in preterm and very low birth weight infants. For instance, levels of the hormone, cortisol, were found to show different patterns of correlation with stress reactions in cocaine-exposed and preterm infants.[25]

2. Cry Characteristics

Crying is one of the most evident of infant behaviors. While a clinical assessment of the infant's cry is usually included in the neurobehavioral assessment, more refined methodologies also can be used to measure status in the neonatal period.[26] Physiologically, crying involves the nervous system arousal and inhibitory mechanisms as well as the coordination of cardiorespiratory activity and the muscles involved in vocalization. A number of aspects of the cry have been studied, including phonation, spectrographic characteristics, and the latency to respond to a pain stimulus (i.e., a rubber band snap on the foot). Number of "snaps" (response threshold) and latency of response in seconds are thought to be measures of the child's arousal and state control. The spectrographic characteristics of the cry are examined because the frequency of the cry (low pitched/high pitched) is related to the intactness of the autonomic nervous system as well as to the infant's arousal level.[26]

Crying is also of interest because it is aberrant in infants with neurological damage and in those with genetic disorders.[27] The quality of the cry may also have implications for the child's future well being since it has been established that abnormal and high pitched cries are particularly annoying to caregivers.[28] For this reason, unusual cries may place a child at risk for future abuse and neglect.

3. Neonatal Behavior
a. States/State Changes

Another important set of behaviors which has been measured during early infancy result from the ability to regulate "state." Prechtl[13] was among the first to note the importance of state in the measurement of infant status. He pointed out that the measurement of other functions (e.g., motor tone) could be inaccurate if the infants' behavioral state was not taken into account. For instance, a sleeping infant has a significantly lower motor tone that the highly aroused, crying baby. Accurate assessment of many other characteristics involved in optimality requires a quiet but alert infant. State is also theoretically important in that the ability to regulate state or achieve "homeostasis"[29] ("state control") is often seen as the first challenge of the developing infant and as a precursor of further cognitive and social development.

State has been measured differently by different theorists. Prechtl[13] proposed five states (see Table 2) ranging from deep sleep to active crying, plus an "other" category to describe abnormal conditions while Brazelton[14] and most other developers of neurobehavioral measures[30] use six states to characterize the typical range of states.

TABLE 2

MEASUREMENT OF STATE IN THE NEONATAL PERIOD

Prechtl's Classification[13]

State 1: Eyes closed, regular respiration, no movements
State 2: Eyes closed, irregular respiration, no gross movements
State 3: Eyes open, no gross movement
State 4: Eyes open, gross movement, no crying
State 5: Eyes open or closed, crying
State 6: Other state-describe (e.g., coma)

Brazelton's Classification[14]

State 1: Deep sleep
State 2: Light sleep, rapid eye movement is present
State 3: Drowsy: eyes closed by stirs and moves
State 4: Awake and alert; no gross motor activity
State 5: Active alert state: eyes open and gross motor activity is present
State 6: Crying

b. Components of "Neurobehavioral Status"

The term "neurobehavior" implies that the observed behavior results from the activity or status of the nervous system, usually the CNS, which underlies the behavior. Of course, all behavior could be so designated; however, by convention, the term is used only to describe certain classes of behaviors and activities. These behaviors are those which speak to the intactness or optimality of the CNS. Thus shuffling cards, if it were carried out efficiently, generally would not be described in this way while evidence of a tremor observed during such volitional activity (an "intentional tremor"), would be . Sometimes the term acquires a circular quality as when, for instance, a child is assumed to have a neurologically-based "specific learning disability", inferred to result from a neurological problem simply because problems in learning are observed.

In newborns, who lack both a learning history and the ability for most volitional activity, most behaviors have been designated as signs of neurobehavioral status. As a way of describing the status of the newborn, a number of scales have been developed. The most commonly used tests for full term infants are Brazelton's[14] Neonatal Behavioral Assessment Scale (BNBAS), Prechtl's[13] Neurological Examination of the Newborn Infant, and Amiel-Tisan's Neonatal Neurologic and Adaptive Capacity Scale (NACS).[31] Scales designed for the assessment of the preterm infant include Al's Assessment of Preterm Infant Behavior (APIB)[32] and Korner's Neurobehavioral Assessment of the Preterm Infant (NAPI).[33]

All of these scales rely on the clinical examination of the neonate by a trained examiner who rates the child on a number of dimensions. These dimensions usually include: *State, Motor Tone* (active and passive),

Orientation and *Alertness*, status of *Primitive Reflexes*, and *response to stress*. Some tests include ratings of the child's social behavior and response to the examiner and may include more global "Qualitative" judgements by the examiner describing the infant's performance. Because of the nature of the examination process, the outcome is totally dependent on the skill and training of the examiner. For this reason many of these scales can be administered only by "certified" examiners who are required to undergo an extensive training process as well as "certification" by a training center.

c. Response to Operant Procedures

Since the infants repertoire is limited, most of those behaviors which are present at birth have been investigated. Neonatal sucking is often rated as measure of neurobehavior "intactness."[13] However, it has also been used as the outcome measure in operant procedures.[34] Nutritive and non-nutritive sucking have been used to evaluate infant preferences and learning rates.[35] In studies that have examined drug and alcohol exposure infants, alterations in sucking rate and pattern have been noted to be related to maternal substance use.[36-37]

Novelty preference has also been used to assess infant status. In this procedure, infants are presented with stimuli which are either familiar or novel and their responses measured either through judgement of the direction of their gaze or through measurement of some other response, usually heart rate or sucking behavior. While this procedure is most often used later in infancy, it can be employed during the neonatal period. For instance, Karmel, Gardner, and Magnano[38] investigated outcomes in very low birth weight (VLBW) babies (<1500 grams) who were evaluated for the effects of cocaine exposure on orientation (stimulus seeking).

IV. RESEARCH WITH ALCOHOL EXPOSED NEONATES

Using the techniques described above, a number of studies of the effects of prenatal alcohol exposure have been carried out. While there are difficulties, there are also some advantages in doing research in the first weeks of life. Because so little time has passed since the child was exposed to the teratogen, there is some limitation on the effect of the confounding factors that can make interpretation difficult later in childhood. In addition, in the newborn nursery and the first few weeks of life, the child may be accessible to investigators. Later in infancy and childhood, parents and infants are involved in other activities and may not be available to continue participation in research. Finally, the argument could be made that, if behavioral effects of teratogens exist, evidence of them should be most apparent at this early stage which is closest in time to the presumed insult.

Those behaviors which have been examined during the neonatal period in alcohol-exposed infants include the cluster of behaviors that constitute neonatal withdrawal syndrome (NWS), the "neurobehavioral" characteristics measured by neonatal tests, cry characteristics, and a few other behaviors.

A.   NEONATAL WITHDRAWAL SYNDROME (NWS)

Neonatal withdrawal or abstinence syndrome is usually observed in neonates who have developed a dependency on a CNS depressant due to maternal use of such drugs during gestation.[18] The signs include those associated with CNS irritability and autonomic nervous system dysfunction. That is: gastrointestinal dysfunction, respiratory distress, agitated, hyperactive behavior, including frantic sucking and rooting, and hyperactive reflexes. Tremors are common as are sneezing, yawning and skin mottling. Frequently, high pitched crying and disturbed sleep are also observed. Infants often suffer feeding difficulties due to gastrointestinal dysfunction and poorly coordinated sucking. As a result of the feeding difficulties and gastrointestinal irritability, failure to gain weight is also a problem. These behaviors begin when the drug to which the child has developed a tolerance is no longer being supplied and may persist for some time--from days to weeks. The extent and seriousness of the NWS depends on a number of factors including dose size, recency of drug use, infant health status and type of drug.[18] Drugs which have different pharmacological effects (i.e., stimulants, hallucinogens) do not cause the same kind of withdrawal syndrome. Thus, the classic form of NWS is not observed in children with a primary exposure to cocaine, cigarettes or marijuana.

Like other CNS depressants, alcohol is associated with dependence and withdrawal in adults and signs of neonatal withdrawal syndrome have been noted occasionally in neonates. Pierog, Chandavasu and Wexler[39] examined six newborns diagnosed with FAS and compared their behavior to that seen in narcotics dependent neonates, finding that signs of withdrawal could be observed in the first 24 hours. These signs included irritability, tremors, alterations in motor performance, increased respiratory rate and evidence of seizure activity.   Gastrointestinal symptoms (abdominal distention and vomiting) were also observed.

Robe, Gromisch and Iosub[40] did a meta-analysis of 15 cases of neonates diagnosed with fetal alcohol syndrome whose behavior was reported in the literature. Infants born to mothers with significant evidence of alcoholism were compared to those whose mothers were addicted to narcotics. They reported finding similar symptoms in each group but the infants with FAS were more likely to have signs associated with seizures, apnea and weight loss while those in the narcotics group had more gastrointestinal symptoms and irritability. Similar results were reported by Bohlin and Larsson[41] who found that children born to women with identified alcohol problems had significantly higher levels of hyperexcitability and seizure activity.

Coles *et al.*[42] examined 8 newborns *without* a diagnosis of FAS whose mothers were heavy alcohol users[a] (Mean alcohol use: 21.0 oz AA/wk or 42 drinks/wk) and who continued this use throughout their pregnancies. These children were compared to 29 infants whose mothers did not use alcohol at all and 15 infants whose heavily-drinking mothers (17.6 oz AA/wk or 35.2 drinks) stopped drinking during the second trimester of pregnancy. Infants were examined "blind" (without knowledge of their mother's drinking history) and rated on 10 categories of signs of NWS: tremor/clonus, wakefulness/restlessness, unusual or excessive crying, hypertonia (excessive motor tone), abnormal or hyperactive reflexes, excessive mouthing, gastrointestinal signs (e.g., diarrhea, distended abdomen, vomiting, poor feeding), autonomic instability (e.g., startling, sweating) and other miscellaneous signs. The nondrinkers' children and those of the women who had stopped drinking both showed minimal signs of NWS. However, there was significant evidence of such signs among the neonates whose mothers continued to drink. These infants showed higher frequencies of tremoring (75%), sleep disturbances and restlessness (88%), exaggerated motor tone (88%), and excessive mouthing (88%). Unlike the children reported on by Robe *et al.*,[40] none of these children required medical intervention for their symptoms. This lesser severity of symptoms may be the result of mothers' level of drinking or the absence of the full FAS symptomology in these children.

These studies suggest that infants of alcohol abusers may show signs associated with NWS during the first day or so of life. Infants with the physical signs of FAS appear to be more likely to have such a pattern. That these signs are associated with withdrawal rather than neurological damage sustained earlier in pregnancy is suggested by the lack of symptoms in the children whose mothers quit drinking in midpregnancy despite heavy use earlier in pregnancy.

B.   BEHAVIORAL ALTERATIONS

The neurobehavioral characteristics of neonates exposed to alcohol have been reported by a number of investigators. Although several neonatal tests exist, infant reflexive behavior and behavioral characteristics have most often been tested using the Brazelton Neonatal Behavioral Assessment Scale (NBAS).[14] This individually-administered test of infant status and behavior measures 18 reflexes (e.g., rooting, incurvation, placing), rated on 4 point

---

[a]In describing maternal alcohol use, several conventions are used. Many investigators report alcohol use in terms of ounces of absolute alcohol (oz AA) per day. One ounce of absolute alcohol is equivalent to approximately two regular "drinks" which traditionally contain a half ounce of alcohol. Others prefer to report "oz AA per week" assuming that most drinkers confine their use to one or two days rather than drink equal amounts daily. Since studies usually report the average or mean amount for different groups, the difference between these two methods is simply stylistic. This report will use the "oz AA/wk" convention.

scales, and 28 behavioral traits (e.g., orientation to inanimate stimuli; cuddliness) which are rated on 9 point scales. These items are generally grouped into clusters which reflect aspects of the infants neurobehavioral status[3] (see Table 3). In addition, there are 9 Supplementary scales (Qualifiers) which allow the examiner to rate the quality of the infant's performance. The NBAS, and similar tests, have been used to compare the behavior of alcohol-exposed infant to that of nonexposed infants from the same populations.

These studies have yield a variety of results which can be seen as inconsistent. For instance, clinical studies which identify infants of alcoholics or dysmorphic infants most often report behavioral alterations while those who evaluate infants of moderate drinkers and nondysmorphic infants may report no effects. Because there are biases inherent in most clinical studies, particularly those which do not rely on experimental controls, the studies on which most weight can be placed are probably those which have employed a prospective research design, use appropriate contrast groups, and controlled for confounding factors. Even when such a design is used, attention must be paid to methodology in interpreting results. Important considerations for interpretation include: amount of alcohol used by mothers, duration (in pregnancy) of alcohol use, effects of other drug use, and factors such as age of infant at assessment, and examiner effects. Finally, different investigators have interpreted similar results in different ways.

Streissguth, Barr and Martin[43] examined 417 infants using the NBAS as part of a prospective study of middle class, predominantly white, moderately-drinking women and their offspring. This Seattle sample, which was recruited in the middle 1970's, has been followed since that time to investigate the effects of prenatal alcohol exposure. The investigators were able to collect information about many potentially confounding factors including other psychoactive substances (e.g., tobacco, caffeine) as well as economic and social factors. Women were recruited in the fifth month of pregnancy and information about substance use was collected only at that time. The average amount of alcohol reported by pregnant women who used alcohol at all was .38 ounces of absolute alcohol per day (oz. AA/day) or about 2.5 ounces per week. This is equivalent to about a three fourths of a drink per day or 5 drinks per week. A number of women were included who report no alcohol use.

Infants were examined in the nursery by one of eight certified examiners between 9 and 35 hours postpartum (mean: 27 hours) taking care to conduct the examination between feedings as recommended by Brazelton.[14] Since infants commonly cannot be tested on some NBAS items, only those who completed particular items were included in comparisons of the 6 factors into which the items grouped. In these analyses, those factors were found to be: *Orientation, reactivity/irritability, habituation, tremulousness/motor immaturity, low arousal* (easy to console, low excitability), and *activity/muscle tone*. Other variables which were controlled statistically in these analyses were: Maternal (age, education, parity) and infant characteristics (birth weight, gestational age, sex) and examiner.

Maternal alcohol use was found to be significantly related to two of the NBAS factor scores, *habituation* and *low arousal*. That is, these investigators found that higher maternal alcohol use was associated with poorer habituation to visual (light) and auditory (rattle) stimuli. These results suggest that infants are more responsive to these stimuli (that is, they startle more) and that these responses are maintained over time without the appropriate "habituation" which usually occurs after repeated stimuli. In contrast, differences were also found on a *low arousal* factor which meant that the alcohol-exposed infants were is easier to console, frequently self quieting and did not get upset or excited. Individual examination of the items making up this low arousal factor indicated that it was "state lability" only that was related to maternal alcohol use with those children with higher alcohol exposure showing a restricted range of states. The authors suggest that the *habituation* finding resulted from "mild compromising" (p.1116) of the CNS in a group of otherwise healthy infants. They did not speculate about the *low arousal* factor which seems somewhat inconsistent with the *habituation* results.

Similarly, Jacobson et al.,[44] who examined the effects of tobacco, caffeine and alcohol, reported that maternal alcohol use was associated with a depression of the infants *range of states* during the NBAS but could not establish whether this relationship was with prenatal use or use during pregnancy. In this study, 166 newborns were enrolled postpartum and their mothers questioned retrospectively about their use of these drugs. In this sample, the majority were white (all but one infant), middle class and married (92%). Alcohol users were classified as Abstainers, who used no alcohol, Light drinkers, who reported use of 0.01 to 0.99 oz AA/day (0.07 to 6.93 oz AA/wk or 0.14 to 13.86 drinks/wk) and Heavy drinkers, 1.00 to 1.99 oz AA/day (7 to 13.93 oz AA/wk or 14 to 27.86 drinks/wk). The NBAS[14] was administered 48 to 96 hours after birth by one of four certified examiners. The items were clustered using Lester's et al.[45] procedure but, in order to discriminate between high and low arousal, the *range-of-state* cluster was not recoded as suggested by those authors. Rather the distinction between high and low arousal was maintained. Demographic and medical variables were controlled statistically in a multiple regression procedure that examined the effects of smoking, caffeine and alcohol both prior to and during pregnancy. While smoking was found to affect *Auditory Orientation* and *General irritability* and caffeine consumption, *Orientation, Range of State* and *Reflexes*, Alcohol exposure was related only to *Range of State*. Thus, the exposed offspring were reported to be more placid than nonexposed infants at 3 days of age.

TABLE 3

COMPOSITION OF SEVEN NBAS CLUSTERS[45]

Cluster Name	NBAS Scale Item
Habituation	Light
	Rattle
	Bell
	Tactile Stimulation of Foot
Orientation	Inanimate Visual
	Inanimate Auditory
	Animate Visual
	Animate Auditory
	Animate Visual and Auditory
	Alertness
Motor Performance	General Tonus
	Maturity
	Pull-to-Sit
	Defensive Movements
	Activity
State Range	Peak of Excitement
(Range of State)	Rapidity of Buildup
	Irritability
	Lability of State
State Regulation	Cuddliness
	Consolability
	Self-quieting
	Hand-to-Mouth Facility
Autonomic Regulation	Number of Tremors
	Number of Startles
	Lability of Skin Color
Reflexes	Abnormal Reflexes (number)

Ernhart *et al.*[46] assessed neurobehavioral outcome in 359 infants in Cleveland. Mothers were recruited prenatally from a low income population and approximately a third of the sample was African-American, the rest white. Women were classified as MAST+ or MAST- based on their responses to the Michigan Alcoholism Screening Test (MAST),[47] a reliable measure of problem drinking. MAST+ women who reported drinking in pregnancy averaged about 0.20 oz AA/day (3 drinks/wk) while the MAST- group averaged about 0.08 oz AA/day (1 drink/wk). Infants were assessed using both the NBAS[14] and the Graham/Rosenblith Behavioral Examination of the Neonate (G/R)[48] which has the following summary scores, *General Maturation*, *Soft Sign Score* and *Muscle Tonus*. Tests were administered by one of two nurses certified in their administration. Infants were examined in the second day of life midway between feedings. Male infants were not examined until six hours after circumcision. In this sample, although there was a significant relationship between birth weight and the presence of physical anomalies and Mast+ scores, there were no effects seen on the neurobehavioral measures when potentially confounding factors were controlled statistically. The authors suggested that these neurobehavioral tests were not sensitive to effects at this low level of maternal alcohol use.

Coles and her colleagues in Atlanta have examined several samples of infants exposed to alcohol prenatally.[19,49-52] Low income, predominantly African-American women were recruited prenatally during the second trimester of pregnancy. Three groups of women were identified at delivery, those who continued to drink until delivery despite an educational intervention (Mean: 12.6 oz AA/wk , about 25 drinks a week), those who were drinking at recruitment but who stopped during the second trimester (mean:14.4 oz AA/wk, about 29 drinks/wk) and those who never drank during pregnancy. After controlling for infant health status and other confounding factors, 149 Infants were examined using the NBAS[14] and Precthl's scale[13] on the third day in the neonatal nursery 1 to 2 hours after a feed by the same certified examiner who was blind to mother's drinking status. NBAS data were clustered using the method recommended by Lester *et al.*[45] (see Table 3) and significant group differences were found in *Orientation* and *Autonomic Regulation* (number of tremors, startles)[50] as well as on a number of individual NBAS items, particularly the reflexive items.[49] Examination of cluster scores indicates that nondrinkers children were always perceived as more "optimal" in their behavior than both groups of drinkers children but that the stopped drinkers infants performed better than those whose mothers continued to drink. In contrast to the results of the NBAS,[14] the scores on the Prechtl[13] did not discriminate among these groups.

When a subset of these infants (n=31) was followed up at 14 and 30 days and the NBAS readministered, there were persistent differences as a function of maternal alcohol use.[51] In this sample, the average amount of drinking reported for the stopped-drinking group was 16.25 oz AA/wk (32.5 drinks/wk) and for the continued-to-drink group, 13.34 oz AA/wk (26.68 drinks/wk) classifying these women as heavy drinkers. In addition, about a third of these women reported social or physical complications due to their drinking suggesting that they might be appropriately classified as alcohol abusers.[17] At 30 days, the alcohol-exposed infants did not perform as well as the nonexposed infants on *Autonomic Regulation* and on *Abnormal Reflexes* suggesting some persistent effects of their exposure which could not be accounted for by neonatal withdrawal.

Several years later, these investigators collected and followed a second sample of infants from the same low SES population[52] whose mothers were drinking less heavily.   Sixty infants were seen at birth and at 28 days postpartum and were also classified as: Continued-to-drink (Mean: 7.55 oz AA/wk or 15 drink/wk) and Stopped drinking (Mean: 4.65 oz AA/wk or 9.3 drinks/wk) and Abstainers. Different certified examiners administered the NBAS at 3 and 28 days and were blind both to the mother's drinking status and, at 28 days, to the previous examiner's results. In this sample, at 3 days, significant differences were found between drinkers children and controls on *Habituation, Orientation, Motor Performance* and *Autonomic Regulation*. At 28 days, differences were found on *Motor Performance* and *Abnormal Reflexes*. Differences all favored the nondrinkers infants. The ratings of the independent examiners of the infants at the two different time points were highly correlated indicating that these experienced examiners rated the same infants similarly. The larger number of infants who were included in this follow-up sample may account for the higher number of significant effects than were seen in the more heavily exposed but smaller sample which was seen previously.

In the late 1980's, Coles *et al.*[19] collected a third sample of infants who were exposed to both alcohol and cocaine was well as marijuana and tobacco. One hundred and seven infants were recruited postpartum and seen in the nursery (Mean age: 39.37 hours) and at 14 days (Mean age: 13.55) and 28 days (Mean age: 28.54) for evaluation with the NBAS using the standard methodologies. In this sample, collected when cocaine use was at a high point, the inclusion of cocaine as a variable resulted in clinically significant changes in the pattern of reported drug use from that seen previously in this population. Among that group of women who reported alcohol but not cocaine use, the average alcohol amount reported was 24.17 oz AA/wk (48.34 drinks/wk) and these women continued to drink through out pregnancy. Among the women who reported cocaine use and had a positive urine screen, the average amount of alcohol per week was 4.31 oz AA/wk (8.62 drinks/wk) while among self-reported cocaine users without positive urine screens, the average alcohol amount was 6.97 oz AA/wk (13.94 drinks/wk). All groups of drug-using women reported cigarette and marijuana use as well. Because this polydrug use made it difficult to interpret statistical comparisons between groups, regression procedures were used to identify the effects of the amount and duration of use of each of these drugs. A number of confounding factors were controlled either through the experimental design or statistically, including gestational age, infant and maternal health status, prenatal care and SES. The results suggested that duration (in pregnancy) of alcohol, cigarette and marijuana use affected infants at 2 days with alcohol accounting for significant variance on *Motor Behavior*, and *Abnormal Reflexes*. At 14 days, duration of alcohol use (with cigarettes) affected *Orientation* and *Range of State* and at 28 days, *Orientation* (with marijuana) and *Abnormal Reflexes*. Cocaine contributes to the variance on *Motor Behavior*, *State Regulation*, and *Abnormal Reflexes* only at 28 days. Variances (R^2) accounted for by these variables range from 5 to 29%.

Richardson, Day and Taylor[53] examined 373 full-term newborns on the second day of life (average age: 46.8 hours) in the newborn nursery approximately 2.6 hours after a feeding. Only infants born in uncomplicated deliveries were included. Five examiners were certified in the administration of the NBAS and were blind to maternal drug and alcohol use. Mothers were identified by the fourth month of pregnancy and were repeatedly interviewed about their use of alcohol, marijuana and tobacco as well as other drugs. Use prior to pregnancy as well as in each trimester was assessed through interviews at seven months and postpartum. Demographic, life-style and psychological characteristics were also repeatedly assessed. For the purposes of analysis, the NBAS clusters recommended by Lester *et al.*[45] were used.

Families in this Pittsburgh sample were predominantly of low socioeconomic status (SES) and divided evenly as to race (white: 51%; African-American: 49%). The Mean oz AA/day in pregnancy were: 0.64 in the first trimester (5 to 6 drinks per week), 0.13 in the second trimester (2 to 3 drinks per month) and 0 .15 in the third trimester (1 to 2 drinks per week) making this a light drinking group of women. None of the children in the sample had symptoms of FAS and the mean birth weight for the sample was 3337 grams. Both alcohol and marijuana use was reported to decrease over the course of the pregnancy. In contrast, tobacco use increased slightly with the majority smoking about a half a pack a day.

The effect of alcohol use on infant behavior was examined using multiple regression procedures. Separate regressions were done for use during each trimester of pregnancy. In each analysis, examiner effects were found most consistently. When these were controlled, alcohol effects were found for first trimester exposure on *Habituation*, for second trimester exposure on *Orientation* and for third trimester exposure on *Habituation* and *Orientation*. The authors cautioned, however, that 75% of subjects had missing data on the *Habituation* cluster and that the variance accounted for by any of these factors was small (4 to 6%). Based on these findings, the authors suggest that, in their sample, moderate use of alcohol (as well as marijuana and tobacco) was not predictive of changes in neonatal in any clinically significant manner.

Staisey and Fried[54] used the Prechtl scale[13] to investigate the effects of moderate alcohol and tobacco use in a middle class, Canadian sample of 59 newborns who were seen at 9 and 30 days postpartum. The average alcohol use by women was 0 .23 oz AA/day or about 3 drinks per week. At 9 days, maternal alcohol use was found to be related to decreases in *motor tone* and *reflex optimality* as well as to an increase in *startle reactions*. At 30 days, these relationships were no longer apparent.

In a study of "social drinking" in Australia, Walpole et al.[55] used the Einstein Neonatal Behavioral Assessment Schedule which, although similar to the NBAS and other neonatal behavior scales, focuses on sensorimotor impairment and neurobehavioral organization. Of eight factors associated with neurobehavioral development, only *Tonus* (motor tone) was significantly related to alcohol exposure when potentially confounding factors were controlled. Cigarette use was not related to any of the infant behavioral outcomes. The authors caution that the amount of variance (1%) accounted for by alcohol exposure was very low and it was unlikely to be related to developmental sequelae.

C.   INVESTIGATIONS USING OTHER MEASURES OF NEUROBEHAVIORAL OUTCOME

In addition to the neonatal tests, investigators have used a variety of other measures in the neonatal period to identify behavioral differences in neonates associated with maternal alcohol use.

1. Crying

Crying appears to be a sensitive measure of the effects of exposure to drugs of abuse during the neonatal period. Cries of infants who have developed a dependency on narcotics tend to be high pitched and piercing.[56] Similarly, Nugent, Lester, and Greene[57] reported that, in a sample of otherwise "normal" Irish neonates exposed to alcohol as a result of "social" drinking during pregnancy, differences could be observed which were related to alcohol exposure.

Zeskind et al.[58] examined the pain cries of 30 alcohol-exposed newborns at 2, 14, and 28 days using a spectographic analysis of fundamental and peak frequency (F_0) as well as measures of threshold (number of snaps to the foot, latency to respond). These infants were drawn from the samples reported on by Coles et al.[19,52] At 2-days, alcohol-exposed infants had a lower Peak F_0 and a higher Cry Threshold than nonexposed infants. That is, their cries were lower pitched and they required more snaps to respond. At 14 days, the peak F_0 was higher than the controls and the Cry Latency longer. That is, the cries were now more high pitched and the child took longer to begin crying than the control infants. At 28-days, the alcohol-exposed infants continued to show a higher Peak F_0 (more high pitched cries) but other factors had normalized. The authors suggest that the alcohol exposed-infants were depressed in functioning at the initial data collections due to the effects of prenatal exposure to alcohol which is a CNS depressant. By 14 days, however, they showed the higher pitched cry which is characteristic of infants with CNS insults.

Thus, using the characteristics of infant cries as sensitive measures of infant status, it appeared that prenatal alcohol exposure was related to differences in neonatal behavior and that distinct patterns of response could be identified which appeared to be related to the pharmacological actions of the drug, both direct and indirect (NWS).

2. EEG Studies

Psychophysiological studies of alcohol-exposed infants using the electroencephalogram (EEG) have been done in the newborn period. Chernick, Childiaeva and Ioffe[22] reported significant effects using this technique in infants born to women who drank heavily during pregnancy and these effects were found to be predictive of later development in infancy.[59] Olegard et al.[23] also found that the EEG identified effects due to exposure to alcohol. Sher et al.[24] examined sleep EEG effects of marijuana and alcohol in neonates. They found that alcohol exposure in the first and second trimesters was associated with increased arousal and disturbances of sleep while marijuana exposure during each trimester was associated with increased motility and decreased quiet sleep.

3. Observational Studies

Landesman-Dwyer, Keeler, and Streissguth[60] used observational methods to study behavior in neonates exposed to low to moderate amounts of alcohol (see above for description of the sample). These infants showed increased tremors and diminished spontaneous movements. State regulation was examined also by Rosett et al.[61] in 31 infants who were monitored for 24-hour sleep-wake cycles on the third day of life. Fourteen of the infants were born to very heavily drinking mothers (Mean: 160cc AA/day or 10 drinks) who continued to drink throughout pregnancy. Eight infants were born to heavily drinking mothers (Mean:170cc AA/day or 11drinks) who abstained during the third trimester, and nine infants were born to women who did not drink heavily. Among these three groups, no differences were found in the percentages of sleep time spent in active, quiet and indeterminant sleep. However, the continued-to-drink group's infants slept less during the 24 hours of observation and showed a poorer quality of sleep characterized by episodes of wakefulness, greater restlessness and more frequent body movements. These results seem consistent with those reported in the EEG studies cited above. In contrast, Platzman et al.[62] compared spontaneous movements and sleep/wake patterns in infants exposed to alcohol and cocaine and to those of nonexposed infants, finding no differences as a function of drug exposure. However, in this study, infants were observed for only two hours rather than for 24 hours and they had been exposed to cocaine as well as alcohol. It seems likely that this difference in methodology as well as the combination of drugs and the amount used may account for the different outcomes.

V. SUMMARY

Examination of these studies of the behavior of alcohol-exposed neonates over the first month of life suggests several conclusions. First, there is a general relationship between the amount of alcohol used by the mother and the number and kind of behavioral signs that can be observed in the newborn. Those studies in which the infants were heavily exposed[49-51,61] consistently report behavioral effects while those in which women were moderate[53,55] or light[46] users find fewer or no effects. However, this relationship is not always the same. Streissguth *et al.*[43] and Staisey and Fried,[54] using low-risk, middle class samples, both report effects in children of light to moderate drinkers. Because the size of the sample used in a particular study could contribute to the probability of finding significant effects, the reported data were examined to determine whether sample size accounted for these differences. The results do not support this assumption since some small samples of infants report significant findings[42,51,54] while some large samples[46] did not. Nevertheless, it is probable that there may be an interaction between sample size and severity of maternal alcohol use which may contribute to the pattern of results reported in these studies.

A second result is that there are more behavioral differences associated with alcohol observed in the first few days postpartum than are reported later in the first month, even taking into account the relatively few studies which were done at the later time. Based on observation during the first few days, several studies report differences in *State Control, Orientation* and *Habituation*, factors which are all related to the infant's "arousal," as well as some that have noted problems with *Motor Tone.*[52,55] That there may be alterations in arousal are confirmed by the results of the studies which have focused on EEG and sleep states [22-24,61] as well as the Cry studies.[57-58] Studies done several weeks later[19,51,52,54] have found either no effects or a different pattern of outcomes. For instance, at this time, alcohol-exposed infants are found to be relatively immature motorically (*motor tone*) and to have a higher number of unusual *reflexive* responses. These data suggest that some of the behavior observed in the first few days may be acute and transitory, related to the immediate effects of alcohol exposure, while the more persistent effects may reflect a more permanent alteration of the nervous system. However, given the many confounding factors present in these clinical studies, such conclusions are preliminary.

Those few studies which have been carried out point out how difficult it is to evaluate all the factors which are important in interpretation of the children's behavior. For instance, the different kinds of arousal patterns that are seen in the different studies--sometimes, low arousal, sometimes, high--suggest that different factors are at work. Infants who are experiencing some aspects of NWS may be hyperaroused, while infants whose mothers stopped drinking earlier in pregnancy may show a low arousal due to other factors like inadequate nutrition, poor prenatal care or other drug use.

In addition, these outcomes point out, once again, the relationship between what is observed and the observer. In those studies in which alcohol use is heavy and effect size is relatively large, examiner effects are not found to be a problem. However, where there is little behavioral effect to be noted due to a low rate of exposure, examiner bias is often the outcome most reliably seen. Examination of these studies also reinforces understanding of another phenomenon. That is, that women who use alcohol heavily during pregnancy use many other psychoactive drugs as well. The presence of these other drugs also affect the behavior of the neonate and these effects, whenever present, obscure the observations of the effect of alcohol. Although we can "statistically" control these other drugs, in actuality, it is unlikely that such clarity is possible.

In summary, the effects maternal alcohol use in pregnancy on the offspring can be noted during the neonatal period. However, existing research suggests that these effects are most obvious when use has been heavy and has continued through out pregnancy. Whether such effects are significant remains unclear without more research to establish the persistence of effects and the relationship between effects seen in the neonatal period and those shown in later childhood.

REFERENCES

1. **Jones, K.L., Smith, D.W., Ulleland, C.H., and Streissguth, A.P.,** Pattern of malformations in offspring of chronic alcoholic mothers, *Lancet,* 1, 1267, 1973.

2. **Wilson, J.G.,** Current status of teratology: General principles and mechanism derived from animal studies, in *Handbook of Teratology, General Principles and Etiology,* Vol. 1, Wilson, J.G. and Frase, F.C., Eds., Plenum Press, New York, 1977, 74.

3. **Vorhees, C.V.,** Principles of behavioral teratology, in *Handbook of Behavioral Teratology*, Riley, E.P. and Vorhees, C.V., Eds., Plenum Press, New York, 1986, 23.

4. **Streissguth, A.P., Bookstein, F.L., Sampson, P.C., and Barr, H.M.,** *The Enduring Effects of Prenatal Alcohol Exposure on Child Development: Birth Through Seven Years, A Partial Least Squares Solution*, University of Michigan Press, Ann Arbor, MI, 1993.

5. **Ulleland C.N.,** The offspring of alcoholic mothers, *Ann. N.Y. Acad. Sci.,* 197, 167, 1970.

6. **Church, M.W.,** Chronic in utero alcohol exposure affects auditory function in rats and in humans, *Alc. Clin. Exp. Res.,* 4, 231, 1987.

7. **Stromland, K.,** Eyeground malformations in the fetal alcohol syndrome. *Neuropediatrics,* 12, 97, 1981.

8.	**Abel, E.L. and Sokol, R.J.,** A revised conservative estimate of the incidence of FAS and its economic impact, *Alc. Clin. Exp. Res.,* 15, 514, 1991.

9.	**Streissguth, A.P.,** The behavioral teratology of alcohol: Performance, behavioral and intellectual deficits in prenatally exposed children, in *Alcohol and Brain Development,* West, J., Ed., Oxford University Press, New York, 1986, 3.

10.	**Aylward, G.P.,** The relationship between environmental risk and developmental outcome, *Dev. Behav. Peds.,* 13, 222, 1992.

11.	**Bryant, D.M. and Ramey, C.T.,** An analysis of the effectiveness of early intervention programs for environmentally at-risk children, in *The Effectiveness of Early Intervention for At Risk and Handicapped Children,* Gualnick, M.J. and Bennet, F.C., Eds., Academic Press, Orlando, FL, 1987, 33.

12.	**Institute of Medicine Committee to Study Fetal Alcohol Syndrome,** *Fetal Alcohol Syndrome: Diagnosis, Epidemiology, Prevention and Treatment,* National Academy Press, Washington, D.C., 1995.

13.	**Prechtl, H.F.R.,** *The Neurological Examination of the Full Term Newborn Infant,* 2nd edition, Wm Heinemann Medical Books, Ltd: Spastics International Medical Publications, London, 1977.

14.	**Brazelton, T.B.,** *Neonatal Behavioral Assessment Scale, 2nd Edition: Clinics in Developmental Medicine 88,* Lippincott, Philadelphia, Pennsylvania, 1984.

15.	**Korner, A.F.,** Individual differences at birth: Implications for early experience and later development, *Am. J. Orthopsychiat.,* 41, 608, 1971.

16.	**McCall, R.B.,** The development of intellectual functioning in infancy and the prediction of later I.Q., in *Handbook of Infant Development,* J.D. Osofsky, Ed., Wiley, New York, 1979, 707.

17.	**American Psychiatric Association,** *Diagnostic and Statistical Manual,* 4th edition, (DSM-IV), American Psychiatric Association, Washington, D.C., 1994.

18.	**Finnegan, L.P. and Kaltenbach, K.A.,** Neonatal abstinence syndrome. In *Primary Pediatric Care,* 2nd edition, Hoekelman, R.A., Friedman, S.B,. Nelson, N.M., and Seidel, H.M., Eds., Mosby, St. Louis, Missouri, 1992, 1367,

19.	**Coles, C.D., Platzman, K.A., Smith, I.E., James, M.E., and Falek, A.,** Effects of cocaine and alcohol use in pregnancy on neonatal growth and neurobehavioral status, *Neurotoxicol. Teratol.,* 14, 23, 1992.

20.	**Von Bargen, D.M.,** Infant heart rate: A review of research and methodology. *Merrill-Palmer Quart.,* 29, 115, 1983.

21.	**DeGangi, G.A., DiPietro, J.A., Greenspan, S.I., and Porges, S.W.,** Psychological characteristics of the regulatory disordered infant, *Inf. Behav. Dev.,* 14, 37, 1991.

22. **Chernick, V., Childiaeva, R., and Ioffe, S.,** Effects of maternal alcohol intake and smoking on neonatal EEG and anthropometric measurements, *Am. J. Obstet. Gynecol.,* 146, 41, 1983.

23. **Olegard, R., Sobel, K.-G., Aronson, M., Sandin,B., Johansson, R.R., Carlsson, C., Kyllerman, M., Iverson, K., and Hrbeck, A.,** Effects on the child of alcohol abuse during pregnancy, *Acta Paediatr. Scand. Suppl.,* 275, 112, 1979.

24. **Sher, M.S., Richardson, G.A., Coble, P.A., Day, N.L., and Stoffer, D.S.,** The effects of prenatal alcohol and marijuana exposure: Disturbances in neonatal sleep cycling and arousal, *Pediatr. Res.* 24, 101, 1988.

25. **Magnano, L.L., Gardner, J. M. and Karmel, B.Z.,** Differences in salivary cortisol levels in cocaine-exposed and noncocaine-exposed NICU infants, *Dev. Psychobiol.,* 25, 93, 1992.

26. **Thoden, C.J., Jarvenpaa, A-L, and Michelsson, K.,** Sound spectrographic cry analysis of pain cry in prematures, in *Infant Crying: Theoretical and Research Perspectives,* Lester, B.M. and Boukydis, Z., Eds., Plenum, New York, 1985, 105.

27. **Wasz-Hockert, O., Michelsson, K., and Lind, J.,** Twenty-five years of Scandinavian cry research, in *Infant Crying: Theoretical and Research Perspectives,* Lester, B.M. and Boukydis, C.F.Z., Eds., Plenum, New York, 1985, 83.

28. **Donovan, W.L. and Leavitt, L.A.,** Physiology and behavior: Parents' response to the infant cry, in *Infant Crying: Theoretical and Research Perspectives,* Lester, B.M. and Boukydis, C.F.Z., Eds., Plenum, New York, 1985, 241.

29. **Greenspan, S.I., and Wieder, S.,** Regulatory disorders, in *Handbook of Infant Mental Health,* Zeanah, C.H., Ed., Guilford Press, New York, 1993, 280.

30. **Dubowitz, L.M.S., Dubowitz, V., Palmer, P., and Verghote, M. A.,** A new approach to the neurological assessment of the preterm and full-term newborn infant, *Brain Dev.,* 2, 3,1980

31. **Amiel-Tison, C.,** A method for neurological evaluation within the first year of life, in *Current Problems in Pediatrics,* Book Medical Publishers, Chicago, 1976.

32. **Als, H. Lester, B.M., Tronick, E., and Brazelton, T.B.,** Toward a research instrument for the assessment of preterm infants behavior (APIB), in *Theory and Research in Behavioral Pediatrics* ,Vol. 1, Fitzgerald, H.E. *et al.,* Eds., Plenum, New York, 1982, 35.

33. **Korner, A.F, Kraemer, H.C. Reade, E.P., Forrest, T., and Dimiceli, S.,** A methodological approach to developing an assessment procedure for testing the neurobehavioral maturity of preterm infants, *Child Dev.,* 58, 1478, 1987.

34. **Stock, D.L., Streissguth, A.P., and Martin, D.C.,** Neonatal sucking as an outcome variable: Comparison of quantitative and clinical assessments, *Early Human Dev.*, 10, 273, 1985.

35. **Kron, R.E., Stein, M., and Goddard, K.,E.,** A method of measuring sucking behavior in newborn infants., *Psychosom. Med.*, 25, 181, 1963.

36. **Kron, R.E., Finnegan, L. P., Kaplan, S.L., Litt, M., and Phoenix, M.D.,** The assessment of behavioral change in infants undergoing narcotic withdrawal: Comparative data from clinical and objective methods, *Addictive Dis.*, 2, 257, 1975.

37. **Martin, D.C., Martin, J.C., Streissguth, A.P., and Lund, C.A.,** Sucking frequency and amplitude in newborns as a function of maternal drinking and smoking, *Curr. Alcohol.*, 5, 359, 1979.

38. **Karmel, B.Z., Gardner, J.M., and Magnano, C.L.,** Neurofunctional consequences of in utero cocaine exposure, in *NIDA Res Mongr: Problems of Drug Dependency, Proceedings of the 52nd Annual Meeting (NIDA Res Mongr 105)* Harris, L. Ed., NIDA, Rockville, MD, 535.

39. **Pierog, S., Chandavasu, O., and Wexler, I.,** Withdrawal symptoms in infants with the fetal alcohol syndrome, *J. Ped.*, 90, 630, 1977.

40. **Robe, L.B., Gromisch, D.S., and Iosub, S.,** Symptoms of neonatal ethanol withdrawal, *Curr. Alcohol*, 8, 485, 1981.

41. **Bohlin, A-B. and Larsson, G.,** Early identification of infants at risk for institutional care, *J. Advanced Nursing*, 11, 493, 1986.

42. **Coles, C.D., Smith, I.E., Fernhoff, P.M., and Falek, A.,** Neonatal ethanol withdrawal: Characteristics in clinically normal, nondysmorphic neonates, *J. Ped.*, 105, 445, 1984.

43. **Streissguth, A.P., Barr, H.M., and Martin, D.C.,** Maternal alcohol use and neonatal habituation assessed with the Brazelton scale, *Child Dev.*, 54, 1109, 1983.

44. **Jacobson, S.W., Fein, G.G., Jacobson. J.L., Schwartz, P.M., and Dowler, J.K.,** Neonatal correlates of prenatal exposure to smoking, caffeine and alcohol, *Inf. Behav. Dev.*, 7, 253, 1984.

45. **Lester, B.M., Als, H., and Brazelton, T.B.,** Regional obstetrics anesthesia and newborn behavior: A reanalysis toward synergistic effects, *Child Dev.*, 53, 687, 1982.

46. **Ernhart, C.B., Wolf, A.W., Lien, P.L., Sokol, R.J., Kennard, M.J., and Filipovich, H.F.,** Alcohol-related birth defects: Syndrome anomalies, intrauterine growth retardation and neonatal behavioral assessment., *Alc. Clin. Exp. Res.*, 9, 447, 1985.

47. **Selzer, M.L.,** The Michigan alcoholism screening test: The quest for a new diagnostic instrument, *Am. J. Psychiatry*, 127, 12, 1971.

48. **Rosenblith, J.,** The Graham/Rosenblith behavioral examination for newborns: Prognostic value and procedural issues, in *Handbook on Infant Development*, Osofsky, J.D., Ed., New York, Wiley, 1979, 216.

49. **Coles, C.D., Smith, I.E., Fernhoff, P.M., and Falek, A.,** Neonatal neurobehavioral characteristics as correlates of maternal alcohol use during gestation, *Alc. Clin. Exp. Res.,* 14, 650, 1985.

50. **Smith, I.E., Coles, C.D., Lancaster, J., Fernhoff, P.M., and Falek, A.,** The effect of volume and duration of prenatal ethanol exposure on neonatal physical and behavioral development, *Neurobehav. Toxicol. Teratol.,* 8, 375, 1986.

51. **Coles, C.D., Smith, I.E., Lancaster, J.A., and Falek, A.,** Persistence over the first month of neurobehavioral differences in infants exposed to alcohol prenatally, *Inf. Behav. Dev.,* 10, 23, 1987.

52. **Coles, C.D., Platzman, K.A., Smith, I.E., and Falek, A.,** Effects of prenatal alcohol exposure on maternal behavior and infant perception, Unpublished manuscript, available from the Human and Behavior Genetics Laboratory, Emory University, Atlanta, GA.

53. **Richardson, G.A., Day, N.L., and Taylor, P.M.,** The effect of prenatal alcohol, marijuana, and tobacco exposure on neonatal behavior, *Inf. Behav. Dev.,* 12, 199, 1989.

54. **Staisey, N.L. and Fried, P.A.,** Relationships between moderate maternal alcohol consumption during pregnancy and infant neurological development, *J. Stud. Alcohol.,* 44, 262, 1983.

55. **Walpole, I., Zubrick, S., Pontre, S., and Lawrence, C.,** Low to moderate maternal alcohol use before and during pregnancy and neourobehavioural outcomes in the newborn infant, *Dev. Med. Child Neurol.,* 33, 875, 1991.

56. **Blinick, G., Travolga, W.N., and Antopoc, W.,** Variations in birth cries of newborn infants from narcotic addicted and normal mothers, *Am. J. Obstet. Gynecol.,* 120, 948, 1971.

57. **Nugent, J.K., Lester, B.M., and Greene, S.,** Maternal alcohol consumption during pregnancy and acoustic cry analysis, Presented at the 7th International Conference on Infant Studies, Montreal, Canada, April 2, 1990.

58. **Zeskind, P.S., Platzman, K.A., Coles, C.D., and Schuetze, P.A.,** Brief Report: Cry analysis detects subclinical effects of prenatal alcohol exposure in newborn infants, *Inf. Behav. Dev.,* (in press).

59. **Ioffe, S. and Chernick, V.,** Prediction of subsequent motor and mental retardation in newborn infants exposed to alcohol *in utero* by computerized EEG analysis, *Neuropediatrics, 21,* 11, 1990.

60. **Landesman-Dwyer, S., Keeler, S., and Streissguth, A.P.,** Naturalistic observation of the newborn: Effects of maternal alcohol intake, *Alc. Clin. Exp. Res.,* 2, 171,1978.

61. **Rosett. H.L., Snyder, P., Sander, L.W., Lee, A., Cook, P., Weiner, L., and Gould, J.,** Effect of maternal drinking on neonate state regulation, *Dev. Med. Child Neuro.,* 21, 464, 1979.

62.   **Platzman, K.A., Coles, C.D., and Raskind-Hood, C.L.,** State Organization in Neonates Prenatally Exposed to Cocaine, Presented at the International Society of Infant Studies, Miami, Florida, May 7-10, 1992.

Chapter 8

NEUROTRANSMITTER FUNCTION: CHANGES ASSOCIATED WITH *IN UTERO* ALCOHOL EXPOSURE

Mary Druse Manteuffel

I. INTRODUCTION

The incidence of fetal alcohol syndrome (FAS) is ~1.9 cases/1000 live births,[1] and as such it ranks as the leading preventable cause of mental retardation in the U.S. In addition to mental retardation, FAS children frequently exhibit signs of hyperactivity, attention and perceptual deficits, motor abnormalities, behavioral problems, and slower reaction times.[2-13] Neuroanatomical malformations have been documented in FAS children both by autopsies and by use of magnetic resonance imaging.[14-15]

Animal models of FAS have been useful in elucidating neurochemical and neuroanatomical abnormalities which result from *in utero* ethanol exposure. Studies of animal models of FAS have established that early ethanol exposure markedly impairs the development of most neurotransmitter systems. That is, the development of the serotonergic, dopaminergic, noradrenergic, cholinergic, glutamatergic, GABAergic and histaminergic systems is adversely affected by ethanol.[16-17] In addition, the concentration of opiate peptides is altered in ethanol-exposed offspring.[18-19] A previous review[16] emphasizes that most neurotransmitter system abnormalities were detected by analyses of brain regions in offspring of rats or mice which received ethanol either in a liquid diet or through gastric intubation. Quantitation of neurotransmitters in whole brains often masked differences which could be detected by regional analyses. In addition, studies which used a low ethanol dose (e.g., that administered in drinking water) did not consistently report significant changes.

This review summarizes recent reports of the effects of prenatal and early postnatal ethanol exposure on developing neurotransmitter systems. Additional information is provided regarding the components of the adenylate cyclase and phosphoinositide second messenger systems and the G proteins which link many neurotransmitter systems to these second messenger systems. Potential mechanisms by which ethanol may exert its deleterious effects are considered.

II. NEUROTRANSMITTER SYSTEMS

A.   SEROTONIN

The influence of ethanol on the development of 5-HT containing neurons and their projections has been studied by assessing neurotransmitter and metabolite content and the concentration of reuptake sites. Serotonin receptors have also been examined. Such work in this and other laboratories has demonstrated that *in utero* ethanol exposure seriously impairs the development of the serotonergic system. The concentration of serotonin (5-HT) and its acid metabolite 5-hydroxyindoleacetic acid (5-HIAA) were significantly decreased in whole brain and brain regions of ethanol-exposed offspring.[20-24] A 5-HT deficit can be detected in the brain stem as early as gestational day 15 (G15).[24] Low 5-HT levels persist in this region until at least postnatal day 5 (PN5). Decreased 5-HIAA was found in whole cortex on G19 and PN5; G19 is an age when the normal distribution of serotonergic neuronal projections to cortical target areas is similar to that in the adult.[25] Lower 5-HT and/or 5-HIAA were noted on PN19 and PN35 in cortical regions (e.g. motor and somatosensory cortex). Thus, *in utero* ethanol exposure impairs the development of both the cell bodies of serotonergic neurons and their projections to target areas. Three-month-old ethanol-exposed offspring exhibited a deficiency of whole brain 5-HT;[22] whole brain analyses were unable to detect the 5-HT deficit at 4-5 months of age.[26] Regional 5-HT analyses were not performed in the older animals.

In addition to a lower concentration of 5-HT, the number of 5-HT reuptake sites was significantly reduced in several target areas of ethanol-exposed offspring. Since 5-HT reuptake sites are located on nerve terminals, their concentration has been used as an index of serotonergic innervation. Tissue homogenate studies detected a significant decrease in [³H]5-HT reuptake in the motor cortex of PN19 and PN35 rats.[27] More recent quantitative autoradiographic (QAR) analyses demonstrated lower binding of [³H]citalopram to 5-HT reuptake sites in the frontal cortex, parietal cortex, lateral hypothalamus, substantia nigra, medial septum and striatum of PN19 and/or PN35 offspring of pair-fed control and ethanol dams.[28] These observations provide additional evidence that *in utero* ethanol exposure impairs the development of serotonergic projections to target areas. However, in contrast to the lower [³H]citalopram binding in many target areas, binding was increased in the dorsal and median raphe (cell body region) on PN5. The latter finding could indicate a transient 5-HT hyperinnervation or sprouting due to an early ethanol-associated 5-HT deficit in these regions; a similar hyperinnervation of 5-HT containing neurons was found in the brain stem of neonatal rats, in which 5-HT had been depleted by prior treatment with the 5-HT neurotoxin, 5,7-dihydroxytryptamine.[29]

Both homogenate binding[24] and QAR studies have been used to assess 5-HT_{1A} receptors. These investigations demonstrated that 5-HT_{1A} receptors were decreased in the cortex, and cortical regions, and transiently increased in the dentate gyrus of ethanol-exposed offspring.[24,30] In contrast, no significant differences were noted in [^{3}H]ketanserin binding to 5-HT_2 receptors in the motor or somatosensory cortex.[31] It is interesting that both the 5-HT_{1A} receptors in cortical and dentate gyrus projection areas[32-33] and the cortical 5-HT_2 receptors[34] are located postsynaptically on neurons innervated by serotonergic neurons. Thus, it appears that the effects of early ethanol exposure on serotonergic target neurons are not general. Rather, the effects may be selective for a specific receptor type, or a particular neuron type on which the receptors are located.

The early development of serotonergic neurons is markedly impaired by *in utero* ethanol exposure. This is shown by the fact that the 5-HT deficit was detected in the brain stem of ethanol-exposed offspring on G15.[24] This finding is important because the brain stem contains the serotonin-producing cell bodies of the raphe neurons, and the age (G15) is within days of the first appearance of 5-HT immunopositive neurons.[35-36] Furthermore, fetal 5-HT regulates the normal development and maturation of serotonergic neurons.[37-40] 5-HT modulates neurite outgrowth to target areas,[41-43] and promotes formation of collateral connections between serotonergic neurons[40] Many of these trophic actions of 5-HT are mediated by 5-HT_{1A} receptors, located on the cell bodies of the 5-HT producing raphe neurons.[39-40] However, fetal 5-HT also acts on astroglial 5-HT_{1A} receptors to promote the synthesis and release of trophic factors, essential for normal serotonergic development.[44]

In light of the evidence that *in utero* ethanol exposure decreased fetal 5-HT in the brain area containing the developing raphe neurons, and that fetal 5-HT functions as an essential trophic factor, we hypothesized that this 5-HT deficit could contribute to further CNS developmental abnormalities in ethanol-exposed offspring. In an attempt to overcome the low concentration of fetal 5-HT and the presumed decreased stimulation of fetal 5-HT_{1A} neuronal and astroglial receptors, we administered a 5-HT_{1A} receptor agonist, buspirone, to ethanol-fed and control dams from the 13th to the 20th day of gestation. This treatment appeared to reverse or prevent many of the developmental abnormalities in the serotonergic system of ethanol-exposed offspring. Specifically, maternal buspirone treatment prevented postnatal deficits of 5-HT/5-HIAA and 5-HT reuptake sites in cortical regions of ethanol-exposed offspring. While the offspring of untreated, ethanol-fed dams had a 5-HT and/or 5-HIAA deficiency in whole cortex on PN5, and in the motor cortex on PN19 and PN35, there were no significant differences in these regions of age-matched offspring of buspirone-treated, ethanol-fed dams.[45] Similarly, maternal buspirone treatment prevented the decline in [^{3}H]-citalopram binding to reuptake sites in the frontal cortex, lateral hypothalamus, substantia nigra, and medial septum, and the transient increase in the dorsal and median raphe.[28]

This treatment also prevented postnatal ethanol-associated changes in 5-HT$_{1A}$ receptors in the dentate gyrus, parietal cortex, and lateral septum.[30]

At present, it is not known whether buspirone's protective effects were mediated solely by its actions on raphe 5-HT$_{1A}$ neuronal receptors, or also by its actions on astroglial receptors. Serotonin reportedly stimulates astroglial proliferation,[46] as well as synthesis and release of essential astroglial trophic factors.[40] Specifically, serotonin stimulates astroglial 5-HT$_{1A}$ receptors to release S100β,[44] a protein which promotes serotonergic neuron development.[47] Additional studies are needed to determine the mechanism by which buspirone exerted its protective effects and to establish whether this treatment affected other neurotransmitter systems as well.

Cell culture studies provide evidence that the production of essential astroglial neurotrophic factors is impaired by ethanol exposure. Conditioned media produced by ethanol-exposed astroglia (ECM) is less able to sustain normal development of cultured fetal rhombencephalic neurons than control astroglial conditioned media (CCM). That is, there was decreased DNA content, as well as decreased 5-HT immunopositive neurons and 5-HT reuptake, and altered neurite growth in fetal rhombencephalic neurons cultured in ECM.[48] In addition, there is evidence that ethanol-treated astroglial cells exhibit decreased protein content and decreased synthesis of DNA, RNA and protein.[48-53] In contrast, when fetal rhombencephalic neurons were cultured in the presence of 150 - 300 mg/dl ethanol but in a media rich in serum growth factors, the content of DNA, protein and 5-HT, as well as the number of 5-HT reuptake sites and 5-HT immunopositive neurons was unchanged.[54]

B.   DOPAMINE

Prenatal ethanol exposure also impairs the development of the dopaminergic system. The offspring of ethanol-exposed dams reportedly have a decreased concentration of dopamine (DA) in brain areas which are targets of dopaminergic projections --- namely, the cortex, striatum, and hypo-thalamus.[23,55,58] A DA deficit was noted as early as PN5[56] in brain regions which contain the substantia nigra and ventral tegmental area, and hence in areas which contain the cell bodies of dopaminergic neurons.[56] The lack of DA in the noted target areas, as well as the decreased concentration of reuptake sites indicate that *in utero* ethanol exposure impairs the development of DA projections. However, although basal DA levels were unchanged in the nucleus accumbens of ethanol-exposed rats, these animals exhibited attenuated release of dopamine following cocaine administration. Although not specifically linked to DA or NE changes,[57] catecholaminergic differences reportedly explain the observed altered sensitivity of ethanol-exposed rats to low doses of ethanol.[58]

Ethanol adversely impacts on the development of dopamine reuptake sites and receptors. Fewer dopamine reuptake sites and D$_1$ receptors were detected in the striatum; less D$_1$ receptors in the frontal cortex of ethanol-exposed offspring.[56]   A lowered concentration of D_1 receptors indicates that post-synaptic targets may also be affected. There are conflicting reports regarding the effects of *in utero* exposure on striatal D_2 receptors.[56,59-60]

Like the fetal 5-HT deficit, an early lack of dopamine may adversely affect subsequent neural development. Dopamine is another neurotransmitter which reportedly plays a role in neuronal differentiation,[61] and on neurite elongation.[43] Some of these actions are mediated by D_1 receptors.[61] Consequently, an early DA deficit could contribute to additional developmental abnormalities in the dopaminergic system.

C.   NOREPINEPHRINE

There is considerable evidence that the developing noradrenergic system in brain is markedly impaired by early ethanol exposure. The concentration of brain norepinephrine (NE) was reduced in the offspring of ethanol-fed dams.[18,62-64] Regional analyses demonstrated that the NE deficiency was present in the hypothalamus, striatum, and septal area;[53,62,64] the hypothalamic deficit reportedly persisted for at least 26 weeks.[64] Hypothalamic norepinephrine turnover was decreased in ethanol-exposed offspring. A recent investigation reported that despite normal basal levels of cortical NE in young adult ethanol-exposed offspring, cortical NE content was decreased following a single acute restraint and repeated restraint stress.[65] In addition,sensitivity to the stimulatory effects of a low ethanol dose was altered.[58] In terms of receptors, there is evidence that hippocampal β-adrenergic receptors were also reduced in ethanol-exposed offspring.[66] Additional work indicates that the sympathetic nervous system is also affected by *in utero* exposure in terms of NE content and β_1-adrenergic receptors.[67]

D.   ACETYLCHOLINE

The developing cholinergic system in rats is sensitive to *in utero* ethanol exposure. Acetylcholine concentration was significantly reduced in fetal and neonatal rat brain.[68] However, in PN20 ethanol-exposed rat offspring the cortical activities of choline acetyltransferase (ChAT), a cholinergic biosynthetic enzyme, and acetylcholinesterase (AChE), the degradative enzyme, were unchanged.[69] Muscarinic QNB (quinuclidinyl benzilate) receptors were transiently altered in ethanol-exposed rat offspring; these receptors were increased in the cortex at PN8, but not PN20[70] or at 4-5 months.[26] Hippocampal muscarinic receptors were reportedly increased on PN4 and PN30.[58] Studies with chick embryos measured the development of cholinergic neurons, by assessing ChAT activity. ChAT activity was decreased in brains of ethanol-treated embryonic chicks.[71-74] Interestingly, the cholinotoxic effects of ethanol in the chick embryo could be reversed or prevented by treatment with nerve growth factor (NGF) or epidermal growth factor.[61,72,74-75] These observations may be physiologically significant since ethanol exposure decreases NGF secretion from proliferating astrocytes.[76]

E.   GLUTAMATE

Investigations of the effects of *in utero* ethanol exposure on glutamate concentration have produced conflicting findings. Whereas one report found decreased glutamate at G19,[77] another noted an elevation from G19 to PN10.[68] More consistent observations have been made regarding glutamate receptors. *In utero* ethanol exposure lowers [³H]-glutamate binding sites in whole brain on PN17 offspring.[78] In addition, Savage and his colleagues demonstrated the sensitivity of hippocampal glutamate receptors to *in utero* ethanol exposure. They reported a decrease in [³H]-glutamate binding sites in the hippocampus of PN5 rats,[79] and more specifically of the NMDA receptors in the CA1 and other hippocampal areas of PN45 ethanol-exposed offspring.[80] NMDA-sensitive [³H]-glutamate binding was reduced in offspring of dams exposed during the last half or third of pregnancy, but not during the first half.[81] In addition to NMDA receptor changes, there were less of the kainate-sensitive receptor subtype of glutamate receptors in the entorhinal cortex and ventral hippocampal CA3 stratum lucidum of PN45 rats. However, this effect was noted only in rats that consumed a 3.35% (v/v) but not a 6.7% (v/v) ethanol-containing liquid diet.[82]

F.   GABA

Despite one conflicting report,[68] the majority of studies suggest that prenatal ethanol exposure does not significantly alter whole brain GABA,[83-84] or GABA concentration in the amygdaloid cortex or corpus striatum.[85] However, activity of glutamic acid decarboxylase, a marker of GABAergic neurons, was reduced in brains of ethanol-exposed embryonic chicks,[72] and there was a region specific alteration of GABA-stimulate Cl⁻ flux in response to flunitrazepam and neurosteroids.[86]

G.   OPIATES

In utero ethanol exposure adversely affects the development of opiate containing neurons. β-Endorphin concentration was reduced in both the midbrain and hind brain of the offspring of rats fed an ethanol-containing, low protein diet.[18] In addition, the response of the β-endorphin system to stress is altered in ethanol-exposed offspring.[19] Met- and leu-enkephalin were increased in the globus pallidus of ethanol-exposed adult offspring.[87]

H.   OTHER NEUROTRANSMITTERS

Both glycine and histamine are sensitive to the effects of an early ethanol exposure. Brain glycine is decreased by 30% in G19 ethanol-exposed offspring;[77] there is a 40-80% deficiency of cerebellar histamine receptors on PN8 and PN20.[70]

I. NEUROTRANSMITTER-LINKED SECOND MESSENGER SYSTEMS

As noted, *in utero* ethanol exposure adversely affects the development of receptors for several neurotransmitter systems. An attempt was made to further elucidate the neurochemical correlates by examining potential postreceptor changes. Since most of the affected receptors are G protein-linked receptors, their normal postreceptor function is coupled either to the stimulation or inhibition of adenylate cyclase (AC), stimulation of phosphoinositide (PI) hydrolysis, or ion flux. The second messenger pathways, associated with AC activity and PI hydrolysis, are subsequently linked to the phosphorylation of specific cellular proteins.

The α subunit of several G proteins was quantitated in cortical regions and brain stem using Western blot analysis. The G proteins which were analyzed include those which stimulate ($G\alpha s$) or inhibit ($G\alpha i$) adenylate cyclase, and Go. G protein content was determined using antibodies directed against the α subunit of either Gs, Go, or the combinations of Gi1/Gi2, and Gi3/Go.[88] In addition, mRNA content for the α subunits of each of these G proteins was assessed. These experiments demonstrated that prenatal ethanol exposure did not markedly affect G protein content or synthesis in the brain regions analyzed.[88]

The influence of ethanol on the development of adenylate cyclase activity was determined by assessing basal activity, dopamine-stimulated activity, and the binding of forskolin to the catalytic subunit of adenylate cyclase. These experiments found a lower content of the catalytic subunit of adenylate cyclase in the CA1 region of the hippocampus and occipital cortex of ethanol-exposed offspring.[58] In addition, basal adenylate cyclase activity was decreased in brains of ethanol-exposed embryonic chicks.[89] Nonetheless, in cortical regions and striatum of PN5 and PN19 rats, there were no significant differences in either basal adenylate cyclase or in the enzyme activity, stimulated by 100 μM of dopamine.[88] Thus, despite evidence of decreased cortical and striatal D_1 receptors, stimulation of D_1-linked adenylate cyclase by a high concentration of dopamine was not changed. It is possible that differences in adenylate cyclase activity may have been noted if a lower dopamine concentration were used.

Stimulation of muscarinic cholinergic receptors is often linked to PI hydrolysis. However, although there is reportedly a transient increase in cortical muscarinic receptors,[70] no significant differences in cortical carbachol-stimulated PI hydrolysis were detected in the offspring of rats that consumed an ethanol-containing liquid diet during pregnancy.[88] (Blood alcohol levels in the mother rats were typically 80-120 mg/dl.) In contrast, postnatal exposure to a higher ethanol dose (peak blood alcohol levels from 237 to 283 mg/dl) was associated with decreased carbachol-stimulated cortical PI hydrolysis in rats aged PN7 and PN19.[90] The same authors noted that early postnatal ethanol treatment had its greatest effect on PI hydrolysis during the peak of the brain growth spurt and maximal efficacy of muscarinic receptor agonists to induce PI hydrolysis.[91] The postnatal effects were similar to those observed when brain slices were exposed to high ethanol concentrations.[92] No significant differences were found in 5-HT-stimulated phosphoinositide hydrolysis in the offspring of ethanol-fed rats.[88] The latter finding was not unexpected since one of the receptor subtypes linked to PI hydrolysis (e.g. 5-HT$_2$ receptors) were unchanged in similarly treated rats.[31]

The products of PI hydrolysis are IP$_3$ and diacylglycerol (DAG). Stimulation of IP$_3$ receptors results in an increase of intracellular Ca^{2+}, which subsequently can activate Ca^{2+}-dependent protein kinases to phosphorylate specific cellular proteins. Increased DAG causes stimulation of protein kinase C to phosphorylate cellular proteins. One investigation examined steps downstream of receptor-stimulated PI hydrolysis. It found decreased receptors for IP$_3$ in multiple brain areas, and increased phorbol ester binding sites (presumably as a measure of protein kinase C) in the cortex, striatum and hippocampus of ethanol-exposed offspring.[58]

Protein phosphorylation can be activated by several protein kinases (PK's) (e.g., PKA, PKC, Ca^{2+}-calmodulin dependent PK). The activation of these PK's is associated with the stimulation of adenylate cyclase, PI hydrolysis, and an increase in intracellular Ca^{2+} levels. A recent study demonstrated that basal phosphorylation of MAP-2 (a microtubule associated protein) was reduced by ~23% in frontal cortex of ethanol-exposed offspring, while it was unaffected in the hippocampus. In contrast, basal phosphorylation of several other cellular proteins (e.g., tau, MAP-1, synapsin 1, GAP 43, and others) was not changed.[93] At present, there does not appear to be any information regarding the effects of *in utero* ethanol exposure on agonist-stimulated phosphorylation of important brain phosphoproteins.

J.   SUMMARY OF NEUROTRANSMITTER, G PROTEIN AND SECOND MESSENGER SYSTEM STUDIES

There is now a substantial body of evidence that *in utero* ethanol exposure markedly impairs the development of several neurotransmitter systems. The affected systems include those which use the following neurotransmitters: serotonin; dopamine; norepinephrine; acetylcholine; glutamate; GABA; glycine; and histamine. Neuropeptide levels were also altered. In several systems there is evidence that ethanol impairs the development of neuronal cell bodies and their projections. In most cases, the abnormalities in concentration of neurotransmitters, receptors and reuptake sites were detected at the earliest ages examined. Although some of the observed changes were long-lasting, others were transient. At present, it is not known whether the return to standard levels is associated with normal function. In addition, the impact of transient deficiencies of the neurotransmitters which function as fetal neurotrophic factors is not fully understood.

A limited number of investigations indicate that there are significant postreceptor neurochemical alterations in the adenylate cyclase and phopshoinositide pathways as well as in protein phosphorylation. Many of the observed changes in adenylate cyclase, phosphoinositide hydrolysis and protein phosphorylation were general effects, and not linked to specific neurotransmitter systems. These changes may further contribute to abnormalities in specific neurotransmitter systems. Basal adenylate cyclase levels and the concentration of the catalytic subunit of this enzyme are altered in some brain regions of ethanol-exposed offspring. In addition, some components of the phosphoinositide system may be altered by early ethanol exposure. However, additional work is needed to fully elucidate the ethanol-associated cellular changes associated with altered development of CNS neurotransmitter systems.

III. POTENTIAL MECHANISMS

The mechanism(s) by which *in utero* ethanol exposure impairs the development of multiple CNS neurotransmitter systems is not totally clear. However, there are a number of potential factors which may contribute to the abnormal development Previous reviews have considered factors such as the involvement of ethanol or acetyaldehyde, maternal malnutrition, intestinal and placental nutrient transport, glucose homeostasis, hypoxia, prostaglandins,[99] neurotransmitter trophic factors, cellular and substrate adhesion molecules, retinol levels and neurotoxicity.[16-17] This section will focus on two potential mechanisms that either directly or indirectly involve neurotransmitter levels: maternal hypoxia and the potentially associated neurotoxicity, and; essential neurotrophic factors.

Maternal ethanol consumption can cause fetal hypoxia as a result of an ethanol-induced contraction of the uterine and placental vessels.[94-96] Destruction of select cell types in distinct brain areas may accompany transient or intermittent fetal hypoxia.[97-98] In fact, investigators have noted a similarity in the hippocampal damage which is caused by ethanol and that seen following hypoxia or ischemia.[99] The brain areas most susceptible to hypoxic damage would likely be those utilizing the neurotransmitter glutamate. Consistent with this line of thinking is the evidence that animal models of FAS demonstrated hippocampal damage and alterations in the both NMDA and kainate receptor subtypes.[80] Glutamate has been associated with neurotoxicity and the generation of free radicals.[100-102] The developing ethanol-exposed fetus may be particularly susceptible to the toxic effects of alcohol or the free radicals generated by its metabolism because of decreased brain levels glutathione (GSH); GSH is an important nonprotein thiol which protects cells from damage caused by free radicals.[103]

There is recent evidence that ethanol impairs the synthesis and/or secretion of trophic factors which are essential for normal CNS development, or the ability of such factors to mediate their normal cellular effects. For example, our studies demonstrated that *in utero* ethanol exposure causes decreased fetal concentration of two neurotransmitter trophic factors -- 5-HT and dopamine.[24,56] The potential involvement of the low fetal 5-HT level with subsequent aberrant CNS development is supported by studies showing that maternal treatment with buspirone, a 5-HT$_{1A}$ agonist, prevented or reversed many of the effects of *in utero* ethanol exposure on 5-HT and 5-HIAA content, as well as on the aberrant development of 5-HT reuptake sites (e.g., serotonergic terminals) and 5-HT$_{1A}$ receptors.[28,30,92]

In addition to affecting the fetal concentration of two neurotransmitter trophic factors, *in utero* ethanol exposure impairs the synthesis, secretion or response to several other growth factors, such as nerve growth factor (NGF), epidermal growth factor (EGF), or the insulin like growth factors (IGFs). For example, ethanol's cholinotoxic effects on embryonic chick neurons could be prevented or reversed by treatment with NGF or EGF.[71-75] These observations may be physiologically significant since ethanol exposure can lower both astroglial NGF secretion[76] and the responsiveness of neural tissue to NGF[104] In light of NGF's chemotactic properties, an alteration in NGF levels in response to ethanol may contribute to the aberrant neuronal migration pattern seen in animal models of FAS.

IGF-1 and IGF-2 are additional important neurotrophic factors.[52] The function of these growth factors appears to be impaired in ethanol-exposed offspring. Several laboratories have noted an association of ethanol exposure with decreased content, release and/or expression of peripheral IGF-1.[105-107] In addition, ethanol inhibits the response of glial cells to IGF-1 in terms of cell growth, protein and DNA synthesis; IGF-1 receptor autophosphorylation, and PI-3 kinase activation.[52,108-109]

The synthesis of trophic factors could be affected by ethanol through alterations in the expression of genes. Although this topic has received little prior attention, several studies suggest that ethanol can inhibit protein synthesis.[53,110] However, detailed information regarding the effects of ethanol on the expression of specific genes is limited. To date, only a few laboratories have investigated this topic, and most of the investigations have focused on genes which are present in glial cells. Such studies suggest that ethanol impairs the expression of oligodendroglial genes coding for myelin basic protein (MBP), transferrin, and CNP (2',3' cyclic nucleotide phosphorylase).[111-112] The observed changes in gene expression may be primary effects of ethanol or could reflect a general delay in the development and maturation of oligodendroglia. In contrast, a moderate and brief postnatal ethanol exposure can cause a transient increase in the expression of an astroglial marker, GFAP (glial fibrillary acid protein),[113] particularly in cortical astrocytes. In addition to the evidence that ethanol affects the expression of specific glial genes, the expression of glut-1, the glucose transporter, is decreased by ~50% in the brains of ethanol-exposed offspring; there is a corresponding decrease in the uptake of 2-deoxyglucose.[107]

IV. SUMMARY

In summary, it is clear that *in utero* ethanol exposure markedly impairs the development of several neurotransmitter systems. Many potential mechanisms have been put forth to explain the cause(s) of these devastating actions of ethanol. It is likely that a combination of several mechanisms act in the human situation to produce the disastrous and complex actions of ethanol on multiple neurotransmitter systems. The investigator's challenge is to elucidate means by which this damage can be prevented or reversed.

REFERENCES

1. Abel, E.L. and Sokol, R.J., Incidence of fetal alcohol syndrome and economic impact of FAS-related anomalies, *Drug Alcohol Depend.*, 19, 51, 1987.
2. Jones, K.L., Smith, D.W., Ulleland, C.N., and Streissguth, A.P., Patterns of malformations in offspring of chronic alcoholic mothers, *Lancet*, 1, 1267, 1973.
3. Hanson, J.W., Jones, K.L., and Smith, D.W., Fetal alcohol syndrome: Experience with 41 patients, *JAMA*, 235, 1458, 1976.
4. Streissguth, A.P., Psychologic handicaps in children with the fetal alcohol syndrome, *Ann. N.Y. Acad. Sci.*, 273, 140, 1976.
5. Steinhausen, H.C., Nestler, V., and Spohr, H.L., Development and psychopathology of children with the fetal alcohol syndrome, *Dev. Behav. Pediatr.*, 3, 49, 1982.
6. Spohr, H-L. and Steinhausen, J-C., Clinical, psychopathological and developmental aspects in children with the fetal alcohol syndrome: A four-year follow-up study, *Mechanisms of Alcohol Damage In Utero*, Pitman, London (Ciba Foundation symposium 105), 197, 1984.
7. Aronson, M., Kyllerman, M., Sabel, K-G., Sandin, B., and Olegard, R., Children of alcoholic mothers: Developmental, perceptual and behavioral characteristics as compared to matched controls, *Acta Paediatr. Scand.*, 74, 27, 1985.
8. Streissguth, A.P., Sampson, P.D., and Barr, H.D., Neurobehavioral dose-response effects of prenatal alcohol exposure in humans from infancy to adulthood, *Ann. N.Y. Acad. Sci.*, 562, 145, 1989.
9. Conry, J., Neuropsychological deficits in fetal alcohol syndrome and fetal alcohol effects, *Alc. Clin. Exp. Res.*, 14, 650, 1990.

10. **Nanson, J.L. and Hiscock, M.,** Attention deficits in children exposed to alcohol prenatally, *Alc. Clin. Exp. Res.,* 14, 656, 1990.

11. **Spohr, H.L., Willms, J., and Steinhausen, H.C.,** Prenatal alcohol exposure and long-term developmental consequences, *Lancet,* 341, 907, 1993.

12. **Jacobson, J.L., Jacobson, S.W., Sokol, R.J., Martier, S.S., Ager, J.W., and Kaplan-Estrin, M.G.,** Teratogenic effects of alcohol on infant development, *Alc. Clin Exp. Res.,* 17, 174, 1993.

13. **Jacobson, S.W., Jacobson, J.L., and Sokol, R.J.,** Effects of fetal alcohol exposure on infant reaction time, *Alc. Clin. Exp. Res.,* 18, 1125, 1994.

14. **Clarren, S.K. and Smith, D.W.,** The fetal alcohol syndrome, *N. Engl. J. Med.,* 298, 1063, 1978.

15. **Mattson, S.N., Riley, E.P., Jernigan, T.L., Garcia, A., Kaneko, W.M., Ehlers, C.L., and Jones, K.L.,** A decrease in the size of the basal ganglia following prenatal alcohol exposure: A preliminary report, *Neurotoxicol. Teratol.,* 16, 283, 1994.

16. **Druse, M.J.,** Effects of *in utero* ethanol exposure on the development of CNS neurotransmitter systems, in *Development of the Central Nervous System. Effects of Alcohol and Opiates,* Miller, M.W., Ed., Wiley-Liss, Inc., New York, 1992, 139.

17. **Druse, M.J.,** Effects of maternal alcohol consumption on the developing nervous system, in *Alcohol and Neurobiology. Brain Development and Hormone Regulation,* Watson, R.R., Ed., CRC Press, New York, 1992, 1.

18. **Shoemaker, W.J., Baetgem G., Azad, R., Sapin, V., and Bloom, F.E.,** Effect of prenatal alcohol exposure on amine and peptide neurotransmitter systems, *Monogr. Neural. Sci.,* 9, 130, 1983.

19. **Angelogianni, P. and Gianoulakis, C.,** Prenatal exposure to ethanol alters the ontogeny of the α-endorphin response to stress, *Alc. Clin. E Exp. Res.,* 13, 564, 1989.

20. **Elis, J., Krsiak, M., Poschlova, N., and Masek, K.,** The effect of alcohol administration during pregnancy on the concentration of noradrenaline, dopamine and 5-hydroxytryptamine in the brain of offspring of mice, *Act. Nerv. Super. (Praha),* 18, 220, 1976.

21. **Elis, J., Krsiak, M., and Poschlova, N.,** Effect of alcohol given at different periods of gestation on brain serotonin in offspring, *Act. Nerv. Super. (Praha),* 20, 287, 1978.

22. **Krsiak, M., Elis, J., Poschlova, N., and Masek, K.,** Increased aggressiveness and lower brain serotonin levels in the offspring of mice given alcohol during gestation, *J. Stud. Alcohol,* 38, 1696, 1977.

23. **Rathbun, W. and Druse, M.J.,** Dopamine, serotonin and acid metabolites in brain regions from the developing offspring of ethanol treated rats, *J. Neurochem.,* 44, 57, 1985.

24. **Druse, M.J., Kuo, A., and Tajuddin, N.,** Effects of *in utero* ethanol exposure on the developing serotonergic system, *Alc. Clin. Exp. Res.,* 15, 678, 1991.

25. **Lidov, H.G.W. and Molliver, M.E.,** Immunohistochemical study of the development of serotonergic neurons in the rat CNS, *Brain Res. Bull.* 9, 559, 1982.

26. **Chan, A.W.K. and Abel, E.L.,** Absence of long-lasting effects on brain receptors for neurotransmitters in rats prenatally exposed to alcohol, *Res. Community Subst. Abuse* 3, 219, 1982.

27. **Druse, M.J. and Paul, L.H.,** Effects of *in utero* ethanol exposure on serotonin uptake in cortical regions, *Alcohol,* 5, 455, 1989.

28. **Kim, J-A. and Druse, M.J.,** Protective effects of maternal buspirone treatment on serotonin reuptake sites in ethanol-exposed offspring, submitted.

29. **Pranzatelli, M.R. and Martens, J.M.,** Plasticity and ontogeny of the central 5-HT transporter: Effect of neonatal 5, 7- dihydroxytryptamine lesions in the rat, *Dev. Brain Res.,* 70, 191, 1992.

30. **Kim, J-A. and Druse, M.J.,** Effects of maternal buspirone treatment on 5-HT$_{1A}$ receptors in ethanol-exposed offspring, submitted.

31. **Tajuddin, N. and Druse, M.J.,** Effects of *in utero* ethanol exposure on cortical 5-HT$_2$ binding sites, *Alcohol,* 5, 461, 1989.

32. **Hall, M.D., El Mestikawy, S., Emerit, M.B., Pichat, L., Hamon, M., and Gozlan, H.,** [^{3}H]8-Hydroxy-2-(di-n-propylamino)tetralin binding to pre- and postsynaptic 5-hydroxytryptamine sites in various regions of the brian, *J. Neurochem.,* 44, 1685, 1985.

33. **Verge, D., Davl, G., Marcinkiewicz, M., Patey, A., El Mestikawy, S., Gozlan, H., and Hamon, M.,** Quantitative autoradiography of multiple 5-HT$_1$ receptor subtypes in the brain of control and 5,7-DHT treated rats. *J. Neurosci.,* 6, 3474, 1986.

34. **Leysen, J.E., van Gompel, P., Verwimp, M., Niemegeers, C.J.E.,** Role and localization of serotonin$_2$ (S$_2$)-receptor-binding sites: Effects of neuronal lesions, in *CNS Receptors - From Molecular Pharmacology to Behavior,* Mandel, P., De Feudis, F.V. Eds., Raven Press, New York, 1983, 373.

35. **Lauder, J.M. and Krebs, H.,** Serotonin as a differentiation signal in early neurogenesis, *Dev. Neurosci.,* 1, 15, 1978.

36. **Aitken, A.R. and Tork, I.,** Early development of serotonin- containing neurons and pathways as seen in whole mount preparations of the fetal rat brain, *J. Comp. Neurol.,* 274, 32, 1988.

37. **Budnik, V., Wu, C.F., and White, K.,** Altered branching of serotonin-containing neurons in Drosophila mutants unable to synthesize serotonin and dopamine, *J. Neurosci.,* 9, 2866, 1989.

38. **DeVitry, F., Hamon, M., Catelon, J., Bubois, M., and Thibault, J.,** Serotonin initiates and autoamplifies its own synthesis during mouse central nervous system development, *Proc. Natl. Acad. Sci.,* 83, 8629, 1986.

39. **Whitaker-Azmitia, P.M. and Azmitia, E.C.,** Autoregulation of fetal serotonergic neuronal development: Rrole of high affinity serotonin receptors, *Neurosci. Lett.,* 67, 307, 1986.

40. **Whitaker-Azmitia, P.M., Lauder, J.M., Shenner, A., and Azmitia, E.C.,** Postnatal changes in serotonin$_1$ receptors following prenatal alterations in serotonin levels: Further evidence for functional fetal serotonin$_1$; receptors, *Dev. Brain Res.,* 33, 285, 1987.

41. **Haydon, P.G., McCobb, D.P., and Kater, S.B.,** Serotonin selectively inhibits growth cone motility and synaptogenesis of specific identified neurons, *Science,* 236, 561, 1984.

42. **Haydon, P.G., McCobb, D.P., and Kater, S.B.,** The regulation of neurite outgrowth, growth cone motility, and electrical synaptogenesis by serotonin, *J. Neurobiol.,* 18, 197, 1987.

43. **McCobb, D.P., Haydon, P.G., and Kater, S.B.,** Dopamine and serotonin inhibition of neurite elongation of different identified neurons, *J. Neurosci. Res., 19,* 19, 1988.

44. **Whitaker-Azmitia, P.M., Murphy, R., and Azmitia, E.C.,** Localization of 5-HT$_{1A}$ receptors releases the serotonergic growth factor, protein S-100, and alters astroglial morphology, *Brain Res.,* 528, 155, 1990.

45. **Tajuddin, N.F. and Druse, M.J.,** Treatment of pregnant alcohol-consuming rats with buspirone: Effects of serotonin and 5-hydroxyindoleacetic acid content in offspring, *Alc. Clin. Exp. Res.,* 17, 110, 1993.

46. **Chubakov, A.R., Gromova, E.A., Konovalov, G.V., Sarkisova, E.F., and Chumasov, E.I.,** The effects of serotonin on the morpho-functional development of rat cerebral neocortex in tissue culture, *Brain Res.,* 369, 285, 1986.

47. **Azmitia, E.C., Dolan, K., and Whitaker-Azmitia, P.M.,** S-100$_B$ but not NGF, EGF, insulin or calmodulin is a CNS serotonergic growth factor, *Brain Res.,* 516, 354, 1990.

48. **Kim, J-A. and Druse, M.J.,** Conditioned media from ethanol- exposed astroglia lacks essential trophic factors, submitted.

49. **Babu, P.P., Kumari, L.R., and Vemuri, M.C.,** Differential changes in cell morphology, macromolecular composition and membrane protein profiles of neurons and astrocytes in chronic ethanol treated rats, *Mol. Cell. Biochem.,* 130, 29, 1994.

50. **Davies, D.L. and Vernadakis, A.,** Effects of ethanol on cultured glial cells: Proliferation and glutamine synthetase activity, *Dev. Brain Res.,* 16, 27, 1984.

51. **Guerri, C., Saez, R., Sancho-Tello, M., Martin de Aquilera, and Renau- Piqueras, J.,** Ethanol alters astrocyte development: A study of critical periods using primary cultures, *Neurochem. Res.,* 15, 559, 1990.

52. **Snyder, A.K., Singh, E.P., and Ehmann, S.,** Effects of ethanol on DNA, RNA, and protein synthesis in rat astrocyte cultures, *Alc. Clin. Exp. Res.,* 16, 295, 1992.

53. **Lokhorst, D.K. and Druse, M.J.,** Effects of ethanol on cultured fetal astroglia, *Alc. Clin. Exp. Res.,* 17, 810, 1993a.

54. **Lokhorst, D.K. and Druse, M.J.,** Effects of ethanol on cultured fetal serotonergic neurons, *Alc. Clin. Exp. Res.,* 17, 86, 1993b.

55. **Cooper, J.D. and Rudeen, P.K.,** Alterations in regional catecholamine content and turnover in the male rat brain in response to *in utero* ethanol exposure, *Alc. Clin. Exp. Res.,* 12, 282, 1988.

56. **Druse, M.J., Tajuddin, N., Kuo, A.P., and Connerty, M.,** Effects of *in utero* ethanol exposure on the developing dopaminergic system in rats, *J. Neurosci. Res.,* 27, 233, 1990.

57. **Chen, W.-J. A., Maier, S.E., and West, J.R.,** Prenatal alcohol and pair-fed treatments attenuate postnatal cocaine-induced dopamine elevation in the nucleus accumbens, *Alc. Clin. Exp. Res.,* 19, 52A, 1995.

58. **Becker, H.C., Hale, R.L., Boggan, W.O., and Randall C.L.,** Effects of prenatal ethanol exposure on later sensitivity to the low-dose stimulant actions of ethanol in mouse offspring: Possible role of catecholamines. *Alc. Clin. Exp. Res.,* 17, 1325, 1993.

59. **Lucchi, L., Lupini, M., Govoni, S., Covelli, V., Spano, P.F., and Trabucchi, M.,** Ethanol and dopaminergic systems, *Pharmacol. Biochem. Behav.,* 18, Suppl. 1, 379, 1983.

60. **Nio, E., Kogure, K., Yae, T., and Onoder, H.,** The effects of maternal ethanol exposure on neurotransmission and second messenger systems: A quantitative autoradiographic study in the rat brain. *Dev. Brain Res.,* 62, 51, 1991.

61. **Lankford, K.L., DeMello, F.G., and Klein, W.L.,** D_1-type dopamine receptors inhibit growth cone motility in cultured retina neurons: Evidence that neurotransmitters act as morphogenic growth regulators in the developing central nervous system, *Proc. Natl. Acad. Sci. USA,* 85, 2839, 1988.

62. **Detering, N., Collins, R., Hawkins, R.L., Ozand, P.T., and Karahasan, A.M.,** The effects of ethanol on developing catecholamine neurons. *Adv. Exp. Med. Biol.,* 132, 721, 1980.

63. **Detering, N., Collins, R.M., Hawkins, R.L., Ozand, P.T., and Karahasan, A.,** Comparative effects of ethanol and malnutrition on the development of catecholamine neurons: Changes in norepinephrine turnover, *J. Neurochem.,* 34, 1788, 1980.

64. **Detering, N., Collins, R.M., Hawkins, R.L., Ozand, P.T., and Karahasan, A.,** Comparative effects of ethanol and malnutrition on the development of catecholamine neurons: A long lasting effect in the hypothalamus, *J. Neurochem.*, 36, 2094, 1981.

65. **Rudeen, P.K. and Weinberg, J.,** Prenatal ethanol exposure: Changes in regional brain catecholamine content following stress, *J. Neurochem.* 61, 1907, 1993.

66. **Wigal, S.B.E., Amsel, A., and Wilcox, R.E.,** Fetal ethanol exposure diminishes hippocampal β-adrenergic receptor density while sparing muscarinic receptors during development, *Dev. Brain Res.*, 55, 161, 1990.

67. **Zimmerberg, B. and Wang, G.J.,** Prenatal alcohol exposure alters the functional responsiveness of the SNS in brown adipose tissue, *Alc. Clin. Exp. Res.*, 19, 18A, 1995.

68. **Rawat, A.K.,** Developmental changes in the brain levels of neurotransmitters as influenced by maternal ethanol consumption, *J. Neurochem.*, 28, 1175, 1977.

69. **Light, K.E., Serbus, D.C., and Santiago, M.,** Exposure of rats to ethanol from postnatal days 4 to 8: Alterations of cholinergic neurochemistry in the cerebral cortex and corpus striatum at day 20. *Alc. Clin. Exp. Res.*, 13, 29, 1989.

70. **Serbus, D.C., Stull, R.E., and Light, K.E.,** Neonatal ethanol exposure to rat pups: Resultant alterations of cortical muscarinic and cerebellar H_1-histaminergic receptor binding dynamics, *Neurotoxicology,* 7, 257, 1986.

71. **Brodie, C., Kentroti, S., and Vernadakis, A.,** Growth factors attenuate the choliotoxic effects of ethanol during early neuroembryogenesis in the chick embryo, *Int. J. Dev. Neurosci.*, 9, 203, 1991.

72. **Brodie, C. and Vernadakis, A.,** Ethanol increases cholinergic and decreases GABAergic neuronal expression in cultures dervied from 8-day-old chick embryo cerebral hemispheres: Interaction of ethanol and growth factors, *Brain Res. Dev. Brain Res.*, 65, 253, 1992.

73. **Swanson, D.J., Daniels, H., Meyer, E.M., Walker, D.W., and Heaton, M.B.,** Chronic ethanol alters CNS cholinergic and cerebellar development in chick embryos, *Alcohol,* 11, 187, 1994.

74. **Heaton, M.B., Paiva, M., Swanson, D.J., and Walker, D.W.,** Responsiveness of cultured septal and hippocampal neurons to ethanol and neurotrophic substances, *J. Neurosci. Res.*, 39, 305, 1994.

75. **Rahman, H., Kentroti, S., and Vernadakis, A.,** The critical period for ethanol effects on cholinergic neuronal expression in neuroblast-enriched cultures derived from 3-day-old chick embryo: NGF ameliorates the cholinotoxic effects of ethanol, *Int. J. Dev. Neurosci.*, 12, 397, 1994.

76. **Valles, S., Lindo, L., Montoliu, C., Renau-Piqueras, J., and Guerri, C.,** Prenatal exposure to ethanol induces changes in the nerve growth factor and its receptor in proliferating astrocytes in primary culture, *Brain Res.*, 656, 281, 1994.

77. **Greizerstein, H.B. and Aldrich, L.K.,** Ethanol and diazepam effects on intrauterine growth of the rat, *Dev. Pharmacol. Ther.*, 6, 409, 1983.

78. **Kelly, G.M., Druse, M.J., Tonetti, D.A., and Oden, B.G.,** Maternal ethanol consumption: Binding of L-glutamate to synaptic membranes from whole brain, cortices, and cerebella of offspring, *Exp. Neurol.*, 91, 219, 1986.

79. **Farr, K.L., Montano, C.Y., Paxton, L.L., and Savage, D.D.,** Prenatal ethanol exposure decreases hippocampal ^{3}H-glutamate binding in 45-day-old rats, *Alcohol,* 5, 125, 1988.

80. **Savage, D.D. and Swartzwelder, H.S.,** Effects of perinatal ethanol exposure on hippocampal formation, in *Alcohol and Neurobiology. Brain Development and Hormone Regulation*, Watson, R.R., Ed., CRC Press, New York, 1992, 177.

81. **Savage, D.D., Queen, S.A., Sanchez, C.F., Paxton, L.L., Mahoney, J.C., Goodlett, C.R., and West, J.R.,** Prenatal ethanol exposure during the last third of gestation in rat reduces hippocampal NMDA agonist binding site density in 45-day-old offspring, *Alcohol,* 9, 37-41, 1992.

82. **Farr, K.L., Montany, C.Y., Paxton, L.L., and Savage, D.D.,** Prenatal ethanol exposure decreases hippocampal ^{3}H-vinylidene kainic acid binding in 45-day-old rats, *Neurotoxicol. Teratol.*, 10, 563, 1989.

83. **Mena, M.A., Salinas, M., Del Rio, R.M., and Herrera, E.,** Effects of maternal ethanol ingestion on cerebral neurotransmitters and cyclic-AMP in rat offspring, *Gen. Pharmacol.*, 13, 241, 1982.

84. **Espina, N., Hannigan, J.H., and Martin, D.L.,** Neuroactive amino acid levels following prenatal exposure to ethanol, *Alc. Clin. Exp. Res.*, 13, 319, 1989.

85. **Moloney, B. and Leonard B.E.,** Pre-natal and post-natal effects of alcohol in the rat II. Changes in gamma-aminobutyric acid concentration and adenosine triphosphatase activity in the brain, *Alc. Clin. Exp. Res.*, 19, 137, 1983.

86. **Savage, D.D., Paxton, L., Wu, H., and Allan A.M.,** Prenatal alcohol exposure alters modulation of the $GABA_A$ receptor-chloride channel complex, *Alc. Clin. Exp. Res.*, 19, 18A, 1995.

87. **McGivern, R.F., Clancy, A.N., Mousa, S., Couri, D., and Noble, E.P.,** Prenatal alcohol exposure alters enkephalin levels without affecting ethanol preference, *Life Sci.,* 34, 585, 1984.

88. **Druse, M.J., Tajuddin, N.F., Eshed, M., and Gillespie, R.,** Maternal ethanol consumption: Effects on G proteins and second messengers in brain regions of offspring, *Alc. Clin. Exp. Res.*, 18, 47, 1994.

89.   **Pennington, S.N.,** Molecular changes associated with ethanol-induced growth suppression in the chick embryo, *Alc. Clin. Exp. Res.,* 14, 832, 1990.

90.   **Balduini, W. and Costa, L.G.,** Effects of ethanol on muscarinic receptor- stimulated phosphoinositide metabolism during brain development, *J. Pharmacol. Exp. Ther.,* 250, 541, 1989.

91.   **Balduini, W., Reno F., Costa L.G., and Cattabeni, F.,** Developmental neurotoxicity of ethanol: Further evidence for an involvement of muscarinic receptor-stimulated phosphoinositide hydrolysis, *Eur. J. Pharmacol. Mol. Pharmacol.,* 266, 283, 1994.

92.   **Balduini, W. and Costa, L.G.,** Developmental neurotoxicity of ethanol: *In vitro* inhibition of muscarinic receptor-stimulated phosphoinositide metabolism in brain from neonatal but not adult rats, *Brain Res.,* 512, 248, 1990.

93.   **Tan, S.E., Abel, E.L., and Berman, R.F.,** Brain MAP-2 phosphorylation is decreased following prenatal alcohol exposure in rats, *Alcohol,* 10, 391, 1993.

94.   **Horiguchi, T., Suzuki, K., Comas-Urrutia, A.C., Muleller-Heubach, E., Boyer-Milic, A.M., Baratz, R.A., Morishima, H.O., James, L.S., and Adamsons, K.,** Effect of ethanol upon uterine activity and fetal acid-base state of the rhesus monkey, *Am.J. Obstet. Gynecol.,* 109, 910, 1971.

95.   **Jones, P.J.H., Leichter, J., and Lee, M.,** Placental blood flow in rats fed alcohol before and during gestation, *Life Sci.,* 29, 1153, 1981.

96.   **Altura, B.M., Altura, B.T., Carella, A., Chatterjee, M., Halevy, S., and Tejani, N.,** Alcohol produces spasms of human umbilical circulation and fetal hypoxia in monkeys, *Science,* 218, 700, 1982.

97.   **Jorgensen, M.B. and Diemer, N.H.,** Selective neuron loss after cerebral ischemia in the rat: Possible role of transmitter glutamate, *Acta Neurol. Scand. ,*66, 536, 1982.

98.   **Auer, R.N., Jensen, M.L., and Whishaw, I.Q.,** Neurobehavioral deficit due to ischemic brain damage limited to half of the CA1 sector of the hippocampus, *J. Neurosci.,* 9, 1641, 1989.

99.   **Michaelis, E.K.,** Fetal alcohol exposure: Cellular toxicity and molecular events in toxicity, *Alc. Clin. Exp. Res.,* 14, 819, 1990.

100.   **Choi, D.W.,** Nitric oxide: Foe or friend to the injured brain?, *Proc. Natl. Acad. Sci.,* 9741, 1993.

101.   **Choi, D.Q.,** Glutamate receptors and the induction of excitotoxic neuronal death, *Prog. Brain Res.,* 100, 47, 1994.

102.   **Duggan, L.L. and Choi, D.W.,** Excitotoxicity, free radicals and cell membrane changes, *Ann. Neurol.,* 35, S17, 1994.

103.   **Reyes, E., Ott, S., and Robinson, B.,** Effects of *in utero* administration of alcohol on glutathione levels in brain and liver, *Alc. Clin. Exp. Res.,* 17, 877, 1993.

104. **Heaton, M.B., Swanson, D.J., and Paiva, M., Walker, D.W.,** Ethanol exposure affects trophic factor activity and responsiveness in chick embryo. *Alcohol,* 9, 161, 1992.

105. **Breese, C.R., D'Costa, A., Ingram, R.L., Lenham, J., and Sonntag, W.E.,** Long-term suppression of insulin-like growth factor-1 in rats after *in utero* ethanol exposure: Relationship to somatic growth, *J. Pharmacol. Exp. Ther.,* 264, 448, 1993.

106. **Mauceri, J.H., Lee, W.-H., and Conway, S.,** Effect of ethanol on insulin-life growth factor-II release from fetal organs, *Alc. Clin. Exp. Res.* ,18, 35, 1994.

107. **Singh, S.P., Srivenugopal, K.S., Ehmann, S., Yuan, X-H., and Snyder, A.K.,** Insulin-like growth factors (IGF-I and IGF-II), IGF-binding proteins and IGF gene expression in the offspring of ethanol-fed rats, *J. Lab. Clin. Med.,* 125, 183, 1994.

108. **Resnicoff, M., Sell, C., Ambrose, D., Baserga, R., and Rubin, R.,** Ethanol inhibits the autophosphorylation of the insulin-like growth factor-1 (IGF-1) receptor and IGF-1-mediated proliferation of 3T3 cells, *J. Biol. Chem.,* 268, 21777, 1993.

109. **Resnicoff, M., Rubini, M., Baserga, R., and Rubin, R.,** Ethanol inhibits insulin-like growth factor-1-mediated signalling and proliferation of C6 rat globlastoma cells, *Lab. Invest.,* 71, 657, 1994.

110. **Tewari, S. and Noble, E.P.,** Ethanol and brain protein synthesis, *Brain, Res.* 26, 469, 1971.

111. **Chiapelli, F., Taylor, A.N., de los Monteros, A.E., and de Vellis, J.,** Fetal alcohol delays the developmental expression of myelin basic protein and transferrin in rat primary oligodendrocyte cultures, *Int. J. Dev. Neurosci.,* 9, 67, 1991.

112. **Kojima, H., Mineta-Kitajima, R., Saitoh-Harada, N., Kurihara, T., Takahashi, Y., Furudate, S., Shirataka, M., Nakamura, K., and Tamai, Y.,** Prenatal ethanol exposure affects the activity and mRNA expression of neuronal membrane enzymes in rat offspring, *Life Sci.,* 55, 1433, 1994.

113. **Fletcher, T.L. and Shain, W.,** Ethanol-induced changes in astrocyte gene expression during rat central nervous system development, *Alc. Clin. Exp. Res.,* 17, 993, 1993.

Chapter 9

BEHAVIORAL PHARMACOLOGY IN ANIMALS EXPOSED PRENATALLY TO ALCOHOL

John H. Hannigan and Surilla Randall

I. PHARMACOLOGICAL TREATMENT FOR FETAL ALCOHOL SYNDROME

Alcohol consumption during pregnancy can result in offspring with alcohol-related birth defects (ARBDs) which can include Fetal Alcohol Syndrome (FAS) in children.[1] The widespread abuse of alcohol and difficulty in preventing alcohol abuse in pregnant women will continue to put the health and well-being of children at risk.[2] A diagnosis of FAS requires the minimal criteria of: (1) pre- and/or postnatal growth retardation; (2) a characteristic pattern of facial features; and (3) abnormal functioning of the central nervous system (CNS).[3-4] Infants with ARBDs can have one or more of a range of the defects associated with FAS (see below) including but not limited to failure to thrive, organ and bone abnormalities, and CNS dysfunction.[5] CNS dysfunction is one of the more consistent and persistent outcomes of *in utero* alcohol[1,4] and can be expressed as mental retardation, developmental delay, attention deficits, hyperactive behavior, poor motor coordination, learning disabilities and memory problems. CNS altered function can occur even after relatively modest amounts of alcohol exposure[6-10] and can persist at least into adolescence.[6,12]

At present there are no specific pharmacological treatments which are recommended specifically for children to address the syndromal problems following fetal alcohol exposure. Children with FAS/ARBDs could be treated, as any other children with these various clinical manifestations with medications such as Ritalin® (methylphenidate) for attention deficits, or Dilantin® (phenytoin) for seizures. Because of the wide range of FAS effects, it seems unlikely that any one medication could have a global impact on all expressions of FAS/ARBDs. However, there are ongoing research efforts utilizing animal models that are assessing basic aspects of biobehavioral responses to psychoactive drugs with potential therapeutic value. This chapter will review much of what is known about experiments in psychopharmacology in animals exposed prenatally to alcohol.

II. RECOGNIZING NEUROCHEMICAL DYSFUNCTION IN PSYCHOPHARMACOLOGICAL RESPONSE

Psychopharmacological assessment of prenatal alcohol-exposed animals can provide information about the relationship between teratogen-induced neurochemical and behavioral alterations. Differential behavioral responses to well-characterized drugs by alcohol-exposed animals can indicate functional alterations at one or more physiological levels. One of the first studies of this kind was by Abel,[13] whose perspective was to assess tolerance or cross-tolerance between alcohol (given prenatally) and other drugs, including alcohol, given as challenges (postnatally). Other perspectives are possible. In addition to indicating altered drug sensitivity, efficacy or response, these "drug challenges" also serve to reveal the functional neural sequelae of prenatal alcohol exposure in animals.[14] We and others have argued that assessment of developmental profiles in psychopharmacological responses to drug challenges is a valuable tool in understanding psychobiological development and teratogenic effects.[14-17] Finally, assessing differences in bio-behavioral responses to psychotherapeutic drugs in animals may have implications for treatment efficacy in children.

Prenatal alcohol has altered most neurotransmitters measured in rats, mice and/or monkeys.[18-22] Prenatal alcohol-induced alterations have been reported in CNS dopamine, norepinephrine, serotonin (5-HT), acetylcholine, and amino acid neurotransmitter systems (e.g., glutamate and GABA). Generalizations about prenatal alcohol-induced changes in neurotransmitters are limited because there are substantial variations across studies in animal models, patterns and routes of alcohol administration, age at assessment, gender, and use of whole brain samples versus specific brain areas. It is also not known to what degree effects in one neurotransmitter system (e.g., dopamine) may be secondary to alterations in other interacting systems (e.g., descending GABA-ergic inhibition of dopamine cells).

While the functional relevance of prenatal alcohol-induced neurochemical changes may be difficult to discern in the presence of such variability, much is known about the relationship of selected brain areas to behavior, or behavioral dysfunction. For example, the nigrostriatal dopaminergic projection system from the substantia nigra (area A9) to the caudate nucleus and putamen, normally mediates cyclic motor patterning (such as oral stereotypy), catalepsy, and sensorimotor integration in the rat.[23-24] The mesolimbic dopamine system, in comparison, includes projections from the ventral tegmental area (area A10) to the nucleus accumbens and supra rhinal neocortex. Mesolimbic functioning tends to be associated predominantly with exploratory locomotor activity, emotional responses, and reactions to reinforcement and reward.[25] Rats and mice exposed prenatally to alcohol show alterations in all the behaviors supported by normal dopamine function, including locomotion (i.e., as hyperactivity), cyclic motor responses (such as stereotypy and catalepsy), motor coordination and sensorimotor integration, and altered responses to reward.[15,26] These general changes in dopamine or any other neurotransmitter function can be evaluated further by measuring how affected animals alter these behaviors in response to psychoactive drugs. To the degree that a given drug's neurochemical mechanism of action is known and specific, differential responses by alcohol-affected animals to that drug should indicate a disruption in that specific neural process.

Depending upon how localized receptors sensitive to the drug are, and the method/route of drug administration, results can also specify dysfunction to particular brain areas. Detailed studies of CNS can later validate or clarify these indications. Research using these strategies is discussed below.

III. CNS STIMULANTS AND OTHER DOPAMINERGIC DRUGS FOLLOWING PRENATAL ALCOHOL EXPOSURE

Rats exposed prenatally to alcohol showed enhanced sensitivity to CNS stimulants, demonstrated by increased peak exploratory behavior, stereotypy and unilateral rotational behavior, and/or dose-response shifts to the left. These findings support the hypothesis that prenatal alcohol alters the maturation of mesolimbic, perhaps more than nigrostriatal, dopamine function.[27-29] Earlier findings of behavioral and neurochemical changes, however, suggested that nigrostriatal dopamine function was also affected.[19,30] Among these types of studies, prenatal alcohol exposure appears to alter most profoundly behavioral responses to dopaminergic drugs.

A. METHYLPHENIDATE (RITALIN®) AND AMPHETAMINE (DEXEDRIN®)

Animals exposed prenatally to alcohol tend to show exaggerated responses to CNS stimulants. The differential effects of prenatal alcohol are influenced by age, gender and dose of psychopharmacological drugs. The CNS stimulant amphetamine enhances release and inhibits reuptake of catecholamines, primarily dopamine.[31] Structurally similar to amphetamine, methylphenidate exerts some of the same qualitative effects. In turn, this increased synaptic activity in dopamine systems can alter the density and/or binding capacity of receptor sites. Differential responsiveness to amphetamine in animals exposed prenatally to alcohol would indicate functional alternations in dopamine (and other monamine) release, uptake, and/or receptors. Fetal alcohol-induced changes could reasonably contribute to hyperactivity and other sensorimotor behavioral deficits reported in rats and mice.[27]

1. Acute Effects

The earliest study assessing altered pharmacological responses assessed cross-tolerance between prenatal alcohol-exposure and other postnatal drugs.[13]

Pregnant rat dams were intubated with 6g/kg/day of alcohol throughout gestation. The mean blood alcohol concentrations were 204 mg% one hour after intubation. The offspring were challenged at postnatal day 180 (PN180) with 5 mg/kg d-amphetamine and rectal temperature assessed every hour for 6 hours. There were no significant differences in either a transient amphetamine-induced hyperthermia, or a longer-lasting hypothermia, between alcohol and control female offspring. It was not clear what the effects were in male offspring.[13]

Other earlier studies hypothesized that treatment with methylphenidate would attenuate spontaneous hyperactivity and decrease differences in locomotion activity between control and prenatal alcohol-exposed groups. In contrast, rats exposed prenatally to alcohol via liquid diet, were shown to have long lasting hyperreponsive effects to methylphenidate as neonates and adults.[32-33] Males rats (PN26-38) exposed prenatally to alcohol and given 0, 1, 2, and 4 mg/kg of methylphenidate on four day intervals starting at PN26 to PN38 increased the frequency of ambulation with progressively increasing doses. Adult rats exposed prenatally to alcohol at PN100 to PN184 also showed greater sensitivity to increased open field locomotion than controls with increasing doses of methylphenidate.[32]

Male rats exposed prenatally to alcohol via liquid diet showed increased locomotor activation after 2 mg/kg d-amphetamine at PN28 and PN42, but not lower doses.[34] On the other hand, females at PN28 showed a small significant reduction in behavioral responding at the same dose. Female rats born to either alcohol-exposed or pairfed control dams were less sensitive to the locomotor activating effects of amphetamine at PN42 than chowfed control offspring, suggesting that a gender-influenced nutritional compromise during gestation also contributed to some alcohol-related developmental effects.[34]

Gender may contribute to the differences in susceptibility to, or recovery from prenatal alcohol exposure. For example, in contrast to these findings, Bond,[37-38] reported no differential locomotor effects of 0.5, 1.0 or 4.0 mg/kg of amphetamine or α-methyl-para-tyrosine (α-MPT; 25, 50 or 100 mg/kg) in rats tested from PN16 up to PN22 when gender was not assessed. The studies using methylphenidate noted above[32-33] assessed males only. There were no significant differences among prenatal treatment groups in amphetamine-induced (1.5 mg/kg) turning when only females were assessed in another study.[39] Female offspring appeared to be consistently less affected by prenatal alcohol, or to recover sooner than males from the alcohol-related effects on postnatal acute stimulant pharmacology. A profound influence of alcohol on testosterone during prenatal neural development and/or modulatory influences of testosterone on dopamine function,[36,40] could contribute to the greater disruptive differences that are frequently shown in males than females.

2. Chronic Effects

Because alcohol-exposed male rats showed exaggerated behavioral activation to acute amphetamine,[27] we assessed the effects of chronic postnatal injections of amphetamine given to postweaning rats exposed to alcohol *in utero* via liquid diet. We reasoned that prenatal alcohol-exposed rats may also be more sensitive to the chronic effects of CNS stimulants. FAS children with attentional and other cognitive deficits or behavioral problems are often treated chronically with CNS stimulants. This suggests that if FAS/ARBD children were also differentially sensitive to long-term stimulant administration, they might show different therapeutic profiles and increased susceptibilities to "side effects."

Alcohol-exposed offspring (rats and children) are born growth retarded and remain developmentally delayed. We hypothesized, therefore, that rats exposed prenatally to alcohol, and perhaps FAS children, may be more sensitive to the growth-retarding side effects of chronic amphetamine. Children and rats given CNS stimulants typically show a growth deceleration during chronic treatment, and a rebound in growth rate during "drug holidays."[41-44]

Rats exposed prenatally to alcohol were injected daily with 0, 2, or 10 mg/kg of amphetamine between PN22 and PN42.[28] Alcohol-exposed rats started out smaller than control rats at PN22 and all prenatal treatment groups showed similar amphetamine dose-dependent decelerations in the relative rate of weight gain during 3 weeks of injections. This was consistent with reports in children and animals given various CNS stimulants.[42] During the 3 weeks following termination of chronic daily amphetamine injections, all amphetamine-injected groups, regardless of prenatal alcohol history, showed equivalent rebounds in growth rate, relative to their respective chronic saline-injected counterparts. Interestingly, both during and after the amphetamine injections, the alcohol-exposed offspring gained weight at a relatively faster rate than controls, although they remained significantly lighter up to PN64.[28] These results indicated that prenatal alcohol-exposed offspring were not more sensitive than controls to the growth-retarding side effects of amphetamine.

Alcohol-exposed rats also showed amphetamine dose-, age-, and gender-influenced increases in the magnitude of locomotor activation when tested periodically during the chronic amphetamine administration. Male and female alcohol-exposed animals were more sensitive to the lower amphetamine dose (2 mg/kg) at PN22 and PN28 than at the older test ages (PN36 and PN42). The alcohol-exposed males became more sensitive than controls to the activational effects of 10 mg/kg amphetamine between PN22 and PN28, perhaps indicating greater sensitization to amphetamine. Both male and female alcohol-exposed offspring appeared to be initially more sensitive than controls to 2 mg/kg amphetamine in this study, and all groups decreased locomotor activation to this amphetamine dose between PN22 and PN42. The results indicated that although animals exposed prenatally to alcohol were at no greater risk for stimulant-induced growth retarding side effects than controls, there were large progressive differences in behavioral responses. These response changes were suggestive of enhanced sensitization by males and perhaps tolerance by females challenged with the high-dose amphetamine,[28] but the design of this study did not allow unambiguous interpretation of sensitization versus tolerance.

To explore further the possibility of altered sensitization - or tolerance - to chronic daily amphetamine after alcohol exposure *in utero*, offspring were exposed to 0 or 2 mg/kg of amphetamine each day from PN22 through PN41. On PN42 they were challenged with one of several doses of amphetamine from 0.5 to 8 mg/kg.[45] As in earlier work, alcohol-exposed males again tended to be more active after the first, acute injection with amphetamine. Following a chronic, moderate dose of amphetamine, it appeared that alcohol-exposed animals showed behavioral sensitization similar to controls.

Relative to <u>daily</u> chronic amphetamine injections, repeated <u>intermittent</u> administration has been shown to greatly facilitate the development of behavioral sensitization.[25,46-47] In a recent abstract, prenatal alcohol-exposed and control rats were given amphetamine injections (2 mg/kg) every 3-4 days for 3 weeks beginning an PN22. The behavioral responses to amphetamine after this regime indicated that all groups developed sensitization to repeated, intermittent amphetamine and that the sensitization in prenatal alcohol-exposed groups was greater than that in controls.[45]

B.   OTHER CNS STIMULANTS

Atypical CNS stimulants used to treat some children with attentional problems include pemoline (Cylert®) and caffeine. Pemoline appears to operate by mechanisms related to those of amphetamine, but there may be greater selectivity for nonadrenergic than dopamine systems and smaller peripheral effects.[48] Caffeine acts as an adenosine A_1 receptor agonist. When rats exposed prenatally to alcohol were challenged with 0, 25 or 50 mg/kg pemoline or 0, 50 or 100 mg/kg caffeine every other day between PN22 and PN28, and tested on PN22 and PN28, there were no differential locomotor responses among the various prenatal treatment groups after challenge with either pemoline or caffeine. All groups showed equivalent dose-dependent increases in activity.[40-50]

Pentylenetetrazol (Metrazole®) is a CNS stimulant capable of inducing seizures at low doses. Abel, Berman and Church[51] assessed shifts in sensitivity to metrazole-induced convulsion in female rats exposed prenatally to alcohol. Males were not tested. Alcohol-exposed females were slightly less sensitive to metrazole, but not after 35 or 45 mg/kg metrazole, a dose-response shift to the right reflected in a doubling of the latency (approximately 250 to 500 sec) to convulse after 40 mg/kg metrazole, but not after 35 or 45 mg/kg metrazole - a dose-response shift to the right. The results suggested that GABA-ergic neural mechanisms targeted by metrazole, specifically benzodiazepine binding sites, were altered by prenatal alcohol exposure.[51]

C.   DOPAMINE AGONISTS AND ANTAGONISTS

It has been argued that there is a pharmacological and behavioral selectivity to the influence of prenatal alcohol on the acute effects of the CNS stimulants and dopamine agonists.[15] Low doses of apomorphine (0.1 to 1.2 mg/kg), a mixed D1/D2 receptor agonist, decreased locomotor activity due to stimulation of presynaptic dopamine autoreceptors.[52] In mice, prenatal alcohol exposure decreased relative sensitivity to the locomotor suppressive effects of the higher but not lower doses of apomorphine tested.[53] This may reflect increased sensitivity to the locomotor activational effects of dopamine system stimulation reported in rats.[15]

Adult rats exposed prenatally to alcohol showed no differences in the hyper- or hypothermic effects of chlorpromazine, amphetamine,[13] clonidine,[14] or apomorphine. There were no or inconsistent prenatal alcohol-associated differences in acute amphetamine-induced rotation, stereotypy, and locomotor activity in adult females.[39] There were also no differences in stereotypic responses by adult rats of either sex given acute amphetamine.[27] However, although the gender- and dose-dependent responses to the mixed dopamine agonist apomorphine were often similar to those after amphetamine, there were differences. At PN28, male offspring exposed prenatally to alcohol showed a dose-response shift to the left (increased sensitivity) and female rats exposed to alcohol or pair-fed were again less sensitive to apomorphine.[54] The apparent overall dose-response shift in apomorphine's effects on locomotor activity coincide with earlier findings of increased sensitivity to the effects of amphetamine on locomotor activity after prenatal alcohol exposure.[27] This suggest that there is a functional alternation in dopamine receptor characteristics. Unlike acute amphetamine, challenge with acute apomorphine produced small but significant increases in stereotypy in alcohol-exposed rats relative to controls.[54] Becker, Hale, Boggan and Randall[55] reported no signif- icant effects of prenatal alcohol exposure on locomotor activity changes following acute challenges with up to 400 mg/kg alpha-methylparatyrosine (AMPT), a dopamine synthesis inhibitor, in adult male mice (PN75-PN90). Female mice were not tested. However, there were differences in AMPT effects an ethanol- stimulated locomotion (see below).

Recent research has also studied behavioral responses to selective dopamine receptor agonists. Systemic injections with quinelorane (LY163502; a D2 agonist) produced biphasic age-dependent increases in locomotor activity. At PN22, the age of peak sensitivity, prenatal alcohol-exposed males were more sensitive than controls to the activating effects of quinelorane. Effects of intracranial injections of quinpirole (LY171555) (also a D2 agonist) into the striata of rats exposed prenatally to alcohol, however, did not differ from those in control rats.

Studies which directly assess local neural responses to drugs with neurochemical and/or neurophysiological assessments can elaborate these results. Prenatal alcohol decreased sensitivity to microiontophoretic applications of quinpirole onto nigral neurons and there was a dissociation between firing rate and burst activity in bursting cells.[56] Nigral neurons appeared to phase between bursting and non-bursting modes after prenatal alcohol. Dopamine neurons in the substantia nigra of adult rats that had been exposed prenatally to alcohol, showed a four-fold decrease in the ED50 for systemic (iv) apomorphine-induced inhibition of firing rates after prenatal alcohol exposure.[57] The apomorphine-induced inhibition may be due either to direct stimulation of nigral D2 autoreceptors, or to feedback mediated by postsynaptic dopamine receptors in striatum. Because there was no significant inhibition of dopamine neuron firing rates after direct iontophoretic application of the D2 agonist quinpirole in alcohol-exposed rats, it was concluded that pre- and/or postsynaptic striatal dopamine receptors may both be affected by prenatal alcohol.[57] These changes in apomorphine-induced inhibition of nigral firing rates after prenatal alcohol exposure are consistent with earlier behavioral interpretations effects.[28,58]

These studies with acute or chronic drug challenges suggest that dopamine function is altered in rodents by prenatal exposure to alcohol. Acute challenges suggest there is an increased sensitivity of dopamine receptors that is age and gender influenced. Although it is not yet clear, it appears that there are also alterations in how the alcohol-exposed animals respond to chronic CNS stimulants, perhaps by greater sensitization. Because different responses to dopaminergic[58] but not to noradrenergic[14] or serotonergic agents,[59] were reported, it appears that function of dopamine systems was preferentially affected. From the pattern of behavioral changes after apomorphine challenge[53-54] and from the neurochemical findings,[19] it may be inferred that the dopamine D1 receptors are preferentially involved in prenatal alcohol-induced changes in psychopharmacological response.

To elaborate the role of D1 receptors in fetal alcohol effects, we assessed the ability of the D1 receptor antagonist SCH23390 to induce catalepsy in young rats. Prenatal alcohol exposure reduced the magnitude and delayed the maturation of gender-influenced catalepsy after systemic injections of SCH23390.[58] Specifically, rats showed decreased sensitivity to the cataleptogenic effects of SCH23390. Only at the oldest age tested (PN21) and with the higher dose (1.0 mg/kg) did the rats exposed to alcohol show catalepsy equivalent to controls. Alcohol-exposed female rats were less sensitive to the SCH23390 than male rats, and did not appear to have a development delay in the maturation of catalepsy.[58] The results suggested that sensitivity of D1 dopamine receptors in young rats was changed by prenatal alcohol exposure. In a preliminary study with adult male animals, we found no evidence for differential responses to the relatively non-specific D2 antagonist haloperidol.[60] However, Lucchi et al.,[61] reported decreased sensitivity to neuroleptics. The maturational profiles of D1 receptor function in older offspring and of D2 receptor function with receptor-specific antagonists after prenatal alcohol remain to be determined.

Following chronic amphetamine injections (10 mg/kg/day), there were no significant changes in inhibition of either ventral tegmental or nigral dopamine neuron firing rates with direction iontophoretic application of quinpirole, suggesting that differential changes in response to chronic CNS stimulants were not due to altered autoreceptors on midbrain dopamine neurons.[57,62] However, it was also found that prenatal alcohol exposure reduced sensitivity of glutamate-induced activity in nucleus accumbens to iontophoretically applied SKF38393, a selective D1 agonist. The results to date are entirely consistent with the strong hypothesis that the teratogenic effects of alcohol are seen in postsynaptic D1 receptors in mesolimbic dopamine systems.[54] These findings suggest that receptor-selective dopamine drugs may be useful in treatment of FAS/ARBDs.

Mesolimbic and nigrostriatal function after chronic amphetamine administration in adult male (age ≥ PN100) rats exposed prenatally to alcohol has been assessed.[62] Following chronic amphetamine, there were no changes in inhibition of tegmental or nigral DA neuron firing rates with direct iontophoretic application of the D2 agonist quinpirole, suggesting that differential changes in response to chronic CNS stimulants[28,62] were not due to altered autoreceptors on midbrain DA neurons. However, it was also reported that prenatal alcohol exposure reduced sensitivity of glutamate-induced activity in nucleus accumbens to iontophoretically applied SKF38393, a selective D1 agonist. The results to date are consistent with the hypothesis that the teratogenic effects of alcohol are seen in postsynaptic D1 receptors in mesolimbic DA systems. Although these findings are preliminary, they would suggest that a selective D1 drug may be a preferred treatment choice to a nonselective D1/D2 agent in FAS/ARBD.

D.   OTHER MONOAMINERGIC DRUGS

Clonidine is an α-adrenergic agonist that induces age-characteristic motor activity in young rats. At PN10 clonidine produces dose-dependent "wall climbing" behavior and by PN18, wall climbing has been replaced by locomotion. Prenatal exposure to alcohol via liquid diet increased baseline levels of wall climbing at PN10 and of locomotion at PN18 in male but not female pups.[64] Clonidine produced increases in the age-characteristic responses in all groups although prenatal alcohol exposure produced no differences in responses to clonidine or in the developmental shift in response character.[64] Prenatal alcohol exposure did not influence clonidine-induced hypothermia in rats assessed before and after behavioral measures detailed above[64] or when rectal temperatures were measured periodically over 2 hours following a systemic clonidine (0.0 to 1.0 mg/kg) challenge.[65] Weathersby, Becker and Hale[66] tested adult male mice (PN90) after prenatal alcohol exposure and found that whereas clonidine decreased locomotion in controls, it stimulated locomotion in alcohol-exposed offspring. Further, prenatal alcohol exposed male mice were less sensitive to the ability of clonidine to attenuate alcohol-induced locomotion (see below). These results with clonidine suggested that the early maturation of nonadrenergic function in rats is not disrupted by prenatal alcohol, but that in mice, prenatal alcohol exposure produced long-lasting alterations in nonadrenergic function.[66]

Bond[67] assessed the effects of para-chlorophenylalamine (PCPA), which inhibits tryptophan hydroxylase and leads to a long-lasting depletion of serotonin. In normal rats, PCPA increased locomotor activity substantially at PN16, less so at PN22, but not at PN28. Prenatal exposure to alcohol did not alter dose-response to PCPA at any age tested. In addition, dose-dependent decreases in activity at PN16 after injections of methylsergide, a serotonin antagonist, were unchanged by prenatal alcohol exposure.[67] Finally, some abstracts[59] report no significant effects of prenatal alcohol exposure on the behavioral effects of buspirone or 6-OHDPAT, serotonin agonists. Together, these reports are consistent with the hypothesis that prenatal alcohol does not affect serotinergic function, despite evidence for neurochemical changes.[19] Also, see description of Grace, Rockman and Glavin's[68] study, below.

IV. RESPONSES TO CHOLINERGIC AGENTS

Several studies have explored the role of cholinergic systems in hyperactivity in rats after prenatal alcohol exposure, sometimes with contradictory results. Repeated systemic administration of the acetylcholinesterase inhibitor physostigmine beginning on PN18 reduced hyperactivity in alcohol-exposed rats at a dose (0.2 mg/kg) which did not affect controls.[69] Because the effect of physostigmine is to increase CNS circulating levels of acetylcholine, the results suggested that decreases in cholinergic function mediate behavioral fetal alcohol effects. However, Bond[70] found that physostigmine (0.05 to 0.4 mg/kg) reduced activity in chow fed controls whereas in alcohol-exposed animals 0.1 mg/kg of physostigmine increased activity at PN18. Bond[70] also reported that neostigmine, a quartenary form of physostigmine that acts only on peripheral cholinergic receptors, reduced activity in all groups at PN16, suggesting that central stimulation of cholinergic systems in alcohol-exposed animals increases activity whereas peripheral stimulation in all groups reduce activity. This does not explain why physostigmine decreased activity in the Riley et al.[69] study.

Prenatal alcohol-induced alterations in cholinergic function[71-72] may also contribute to learning deficits. Three studies using physostigmine[73] or the cholinergic antagonist scopolamine[74-76] have assessed drug effects on learning in adult rats after prenatal alcohol exposure. These studies assessed shuttle avoidance[73,75] and spatial learning in a Morris maze.[76] There were consistent prenatal alcohol-induced deficits in avoidance behavior, but no significant difference in escape from the Morris maze. In all studies, the cholinergic drug disrupted performance in the task in dose-dependent fashions, and in all studies, there were no differences in dose-response curves due to prenatal alcohol, suggesting that cholinergic dysfunction is not responsible for learning deficits. Prenatal alcohol-exposed rats showed normal dose-dependent interference with Morris maze performance after scopolamine challenge.[76]

V. SENSITIVITY TO ALCOHOL

Human and animal studies have shown that causes of alcohol abuse are numerous and complex. There is evidence that environmental factors, and heritable genetic traits, as well as the pharmacological actions of alcohol contribute to alcoholic behavior. No single factor determines the development of social or abusive drinking patterns. To date, the link between environmental and genetic factors and their contribution to the initiation and of alcoholism are not fully understood. The influence of maternal alcohol consumption has been shown generally to enhance alcohol preference in offspring. The manifestations of this change in alcohol preference are dependent upon the sensitivity of the testing procedures, as well as upon the species, dose, time and amount of alcohol administered.

A.   ALCOHOL PREFERENCE

Rats exposed prenatally to alcohol tend to have a greater alcohol preference in comparison to controls.[77-80] Alcohol preference is commonly measured with the two bottle home cage preference test, where tap water is the alternative fluid. This paradigm allows the animal free access to water plus a range of concentrations of alcohol. Bond and DiGiusto[77] demonstrated that female Wistar rats exposed to liquid diet containing 6.5% alcohol (95%v/v) during gestation showed an enhanced alcohol preference that was concentration dependent. Rats exposed prenatally to alcohol preferred lower concentrations of alcohol (3-6%) to water more than the control groups, and this preference decreased with higher concentrations (7-8%). Males were not used in this study. Reyes, Garcia and Jones[78] showed in a preliminary study that male Wistar rats exposed prenatally to alcohol demonstrated an increasing alcohol preference over thirty days using the two bottle test. In contrast to Bond and DiGiusto,[77] females did not show the same trend as their male counterparts. Dominguez, Chotro and Molina[80] introduced alcohol into the amniotic fluid of Wistar rat fetuses on the last day of gestation. On PD11 these rats demonstrated an increase in alcohol intake relative to rats not exposed to alcohol when fetuses. Alcohol administered in amniotic fluid prior to birth has not been yet incorporated into the fetus, therefore the memory for alcohol appear to be derived from alcohol's sensory rather than pharmacologic or toxic effects.[80] These studies provide evidence that maternal alcohol consumption can influence offspring preference for, and consumption of, alcohol in multiple ways.

A number of other studies have failed to find detectable differences in drinking preferences in rats exposed to alcohol *in utero* using the two bottle test. Adult offspring of Sprague-Dawley rats exposed prenatally to a liquid diet containing 35% alcohol-derived calories from gestation day 7 to parturition failed to show different alcohol preference.[81] In another study,[79] the female offspring of Sprague-Dawley dams exposed to alcohol *in utero* also failed to demonstrate an alcohol preference using the two bottle test. The alcohol group showed an alcohol preference that was similar to chowfed and pairfed controls. It is not known if strain differences (e.g., Wistar versus Sprague-Dawley) explain these varied preference results.

The two bottle test, which is a common paradigm employed to test for alcohol preference, has been criticized for not being an accurate measure of alcohol's pharmacological or reinforcing effects.[82] The two bottle test may be insensitive to the subtle effects of the pattern and amount of alcohol intake that is the result of prenatal alcohol exposure. In order to overcome the problems associated with the two bottle test, stress was used to "unmask" the effects of prenatal alcohol on later alcohol sensitivity.[79] The female offspring of Sprague-Dawley rats were exposed to an inescapable footshock, and alcohol and total fluid intake were then measured with the two bottle test. After shock, rats given alcohol *in utero* drank more alcohol than water in comparison to chowfed and pairfed controls.[79]

It is unclear how stress may influence alcohol consumption, but animals exposed prenatally to alcohol show profound alterations in physiological, biochemical and behavioral response to stressful situations.[35] Interestingly, adult (PN210) female offspring (males were not tested) of alcohol-treated rat dams showed a 60% greater increase in serum corticosterone levels than control animals when challenged with 20 mg/kg of morphine.[83] Female rats exposed prenatally to alcohol showed greater increases in plasma corticosterone levels than controls after a challenge dose of ethanol (0.75 - 1.5 g/kg; IP;).[84]

In addition to mesolimbic dopamine function,[82] serotonin has been shown to regulate alcohol intake. Grace, Rockman and Glavin[68] administered zimelidine, a serotonin uptake blocker, to male Holtzman rats exposed prenatally to alcohol during the first, second or third week, or throughout pregnancy. Alcohol preference was determined using the two bottle test and was expressed as the percentage of alcohol ingested relative to total daily fluid intake. All prenatal treatment groups injected with zimelidine showed significant decreases in alcohol preference, and rats exposed to alcohol during the first trimester and injected with zimelidine consumed significantly less alcohol than all prenatal treatment groups.

B.   OTHER RESPONSES TO ETHANOL

The adult offspring of pregnant Sprague-Dawley rats maintained on a liquid diet containing 35% ethanol-derived calories were tested for alcohol sensitivity and tolerance.[85] The measure of sensitivity was sleep time, the time interval between the loss of the righting reflex and the regaining of the righting reflex. Following an anesthetic dose of alcohol (3.4 g/kg, IP), rats exposed prenatally to alcohol showed a greater increase in sleep time than controls, even though rats exposed prenatally to alcohol took significantly longer than all other prenatal treatment groups to lose the righting reflex they slept longer than controls.   These results suggest that prenatal administration of alcohol increases postnatal alcohol sensitivity. However, ethanol-induced narcosis, hypothermia and heart-rate depression were unchanged in either Long-Sleep on Short-Sleep mice following prenatal exposure to alcohol.[86] The body temperature of all animals declined during sleep time, but females exposed to alcohol *in utero* demonstrated the greatest decrease in body temperatures among all prenatal treatment groups. The alcohol-exposed males were not significantly different from controls. The rate of alcohol metabolism did not account for differences in sleep time among these treatment groups. Reyes *et al*.[85] suggested that female rats exposed prenatally to alcohol were less tolerant to at least some of the effects of alcohol and less likely to prefer alcohol. These findings also coincide with those of Reyes *et al*.,[78] who also used the two bottle test.

The offspring of Long-Evans rats intubated with 3 g/kg of alcohol twice daily were tested for temperature regulation in response to alcohol and various drugs (see above) as adults.[13] Female rats exposed prenatally to alcohol exhibited less hypothermia over 4 hours after begin injected with 2 or 3 g/kg of alcohol. This group also showed smaller decreases in body temperature to pentobarbital and diazepam in comparison to control. Males also showed less hypothermia only in response to the 2 g/kg of alcohol and did not show significant differences to other drugs.[13] Taylor *et al*.,[84] who did not assess male offspring, reported that prenatal alcohol exposure <u>increased</u> sensitivity to the hypothermic effects of lower doses of ethanol than those used by Abel *et al*.[13] These results showed that prenatal exposure to alcohol can produce differential effects on males and females.

Rockman, Marker, and DelRizzo[76] reported that male Holtzman rats exposed prenatally to alcohol during the second week of pregnancy only showed a significantly greater increase in ethanol-induced (1 g/kg) locomotion than controls at PN30. However, this difference was not significant in offspring when alcohol exposure was limited to the first or third week of gestation, or was given throughout gestation. The small size and inconsistency of this outcome may be because free-choice maternal alcohol intake via drinking water was low (3-4 g/kg/day).

In normal young mice (PN30), lower doses of ethanol (0.75 to 1.5 g/kg) stimulate locomotor activity from about 150%-250% (in males) to 400%-

700% (in females) of baseline activity levels. Becker *et al.*[55] assessed how prenatal alcohol exposure modified ethanol-stimulated locomotion. Interpretation of these studies was difficult because of baseline differences in locomotor activity. Overall, however, alcohol-exposed offspring tended to be hypoactive, compared to controls. Dose-response analyses indicated that prenatal alcohol-exposed females had greater relative increases in activity than controls after an ethanol challenge at PN30 or PN70 when activity was expressed as a percent of baseline.[55] In contrast, according to these authors, male offspring appeared to be relatively less sensitive to ethanol stimulation at PN30 but, that by PN70 males showed normal responses to ethanol.[55]

To assess the role of dopamine function in these differential responses to ethanol challenge, mice were given injections of AMPT with or without 1.5 g/kg ethanol.[55] In the absence of significant baseline differences among prenatal treatment groups in response to AMPT (see above), alcohol-exposed adult (PN75-PN90) male mice showed significantly greater sensitivity to AMPT-induced inhibition of the locomotor response to ethanol.[55] Females were not assessed. These data suggest that the complex changes in responsivity to ethanol challenge may reflect dopaminergic dysfunction. These changes may be gender-influenced.[87]

Similar to the changes in dose-response curves to the dopamine agonist apomorphine given alone to mice,[53] prenatal alcohol-exposed male mice showed decreased sensitivity to the suppression of ethanol-induced locomotor activation by the highest (1.2 g/kg) but not lower doses of apomorphine.[53] Male and female mice (PN80) exposed prenatally to alcohol showed greater increases in locomotion relative to baseline following 40 mg/kg of phenobarbital, but not lower doses (10 or 20 mg/kg).[55]

VI. SUMMARY

Because the long-term objective of identifying potential pharmacological treatments for fetal alcohol effects, including FAS in children is certainly worthwhile, studies in animal models will continue to be valuable. To date, these studies have generally demonstrated altered age- and gender-influenced responses to psychotherapeutic CNS stimulants, dopamine agents, and alcohol in particular for some but not all behaviors. Other agents, for example, agents acting on serotonin, acetylcholine, norepinephrine or GABA systems do not appear to be as affected by prenatal alcohol. There may also be quite specific changes in D1 and D2 dopamine receptors for which there are also well-characterized behavioral distinctions between mesolimbic and nigrostriatal dopamine systems and between D1 and D2 dopamine receptor subtypes.[88-90] The results suggest that prenatal alcohol exposure has a preferential impact on selected dopamine systems and/or receptors. On psychopharmacological evidence alone, it has been proposed that prenatal alcohol exposure causes an increased sensitivity of mesolimbic, postsynaptic D1 receptors,[28] suggesting that selective D1 receptor agonists may have particular therapeutic value.[91] Since the basal ganglia may be particularly affected in FAS children,[92] the results suggest also that a full _functional_ characterization of region- and/or receptor-specific changes in rat dopamine system responses to drugs can help identify effective pharmacotherapeutic interventions for FAS/ARBDs in children.

The exaggerated responses to methylphenidate and amphetamine in rats suggest that prenatal alcohol-exposure altered dopamine systems in functionally significant ways. Although FAS children may also be differentially sensitive to CNS stimulant "therapy," the expression of this relationship in humans would be different. The results imply that dose-response characteristics and predicted efficacy of CNS stimulant therapies may be different for FAS children with attentional deficit disorder (ADD), but that children with FAS who are treated with CNS stimulants may be at no greater risk for deleterious side effects on growth. Differential response to CNS stimulants after prenatal alcohol exposure in rats also implies that FAS/ARBD children receiving CNS stimulant therapy for ADD may respond differently than children with idiopathic ADD or ADD with other etiologies. ADD children in general appear to show idiosyncratic dose-response patterns.[41,44,93] For example, while ~70% of ADD children will respond to Ritalin® (methylphenidate), ~30% may fare better with Dexedrine® (D-amphetamine), Cylert® (pemoline) or, in rarer cases, caffeine.[41,94-95] To our knowledge, there have been no systematic evaluations of either pharmacotherapeutic outcome in children with FAS/ARBDs, or of responses to stimulant therapy as a function of ADD etiology due to alcohol or otherwise.

The changes in responsivity to dopamine agents may also be related to altered preference, intake and responses to ethanol challenges by animals exposed prenatally to alcohol.[53] Similar to results in studies with dopamine agents, changes in reactivity to postnatal ethanol challenges appear to depend upon age, dose, gender, and other variables. For example, Blanchard and colleagues reported gender-influenced alterations in ethanol-induced dopamine release in striatum and nucleus accumbens in rats exposed prenatally to alcohol.[87] As noted by Becker _et al._,[53,55] there are clearly important implications of this research for understanding the role of prenatal alcohol exposure, and more specifically of prenatal alcohol-induced change in mesolimbic dopamine function, in the etiology of alcohol abuse and alcoholism.

ACKNOWLEDGMENTS

Supported in part by grants R01-AA06721 and P50-AA07606 from NIAAA and S06-GM08167 from NIH. Contributions by Drs. B. Blanchard and L. Fitzgerald to an earlier unpublished version of this chapter, and the secretarial assistance of Anissa Poole are gratefully acknowledged.

REFERENCES

1. **Abel, E.L.,** *Fetal Alcohol Syndrome,* Oradell, NJ, Medical Economics Press, 1990.
2. **Abel, E.L. and Sokol, R.J.,** A revised conservative estimate of the incidence of FAS and its economic impact, *Alc. Clin. Exp. Res.,* 15, 514, 1991.
3. **Sokol, R.J. and Clarren, S.K.,** Guidelines for use of terminology describing the impact of prenatal alcohol on the offspring, *Alc. Clin. Exp. Res.,* 16, 378, Abstract #140, 1992.
4. **Hannigan, J. H., Welch, R.A., and Sokol, R.J.,** Recognition of fetal alcohol syndrome and alcohol-related birth defects, in *Medical Diagnosis and Treatment of Alcoholism,* Mendelson, J.H. and Mello, N.K., Eds., McGraw-Hill, New York, 1992, 639.
5. **Coles, C.D.,** Prenatal alcohol exposure and human development, in *Development of The Central Nervous System: Effects of Alcohol and Opiates,* Miller, M., Ed.,Wiley-Liss, New York, 1992, 9.
6. **Streissguth, A.P., Clarren, S.K., Aase, J.M., Randels, S.P., LaDue, R.A., and Smith, D.F.,** Fetal alcohol syndrome in adolescents and adults, *J. Am. Med. Assoc.,* 265, 1961, 1991.
7. **Jacobson, J.L., Jacobson, S.W., Sokol, R.J., Martier, S.S., Ager, J.W., and Kaplan-Estrin, M.G.,** Teratogenic effects of alcohol on infant development, *Alc. Clin. Exp. Res.,* 17, 174, 1993.
8. **Jacobson, J.L., Jacobson, S.W., Sokol, R.J., Martier, S.S., Ager, J.W., and Kaplan-Estrin, M.G.,** Effects of fetal alcohol exposure on infant reaction time, *Alc. Clin. Exp. Res.,* 18, 1125, 1994.
9. **Greene, T., Ernhart, C.B., Ager, J., Sokol, R., Martier, S., and Boyd, T.,** Prenatal alcohol exposure and cognitive development in the preschool years, *Neurotoxicol. Teratol.,* 13, 57, 1991.
10. **Coles, C.D., Brown, R.T., Smith, I.E., Platzman, K.A., Erickson, S., Silverstein, J., and Falek, A.,** Effects of prenatal alcohol exposure at school age. I. Physical and cognitive development, *Neurotoxicol. Teratol.,* 13, 357, 1991.
11. **Coles, C.D., Falek, A., Brown, R.T., Smith, I.E., Platzman, K.A., Silverstein, J., and Erikson, S.,** Effects of prenatal exposure at school age. II. Attention and behavior, *Neurotoxicol. Teratol.,* 13, 369, 1991.
12. **Spohr, H.L., Willms, J., and Steinhausen, H.C.,** The fetal alcohol syndrome in adolescence, *Acta Paediatrica,* 404, 19, 1994.
13. **Abel, E.L., Bush, R., and Dintcheff, B.A.,** Exposure of rats to alcohol *in utero* alters drug sensitivity in adulthood, *Science,* 212, 1531, 1981.

14. **Hannigan, J.H. and Blanchard, B.A.,** Psychopharmacological assessment in neurobehavioral teratology, *Neurotoxicol. Teratol.,* 10, 143, 1988.

15. **Hannigan, J.H.,** Behavioral plasticity after teratogenic alcohol exposure as recovery of function, in *Neurobehavioral Plasticity: Learning, Development, and Response to Brain Insults, Festschrift in Honor of Robert L. Isaacson,* Spear, L.P. and Woodruff, M., Eds., Lawrence Erlbaum Associates Publishers, New Jersey, 1994, 283.

16. **Van Hartesveldt, C.,** Development of dopamine systems and behavior, in *Neurobehavioral Plasticity,* Spear, N.E., Spear, L.P., and Woodruff, M.L., Eds., Lawrence Erlbaum Associates Publishers, New Jersey, 1995, 335.

17. **McDougall, S.A., Crawford, C.A., and Nonneman, A.J.,** Age-related differences in dopamine-medicated behaviors: Effect of irreversible antagonism, in *Neurobehavioral Plasticity,* Spear, N.E., Spear, L.P., and Woodruff, M.L., Eds., Lawrence Erlbaum Associates Publishers, New Jersey, 1995, 311.

18. **Druse, M.J.,** Effects of prenatal alcohol exposure on neurotransmitters, membranes, and proteins, in *Alcohol and Brain Development,* West J.R., Ed., Oxford University Press, New York, 1986, 343.

19. **Druse, M.J.,** Effects of maternal alcohol consumption on the developing nervous system, in *Alcohol and Neurobiology: Brain Development and Hormone Regulation,* Watson R.R., Ed., CRC Press, Boca Raton, 1992, 1.

20. **Middaugh, L.D., Boggan, W.O., and Shepard, C.L.,** Prenatal ethanol effects and dopamine systems of adult C57 male mice, *Neurotoxicol. Teratol.,* 16, 207-212, 1994.

21. **Leydig, M., Ciesielski, L., Similer, S., Lortentz, J.G., and Manadel, P.,** Effect of pre- and postnatal alcohol consumption on GABA levels of various brain regions in the rat offspring, *Alc. Clin. Exp. Res.,* 23, 63, 1988.

22. **Clarren, S.K., Astley, S.J., Bowden, D.M., Lai, H., Milam, A.H., Rudeen, P.K., and Shoemaker, W.J.,** Neuroanatomic and neurochemical abnormalities in nonhuman primate infants exposed to weekly doses of ethanol during gestation, *Alc. Clin. Exp. Res.,* 14, 674, 1990.

23. **Costal, B. and Naylor, R.J.,** Differentiation of dopaminergic mechanisms mediating stereotyped behavior and hyperactivity in the nucleus accumbens and caudate putamen, *J. Pharm. Pharmacol.,* 29, 377, 1977.

24. **Evenden, J.L. and Ryan, C.N.,** Behavioral responses to psychomotor stimulant drugs: Localization in the central nervous system, *J. Pharm. Exp. Toxicol.,* 36, 151, 1987.

25. **LeMoal, M.,** Mesocorticolimbic dopaminergic neurons: Functional and regulatory roles, in *Psychopharmacology: The Fourth Generation of Progress,* Bloom, F.E. and Kupfer, D.J., Eds., Raven Press, New York, 1995, 283.

26. **Meyer, L.S. and Riley, E.P.,** Behavioral teratology of alcohol, in *Handbook of Behavioral Teratology,* Riley, E.P. and Vorhees, C.V., Eds., Plenum Press, New York, 1986, 101.

27. **Blanchard, B.A., Hannigan, J.H., and Riley, E.P.,** Amphetamine-induced activity after fetal alcohol exposure and undernutrition in rats, *Neurotoxicol. Teratol.,* 9, 113, 1987.

28. **Hannigan, J.H. and Pilati, M.L.,** The effects of chronic postweaning amphetamine on rats exposed to alcohol *in utero*: Weight gain and behavior, *Neurotoxicol. Teratol.,* 13, 649-656, 1991.

29. **Druse, M.J., Tajuddin, N., Kuo, A., and Connerty, M.,** Effects of *in utero* ethanol exposure on the developing dopaminergic system in rats, *J. Neurosci. Res.,* 27, 233-240, 1990.

30. **Cooper, J.D. and Rudeen, P.K.,** Alterations in regional catecholamine content and turnover in the male rat brain in response to *in utero* ethanol exposure, *Alc. Clin. Exp. Res.,* 12, 282-285, 1988.

31. **Weiner, N.,** Norepinephrine, epinephrine, and the sympathomimetic amines, in *The Pharmacological Basis of Therapeutics,* Gillman, A.G., Goodman, L.S., Rull, T.W., Murand, F., Eds., 7th ed., McMillan, New York, 1985, 145-180.

32. **Ulug, S. and Riley, E.P.,** The effect of methylphenidate on overactivity in rats prenatally exposed to alcohol, *Neurobehav. Toxicol. Teratol.,* 5, 35-39, 1983.

33. **Means, L.W., Medlin, C.W., Hughes, V.D., and Gray, S.L.,** Rats exposed *in utero* to ethanol are hyperresponsive to methylphenidate when tested as neonates or adults, *Neurobehav. Toxicol. Teratol.,* 6, 187, 1984.

34. **Blanchard, B.A., Riley, E.P., and Hannigan, J.H.,** Deficits on a spatial navigation task following prenatal exposure to ethanol, *Neurotoxicol. Teratol.,* 9, 253-258,1986.

35. **Weinberg, J.,** Prenatal alcohol exposure: Endocrine function of offsprings, in *Alcohol and the Endocrine System,* Zakkari, S., Ed., NIAAA, 1993.

36. **McGivern, R.F. and Riley, E.P.,** Influence of perinatal alcohol exposure on sexual differentiation, in *Alcohol and the Endocrine System,* Zakkari, S., Ed., NIAAA, 1993.

37. **Bond, N.W.,** Prenatal ethanol exposure and hyperactivity in rats: Effects of D-amphetamine and α-methyl-p-tyrosine, *Neurobehav. Toxicol. Teratol.,* 7, 461-467, 1985.

38. **Bond, N.W.,** Fetal alcohol exposure hyperactivity in rats: The role of the neurotransmitter system involved in arousal and inhibition, in *Alcohol and Brain Development*, West, J.R., Ed., Oxford University Press, New York, 45-70, 1986.

39. **Zimmerberg, B., Riley, E.P., and Glick, S.D.,** Differential effects of prenatal exposure to alcohol on activity and circling behavior in rats, *Pharm. Biochem. Behav.*, 25,1021-1025, 1986.

40. **Blanchard, B.A. and Hannigan, J.H.,** Prenatal ethanol exposure: Effects on androgen and nonandrogen dependent behaviors and on gonadal development in male rats, *Neurotoxicol. Teratol.*, 16, 31-39, 1994.

41. **Gittleman-Klein, R.,** Pharmacotherapy of childhood hyperactivity: An update, in *Psychopharmacology: The Third Generation of Progress*, Raven Press, New York, 1987, 1215-1224.

42. **Pizzi, W., Rode, E.C., and Barnhart, J.E.,** Methylphenidate and growth: Demonstration of growth impairment and a growth-rebound phenomenon, *Dev. Pharmacol. Ther.*, 9, 361-368, 1986.

43. **Pizzi, W., Rode, E.C., and Barnhart, J.E.,** Differential effects of methylphenidate on the growth of neonatal and adolescent rats, *Neurotoxicol. Teratol.*, 9, 107-111, 1987.

44. **Rapport, M.D., DuPaul, G.J., Stoner, G., and Jones, J.T.,** Comparing classroom and clinic measures of attention deficit disorder: Differential, idiosyncratic and dose-response effects of methylphenidate. *J. Consult. Clin. Psychol.*, 54, 334-341, 1986.

45. **Hannigan, J.H., Hackett, J.A., and DiCerbo, J.A.,** Behavioral sensitization to amphetamine in rats exposed prenatally to alcohol. *Research Society on Alcoholism*, Annual Meeting, Maui, HI. *Alc. Clin. Exp. Res.*, 1994, 18, 505, Abstract #513.

46. **Robinson, T.E. and Berridge, K.C.,** The neural basis of drug craving: An incentive-sensitization theory of addition, *Brain Res.*, 18, 247-291, 1993.

47. **Paulson, P.E. and Robinson, T.E.,** Sensitization to systemic amphetamine produces an enhanced locomotor response to a subsequent intra-accumbens amphetamine challenge in rats, *Psychopharmacology*, 104, 140-141,1991.

48. **Franz, D.N.,** Central neurons system stimulants, in *The Pharmacological Basis of Therapeutics*, Gilman, A.G., Goodman, L.S., Rull, T.W., and Murand, F., Eds., McMillian, New York, 1985.

49. **Randall, S., Cortese, B.M., DiCerbo, J.A., and Hannigan, J.H.,** Effects *in utero* exposure to alcohol plus caffeine in rats. I. Pregnancy outcome and early offspring development. *Research Society on Alcoholism*, Annual Meeting, San Antonio, TX,

50. **Hannigan, J.H., Cortese, B.M., DiCerbo, J.A., and Lipshutz, B.S.,** Effects of acute pemoline (Cylert®) challenge in young rats exposed prenatally to alcohol. *Research Society on Alcoholism,* Annual Meeting, San Antonio, TX, *Alc. Clin. Exp. Res.,* 1993b, 17, 456, Abstract #90.

51. **Abel, E.L.,** *Fetal Alcohol Syndrome,* Oradell, Medical Economics Press, 1990.

52. **Lynch, M.R.,** Dissociation of autoreceptor activation and behavioral consequences of low-dose apomorphine treatment, *Prog. Neuropsychopharmacol. Biol. Psychiatry,* 15, 689-698, 1991.

53. **Becker, H.C., Weathersby, R.T., and Hale, R.L.,** Prenatal ethanol exposure alters sensitivity to the effects of apomorphine given alone and in combination with ethanol on locomotor activity in adult male mouse offspring, *Neurotoxicol. Teratol.,* 17, 57-64, 1995.

54. **Hannigan, J.H., Blanchard, B.A., Horner, M.P., Riley, E.P., and Pilati, M.L.,** Apomorphine-induced motor behavior in rats exposed prenatally to alcohol, *Neurotoxicol. Teratol.,* 12, 79-84, 1990.

55. **Becker, H.C., Hale, R.L., Boggan, W.O., and Randall, C.L.,** Effects of prenatal ethanol exposure on later sensitivity to the low dose stimulant actions of ethanol in mouse offspring: Possible role of catecholamines, *Alc. Clin. Exp. Res.,* 17, 1325-1336, 1993.

56. **Shen, R.Y. and Chiodo, L.A.,** The effects *in utero* ethanol administration on the electrophysiological activity of rat nigrostriatal dopaminergic neurons, *Dev. Brain Res.,* in press, 1993.

57. **Shen, R.Y., Hannigan, J.H., and Chiodo, L.A.,** The effect of chronic postweaning amphetamine on electrophysiological activity of A10 dopamine neurons in rats exposed prenatally to alcohol, *Alc. Clin. Exp. Res.,* 1992, 16, 378, Abstract #140.

58. **Hannigan, J.H.,** The ontogeny of SCH 23390-induced catalepsy in male and female rats exposed to ethanol *in utero, Alcohol,* 7, 11, 1990.

59. **DiCerbo, J.A. and Hannigan, J.H.,** Effects of buspirone on behavior and biochemistry of rats exposed prenatally to ethanol (EtOH), *Alc. Clin. Exp. Res.,* 1991, 15, 377, Abstract # 155.

60. **Hannigan, J.H. and Fitzgerald, L.W.,** unpublished observation, 1986.

61. **Lucchi, L., Covelli, V., Petkov, V.V., Spano, P.F., and Tracucchi, M.,** Effects of ethanol, given during pregnancy, on the offspring dopaminergic systems, *Pharm. Biochem. Behav.,* 19, 567, 1983.

62. **Shen, R.Y., Hannigan, J.H., and Chiodo, L.A.,** The effect of chronic amphetamine treatment on prenatal ethanol-induced changes in dopamine receptor function: Electrophysiological findings, in press, 1995.

63. **Randall, S. and Hannigan, J.H.,** Prenatal exposure to alcohol increases behavioral sensitivity in response to quinpirone, *Alc. Clin. Exp. Res.,* 1995, 19, 51A, Abstract #287.

64. **Hannigan, J.H., Fitzgerald, L.W., Blanchard, B.A., and Riley, E.P.**, Absence of differential motoric and thermic responses to clonidine in young rats exposed prenatally to alcohol, *Alcohol,* 5, 431, 1988.

65. **Hannigan, J.H. and Zimmerberg, B.**, unpublished observation, 1988.

66. **Weathersby, R.T., Becker, H.C., and Hale, R.L.**, Reduced sensitivity to the effects of clonidine on ethanol-stimulated locomotor activity in adult mouse offspring prenatally exposed to ethanol, *Alcohol*, 11, 517, 1994.

67. **Bond, N.W.**, Prenatal alcohol exposure and offspring hyperactivity: Effects of para-chlorophenylalaine and methysergide, *Neurobehav. Toxicol. Teratol.,* 8, 667, 1986.

68. **Grace, G.M., Rockman, G.E., and Glavin, G.B.**, Effect of prenatal exposure to ethanol an adult ethanol preference and response to zimelidine in rats, *Alc. Alcohol,* 7, 1, 1990.

69. **Riley, E.P., Barron, S., Driscoll, C.D., and Hamlin, R.T.**, The effects of physostigmine on open-field behavior in rats exposed to alcohol prenatally, *Alc. Clin. Exp. Res.,* 10, 50, 1986.

70. **Bond, N.W.**, Prenatal alcohol exposure and offspring hyperactivity: Effects of physostigmine and neostigmine, *Neurotoxicol. Teratol.*, 10, 59, 1988.

71. **Kelly, S.J., Black, A., and West, J.R.**, Changes in the muscarinic cholinergic receptors in the hippocampus of rats exposed to ethyl alcohol during the brain growth spurt, *J. Pharm. Exp. Ther.*, 249, 798, 1989.

72. **Light, K.E., Serbus, D.C., and Santiago, M.**, Exposure of rats to ethanol from postnatal days 4 to 8: Alterations of cholinergic neurochemistry in the cerebral cortex and corpus striatum at day 20, *Alc. Clin. Exp. Res.,* 13, 29, 1989.

73. **Blanchard, B.A. and Riley, E.P.**, Effects of physostigmine on shuttle avoidance in rats exposed prenatally to ethanol, *Alcohol,* 5, 27, 1988.

74. **Bond, N.W.**, Prenatal alcohol exposure and offspring, hyperactivity: Effects of scopolamine and methylscopolamine, *Neurobehav. Toxicol. Teratol.,* 8, 287, 1986.

75. **Rockwood, G.A. and Riley, E.P.**, Effects of scopolamine on spontaneous alternation and shuttle avoidance in rats exposed to alcohol *in utero*, *Alcohol,* 2, 575, 1985.

76. **Rockman, G.E., Marker, L.E., and DelRizzo, M.**, Effects of prenatal ethanol exposure on ethanol-induced locomotor activity in the rat, *Alcohol*, 6, 353, 1989.

77. **Bond, N.W. and DiGiusto, E.L.**, Effects of prenatal alcohol consumption on open-field behavior and alcohol preference in rats, *Psychopharmacologia*, 46, 163, 1976.

78. Reyes, E., Garcia, K.D., and Jones, B.C., Effects of the maternal consumption of alcohol on alcohol selection in rats, *Alcohol,* 2, 323, 1985.

79. Nelson, R.L., Lewis, J.W., Liebeskind, J.C., Branch, B.J., and Taylor, A.N., Stress induced changes in ethanol consumption in adult rats exposed to ethanol *in utero, Proceedings of the Western Pharmacology Society,* 26, 205, 1983.

80. Dominguez, H.D., Chotro, M.G., and Molina, J.C., Alcohol in amniotic fluid prior to cesarean delivery: Effects of subsequent exposure to drug's odor upon alcohol responsiveness, *Behav. Neural Biology,* 60, 129, 1993.

81. McGivern, R.F., Clancy, A.N., Mousa, S., Couri, D., and Noble, E.P., Prenatal alcohol exposure alters enkephalin levels without affecting ethanol preference, *Life Sci.,* 34, 584, 1984.

82. Tolliver, G.A. and Samson, H.H., The influence of early post weaning ethanol exposure on oral self administration behavior in the rat, *Pharm. Biochem. Behav.,* 38, 575, 1991.

83. Nelson, R.L., Taylor, A.N., Lewis, J.W., Poland, R.E.,Redei, E., and Branch, B.J., Pituitary-adrenal responses to morphine and footshock stress are enhanced following prenatal alcohol exposure, *Alc. Clin. Exp. Res.,* 10, 397, 1986.

84. Taylor, A.N., Branch, B.J., Liu, S.H., Wiechmann, A.F.,Hill, M.A., Kokka, N., Fetal exposure to ethanol enhances pituitary-adrenal and temperature responses to ethanol in adult rats, *Alc. Clin. Exp. Res.,* 5, 237, 1981.

85. Reyes, E., Duran, E., and Switzer, S.H., Effects of *in utero* administration of alcohol on alcohol sensitivity in adult rats. *Pharm. Biochem. Behav.,* 44, 307, 1993.

86. Gilliam, D.M., Dudek, B.C., and Riley, E.P., Responses to ethanol challenge in long- and short-sleep mice prenatally exposed to alcohol, *Alcohol,* 7, 1, 1990.

87. Blanchard, B.A., Steindorf, S., Wang, S., LeFevre, R.,Mankes, R.F., and Glick, S.D., Prenatal ethanol exposure alters ethanol-induced dopamine release in nucleus accumbens and striatum in male and female rats, *Alc.Clin. Exp. Res.,* 745, 1993.

88. Clark, D. and White, F.J., D1 dopamine receptor - the search for a function: A critical evaluation of the D1/D2 dopamine receptor classification and its functional implications, *Synapse,* 1, 347, 1987.

89. Johnson, B.L. and Bruno, J.P., D1 and D2 receptors contributions to ingestive and locomotor behavior are altered after dopamine depletions in neonatal rats, *Neurosci. Lett.,* 118, 120, 1990.

90. Johnson, B.L. and Bruno, J.P., D1 and D2 receptor mediation of sensorimotor behavior in rats depleted of dopamine during development, *Behav. Brain Res.,* 47,49, 1992.

91. **Waddington, J.L.,** Therapeutic potential of selective D1 dopamine receptor agonist and antagonist in psychiatry and neurology, *Gen. Pharm.,* 19, 55, 1988.

92. **Mattson, S.N., Riley, E.P., Jernigan, T.L., Ehlers, C.L., Delis, D.C., Jones, K.L., Stern, C., Johnson, K.A., Hesselink, J.R., and Bellugi, U.,** Fetal alcohol syndrome: A case of neuropsychological, MRI, and EEG assessment of two children, *Alc. Clin. Exp. Res.,* 16, 1001, 1992.

93. **Rapport, M.D., DuPaul, G.J., and Kelly, K.L.,** Attention deficit hyperactivity disorders and methylphenidate: The relationship between gross body weight and drug response in children, *Psychopharm. Bull.,* 25, 285, 1989.

94. **Elia, J., Borcherdinging, B.G., Rapport, J.L., and Keysor, C.S.,** Methylphenidate and dextroamphetamine treatments of hyperactivity: Are there true *nonresponders? Psychiatry Res.,* 36, 141, 1991.

95. **Rapport, M.D., Denny, C., DuPaul, G.J., and Garder, M.J.,** Attentional deficit disorder and methylphenidate: Normalization rates, clinical effectiveness, and response prediction in 76 children, *J. Am. Acad. Child Adoles. Psych.,* 33, 882, 1994.

Chapter 10

STRESS REACTIVITY
IN FETAL ALCOHOL SYNDROME

C. Kwon Kim, Jill A. Osborn and Joanne Weinberg

It has been recognized for many years that intrauterine exposure to alcohol has adverse effects on the developing fetus. Lemoine and colleagues[1] in France and Jones and colleagues[2-3] in Seattle independently described a cluster of abnormalities in children whose mothers chronically consumed high doses of alcohol during pregnancy. This cluster of abnormalities was termed the fetal alcohol syndrome (FAS), and was characterized by diagnostic criteria in three categories: prenatal and/or postnatal growth deficiencies, central nervous system (CNS) impairments, and a characteristic facial dysmorphology.[4] Interestingly, FAS does not occur consistently in all infants exposed to high levels of alcohol *in utero*. The full syndrome occurs in approximately one-third of infants born to women who are chronic alcoholics; the remaining two-thirds show effects ranging from severe disabilities to only minimal deficits.[5-6] The terms fetal alcohol effects (FAE) and alcohol related birth defects (ARBD) have been used to describe these cases where all three diagnostic criteria of FAS are not met, yet there are still problems related to prenatal alcohol exposure.[4] The fact that the full syndrome does not occur in all infants exposed to high doses of alcohol suggests that factors other than the dose/duration of alcohol exposure alone are involved. Factors contributing to the pathogenesis may include the developmental period of alcohol exposure, drinking pattern, physiological variables that influence uptake and metabolism of alcohol, general maternal health, nutritional status, maternal age, parity, and the use of other drugs.[7-8]

Recently, with our expanding knowledge of the teratogenic effects of alcohol on the developing organism, effects of maternal alcohol consumption on neuroendocrine and neurobehavioral responses have received considerable attention. This chapter will review data on neuroendocrine responses to stress in fetal alcohol-exposed offspring. Following a description of the hypothalamic-pituitary-adrenal (HPA) axis stress response and its regulation, studies on the effects of prenatal alcohol exposure on responses of the HPA axis and β-endorphin (β-EP) system to stress will be examined. In addition, the possible mechanisms for this altered stress responsiveness will be reviewed. Finally the role of alcohol-induced disturbances in endocrine balance as a possible mediator of alcohol's teratogenic effects on behavior and cognitive function will be discussed.

I. HYPOTHALAMIC-PITUITARY-ADRENAL (HPA) AXIS

Stress can affect the release of virtually every hormone in the body, and thus has widespread effects throughout the whole organism. The stress response allows the organism to withstand immediate threats to its homeostatic balance. It involves a myriad of physiological (e.g., energy mobilization, increase in cardiovascular and respiratory tone, suppression of anabolic processes, suppression of inflammatory/immune function) and behavioral (e.g., sharpened cognition, increased arousal and alertness, focused attention, altered sensory threshold) changes.[9-10] Acute stress responses are advantageous for the survival of the organism; however, prolonged or chronic stress may be maladaptive and can lead to a variety of pathological conditions.[9-11] There are two principal components of the stress response.[9-10] The first is the locus ceruleus (LC)/autonomic (sympathetic) nervous system which mediates the stress response via the release of epinephrine (EP) and norepinephrine (NE). The second component is the HPA axis, which will be the major focus of this chapter.

The HPA axis responds to stressors by releasing a cascade of substances with the final common pathway of the release of corticosterone (CORT) from the adrenal gland (CORT is the major glucocorticoid in rats, cortisol in humans). During the HPA stress response, corticotropin-releasing hormone (CRH) is synthesized and released from the parvocellular division of the paraventricular nucleus (PVN) of the hypothalamus; CRH neurons are widespread throughout the brain but are best characterized in the PVN. CRH reaches the anterior pituitary via the hypothalamic-hypophyseal portal vessels, regulates the synthesis of proopiomelanocortin (POMC), and stimulates the release of the POMC-derived peptides such as adrenocorticotropin (ACTH) and β-EP from the anterior pituitary. Stress also induces release of β-EP-like substances from the intermediate lobe of the pituitary. Although CRH is the main secretagogue of ACTH, it is well recognized that other peptides, especially vasopressin (VP), may facilitate or enhance ACTH release. ACTH is transported via the systemic circulation to the adrenal gland and acts on the adrenal cortex to stimulate the synthesis and release of CORT into the systemic circulation.[11-13]

There are two major classes of intracellular corticosteroid receptors:[14-15] Type I (MR, mineralocorticoid receptor) and Type II (GR, glucocorticoid receptor), which differ in binding affinity to various endogenous and synthetic ligands as well as distribution throughout the brain.[16] MRs bind with high affinity to CORT and aldosterone (ALD), while GRs bind with about 10-fold less affinity to CORT and even less affinity to ALD. GRs are widely distributed throughout the brain with high concentrations in the limbic system (hippocampus, septum), PVN and supraoptic nuclei of the hypothalamus, cerebral cortex, and anterior pituitary. MRs have a more restricted topography than GRs with high densities in the hippocampus, septum and amygdala.

II. FEEDBACK REGULATION OF THE HPA AXIS

CORT exerts negative feedback effects at several sites, the most important being the hippocampus,[17-18] anterior pituitary,[19-20] and prefrontal cortex.[21] The PVN of the hypothalamus was originally thought to be a site of feedback.[22-23] However, recent evidence suggests that the PVN may not be an actual feedback site, but rather the site of termination of neuronal inputs from higher feedback sites.[24]

There are at least three distinct time domains in which negative feedback by CORT operates during and following stress:[12,25] fast feedback (seconds to minutes), early delayed or intermediate feedback (2-10 hr), and late delayed or slow feedback (hours to days). Fast feedback occurs while plasma levels of CORT are increasing and is sensitive to the rate of increase in CORT. It occurs within seconds or minutes of CORT increase and disappears by 20-30 min. Delayed feedback (intermediate and slow) depends on the level of CORT achieved, the amount of CORT exposure, the interval since the stressor, and the duration of exposure to CORT. Intermediate feedback occurs during exposure to CORT for 2-10 hr; slow feedback results during constant CORT exposure for 12 hr or more. Thus, fast rate sensitive feedback probably controls the rate and magnitude of CORT responses to acute stimuli, whereas intermediate feedback may limit the response of the system to repeated stimulation within a relatively short period of time (hours), and slow feedback may limit the response of the system during prolonged stress.[25]

It was originally postulated that MRs were responsible for the permissive or tonic effects of CORT, while GRs mediated the negative feedback action of CORT on the stress response.[14] However, more recent evidence suggests that MRs also play a role in the feedback regulation of CORT.[18,26]

An understanding of the way GRs and MRs mediate feedback effects at the various CNS feedback sites and in the various feedback time domains is far from complete. The anterior pituitary may mediate early and intermediate feedback[19,27] probably via GRs,[27] with a possible role for Mrs.[26] The hippocampus may mediate feedback via GRs, in conjunction with hippocampal MRs and hypothalamic GRs;[18] but hippocampal GRs appear not to play a role in fast feedback.[28] There are suggestions that the PVN of the hypothalamus may mediate fast and intermediate feedback, with GRs in the parvocellular PVN playing the major role in mediating the feedback.[16]

III. EFFECTS OF FETAL ALCOHOL EXPOSURE ON THE STRESS RESPONSE

Although clinical studies have established that alcohol consumption markedly alters HPA function in adults who chronically abuse alcohol, few clinical studies have investigated HPA function in children prenatally exposed to alcohol. A case study of four children with FAS indicated that plasma cortisol levels were within normal limits.[29] However, Binkiewicz and colleagues[30] reported pseudo-Cushing's syndrome in an infant exposed to alcohol via the breast milk, suggesting that alcohol can have stimulatory effects on the HPA axis of the newborn. Recently, Jacobson and colleagues[31] reported that infants with a history of prenatal alcohol exposure demonstrated elevated salivary cortisol levels following an acute stressor (i.e., a routine blood draw).

Animal studies provide evidence of altered HPA axis function of the maternal female, as well as altered HPA axis and β-EP system function in their offspring. Ethanol consumption in pregnant female rats result in increases in maternal adrenal weights, basal CORT levels, and adrenocortical responses to stress without significantly altering the binding capacity of plasma corticosterone binding globulin (CBG).[32-34] The ethanol-induced activation of the maternal HPA axis occurs as early as day 11 of pregnancy and persists throughout gestation, even at low concentrations of ethanol (5.5% w/v) in the diet. In addition, with continued ethanol exposure, stimulatory effects of ethanol on maternal adrenal weights and basal CORT levels may persist through to parturition.[33] Furthermore, this HPA hyperresponsiveness appears to be independent of maternal nutritional status and specifically a result of ethanol exposure.[33] Females consuming diets with varied protein levels but consistently high ethanol content all demonstrated increases in adrenal weights and adrenocortical hyperactivity. Together, these data suggest that ethanol consumption during pregnancy results in hyperactivity of the maternal HPA axis.

During the early neonatal period, fetal ethanol exposed (E) animals have elevated basal levels of brain, plasma, and adrenal CORT and decreased CBG binding capacity,[32,35-37] as well as elevated plasma and decreased pituitary β-EP levels[38] compared to controls. By 3-5 days of age, basal CORT levels in E animals return to normal. However, a transient period of stress hyporesponsiveness follows that lasts until day 15-21 of age. During this period, E animals exhibit suppressed or blunted HPA and β-EP responses to a wide variety of stressors including ether, novel environment, saline injection, and cold, as well as to drugs such as ethanol and morphine.[32,37-39]

As adults, E animals exhibit HPA and β-EP hyperactivity that is evident in response to stressors, but is not apparent in the nonstressed or basal state. Basal levels of CORT, ACTH, and β-EP in E offspring do not differ from those in control offspring.[34,40] However, adult E offspring are hyperresponsive to many physical and neurogenic stressors including cardiac puncture,[40] restraint,[40-42] noise and shaking,[40] ether,[34,38] novel environments,[41] intermittent foot shock,[43,44] and cold.[38] E animals also demonstrate deficits in pituitary-adrenal response inhibition or recovery from stress. For example, E animals show prolonged CORT, ACTH, and β-EP elevations during and following restraint stress,[41,42,45] more prolonged ACTH elevations following footshock stress,[46] and smaller CORT decreases when allowed to perform consummatory behaviors in a novel environment[41] as compared to control animals. Furthermore, the ability to respond to environmental cues in stressful situations also appears to be deficient in E animals; unlike controls, E animals do not respond differentially to predictable versus unpredictable restraint stress.[47]

Interestingly, the HPA hyperresponsiveness may be manifested differentially in males and females depending on the nature and intensity of the stressor, the time course measured, and the hormonal endpoint examined.[48] For example, exposure to a 60 min restraint stress resulted in more prolonged CORT elevations in E than in control females, while E males did not differ from control males.[41] However, exposure to a more prolonged (4 hr) restraint stress resulted in greater and more prolonged CORT elevations in E than in control males, while under these conditions E females did not differ from control females.[42] Furthermore, it was shown that E males and females both exhibited HPA hyperresponsiveness as compared to control animals following repeated exposure to restraint stress and during recovery from restraint. Once again, sex differences in response were observed. E females demonstrated elevated CORT and ACTH but not β-EP levels compared to controls following 5 to 10 daily exposures to 60 min restraint. In contrast, E males demonstrated elevated β-EP levels compared to controls. Following 16 daily exposures to 30 min restraint, E males showed significantly greater ACTH and β-EP levels than controls, whereas E females demonstrated a delayed peak in ACTH and β-EP responses and not in their levels.[45] Together, these data suggest that HPA stress hyperresponsiveness in fetal ethanol-exposed animals is a robust phenomenon, occurring in both males and females, although the nature of the stress response may vary somewhat between the sexes.

IV. MECHANISMS OF FETAL ALCOHOL EFFECTS ON THE HPA AXIS

Ethanol consumed by the pregnant female can readily cross the placenta[49] and have direct effects on the fetal HPA axis, which is functional before birth.[50] Thus, ethanol may produce its effects on the fetus by acting directly on the fetal endocrine glands and/or at brain/pituitary sites. Alternatively, ethanol may affect the fetal HPA axis indirectly through disruption of maternal HPA function.[51] The pregnant female and the fetus constitute an interrelated functional unit and CORT can cross the placenta in both directions.[50] It has been suggested that the ethanol-induced alterations seen in the fetal HPA axis may be a result of ethanol acting as a maternal stressor, elevating maternal CORT levels and indirectly elevating fetal CORT levels.[52] Perinatal administration of glucocorticoids has been shown to result in alterations in cellular growth, neuronal myelination and differentiation, and interfere with normal biochemical, neurochemical, and physiologic processes.[52-53] However, offspring from dams challenged with stressors, ACTH, or adrenalectomy during pregnancy do not display the same pattern of hyperresponsiveness seen in E animals.[37] At present, it appears most likely that a combination of direct and indirect effects of ethanol are likely involved in altering the fetal HPA axis.[48]

The sites and mechanisms underlying the HPA hyperresponsiveness of E offspring are presently unknown. The hyperresponsiveness may be a result of a number of factors including an increase in anterior pituitary and/or adrenal sensitivity to secretagogues, alterations in neurotransmitter systems that regulate HPA function, and deficits in negative feedback control of HPA activity. One or more of these mechanisms may be at work and evidence for one does not preclude the possibility of the other factors.

The anterior pituitary but not the adrenal gland appears to display a greater sensitivity to their secretagogues following prenatal ethanol exposure. No significant differences were found in pituitary sensitivity to CRH[52,54-55] or CRH and VP[55] between E and control animals. However, a recent study in our laboratory[56] in which a range of CRH doses was infused into animals 3 hr following dexamethasone (DEX) blockade found that E female rats displayed higher ACTH levels than controls. DEX is a synthetic glucocorticoid antagonist that acts to block the release of ACTH and subsequently of CORT. Studies have demonstrated no significant differences in CORT levels between E and control groups in response to a wide range of ACTH doses.[40,52,57-58]

Evidence suggests that prenatal ethanol exposure may also result in alterations of neurotransmitter systems that regulate HPA function. Data indicate that ascending adrenergic fibers from the brainstem stimulate CRF neurons[59] and that microinjections of NE stimulate both CRF gene expression and CRF secretion.[60] Furthermore, there appears to be bidirectional input between CRF release and NE release. CRF has been shown to increase medial prefrontal cortex and medial hypothalamic NE and dopamine (DA) release[61] as well as tyrosine hydroxylase levels in the LC.[62] Interestingly, following restraint stress, E animals show altered regional brain catecholamine content compared to control animals.[63] Acute exposure to restraint stress resulted in reduced cortical NE content in E males and females and decreased hypothalamic NE content in E females but not E males, but increased hippocampal NE in E males and females. If the decreased NE content observed in the cortex and hypothalamus of E animals is an indication of depletion of NE by an increase in neuronal activity (turnover), then it is possible that prenatal ethanol effects on catecholamine regulation of CRF secretion may partially mediate the hyperresponsiveness of E animals. It has also been demonstrated that both nonstressed E offspring[52] and E offspring exposed to ether stress[64] have elevated CRF mRNA levels in the PVN of the hypothalamus. It is possible that alterations in the control of CRF synthesis may mediate this elevation.

Finally, data suggest that prenatal ethanol exposure may result in alterations in feedback inhibition of HPA activity. Nelson and colleagues[65] demonstrated that E animals appear to have increased CORT levels following DEX blockade. Recent studies in our laboratory have demonstrated that E animals are less sensitive to DEX suppression than control animals, and that there may be a sex specific difference in response to DEX suppression depending upon the point in the circadian rhythm when testing occurs.[66] During the trough of the CORT circadian rhythm, E females exposed to an ether stress at 3 and 6 hr post-DEX injection showed increased stress levels of CORT but not ACTH compared to controls, whereas there were no significant differences between E and control males. However, at the peak of the circadian cycle, both E females and E males exposed to ether stress 3 hr post-DEX injection demonstrated elevated stress levels of CORT compared to controls. In addition, E females demonstrated elevated stress levels of ACTH. These data support the hypothesis of a deficit in feedback regulation of the HPA axis, and suggests that this deficit occurs in the intermediate feedback time domain. Furthermore, feedback deficits in E animals may also occur in the fast feedback time domain:[55] the ACTH response to multiple footshock stress presented over a 15 min interval was shown to be increased in E animals compared to controls. Moreover, the observed elevation in CRF mRNA levels in the PVN of the hypothalamus in E offspring,[52] can be interpreted as resulting from a deficiency in HPA feedback regulation.

The possibility that deficits in HPA negative feedback might occur as a result of ethanol-induced decreases in hippocampal corticosteroid receptor densities or binding affinities has also been examined in our laboratory.[67] Alterations in corticosteroid receptor densities at CORT feedback sites have been shown to alter efficacy of negative feedback control of the HPA axis.[11] The hippocampus is a major site of CORT feedback,[17-18] has the highest concentration of corticosteroid receptors in the mammalian brain,[16] and is very susceptible to damage following prenatal ethanol exposure.[68] The data demonstrated that there were no significant differences in densities or binding affinities for either GRs or MRs in the hippocampus of male and female E animals compared to controls. Subsequently, it has been shown that prenatal ethanol exposure does not alter GR and MR densities of either sex at other CNS sites involved in CORT feedback, including the anterior pituitary, hypothalamus, and prefrontal cortex.[69-70] However, it is possible that prenatal ethanol exposure may induce alterations in MR or GR densities within specific subfields of a feedback site such as the hippocampus. Furthermore, differential down-regulation of these receptors in E subjects may result following an extended period of CORT elevation; chronic stress or prolonged exogenous glucocorticoid treatment can down-regulate corticosteroid receptors.[71-73] Analogous to the finding that HPA hyperresponsiveness in prenatal ethanol exposed animals is more apparent following a stressor than under basal or nonstressed conditions, it is possible that chronic stress may reveal an underlying vulnerability that may not be apparent under resting conditions. In addition, mRNA levels for the GRs and MRs may display differences following prenatal ethanol exposure. In other words, fetal ethanol exposure could result in changes in receptor densities at the level of transcription and/or at posttranscription processing. These possibilities are currently being examined in this laboratory.

V. IMPLICATIONS OF HPA HYPERRESPONSIVENESS FOLLOWING FETAL ALCOHOL EXPOSURE

A. EFFECTS ON BEHAVIOR

Behavioral abnormalities are very common in children prenatally exposed to alcohol.[7,74-75] These include hyperactivity, poor attention span, distractibility, impaired habituation, perceptual problems, impassivity, lack of inhibition, poor social judgment, and poor sensitivity to social cues. Animal models of prenatal ethanol exposure have replicated many of the behavioral effects found in humans. For example, behaviors reflecting hyperactivity and hyperresponsiveness have been reported, including increases in open field activity,[76-77] wheel running,[78] startle reaction,[79] and exploratory behavior.[80] Behaviors reflecting response inhibition have also been shown, such as deficits in passive avoidance learning,[81-82] taste aversion learning,[83] and reversal learning.[84] In addition, rodents prenatally exposed to ethanol have altered behavioral responses to stressors, including increases in stress-induced analgesia[85] and stress-induced ethanol consumption.[86] CRH, ACTH, and CORT, which are elevated in prenatal ethanol exposed offspring, as discussed above, are known to modulate behaviors during stress,[87] and therefore may play a role in the altered behaviors seen in E offspring.

CRH and its receptors are found in areas outside the hypothalamus.[88] It is now generally accepted that CRH fulfills the requisite criteria to be considered a neurotransmitter[89] and that it plays a major role in coordinating endocrine, behavioral and autonomic responses to stressors. Central administration of CRH at low doses results in behaviors that resemble stress responses, including increases in feeding, locomotion in a novel environment and shock-induced fighting, as well as decreases in social interaction. Administration of high doses results in behaviors reflecting anxiety, such as decreases in feeding, sexual activity, locomotion in a novel environment and shock-induced fighting.[90] It has been demonstrated that local administration of CRH into the LC results in an increase in unstimulated neuronal discharge and decreased or unchanged firing with exposure to foot shock,[91-92] suggesting that elevated CRH disrupts the normal pattern of discharge in the LC. Therefore, it is possible that increased CRH release could result in persistently elevated neuronal discharge rates and decreased responses to phasic sensory stimuli, thus producing alterations in behavior. Such a mechanism could, at least in part, underlie the behavioral changes such as hyperarousal and decreased attention span seen in children prenatally exposed to alcohol.

Furthermore, there has been a considerable amount of research focused on the possibility that hypersecretion of CRH may play a role in the pathophysiology of certain affective and anxiety disorders. Interestingly, individuals with affective or anxiety disorders also demonstrate altered arousal and attention span, as well as altered HPA responses to stressors including elevated CORT and ACTH levels, altered circadian rhythms, and non-suppressiblity of the HPA axis to DEX.[89] Additionally, elevated CRF levels in the cerebrospinal fluid have been found in depressed patients.[93-94] It is possible that increased CRH release may produce persistently elevated neuronal discharge rates and decreased responses to phasic sensory stimuli, and could thus underlie some of the behavioral changes seen in affective and anxiety disorders.[91-92]

B.   EFFECTS ON COGNITIVE FUNCTION

Prenatal ethanol exposure not only results in HPA hyperactivity, but also produces cognitive deficits, a finding well documented in humans[7,74-75] and in many experimental models of spatial[95-97] and nonspatial [83,98-100] learning and memory. Accordingly, the hypothesis that the deficits in cognitive function observed in organisms prenatally exposed to ethanol may result, in part, from the hypersecretion of CORT, will be explored.

Acute stress, which produces high CORT levels, causes impairments in cognitive function. For example, stressors such as exposure to a novel environment,[101] footshock [102] or ether [103] have been shown to impair per-formance on learning/memory tasks in laboratory animals. Similarly, cold stress impaired cognitive function in humans.[104] Interestingly, a dual action of CORT has been demonstrated, with high doses suppressing learning/memory and low doses having a facilitatory effect.[105] Furthermore, CORT insufficiency impairs learning/memory function.[106] Thus, the relationship between CORT levels and cognitive function appears to be U-shaped: learning/memory is impaired by CORT insufficiency and high CORT levels, while it is optimal at intermediate CORT levels.

This U-shaped relationship is also found between CORT levels and the induction of both long-term potentiation (LTP) and primed-burst potentiation (PBP) in the hippocampus. LTP is a long lasting enhancement in synaptic efficacy following high frequency electrical pulse stimulation of afferent fibers.[107-108] This form of neuroplasticity is the most widely studied physiological model of learning and memory. It can be induced in the CA1, CA3 and dentate gyrus subfields of the hippocampus,[107-108] a structure associated with aspects of learning and memory, especially spatial learning/memory.[109] PBP is a low threshold form of LTP in which physiological patterned electrical stimuli mimic the normal cellular firing patterns within the hippocampus.[110] Acute stress impairs LTP[111] and PBP;[112] in fact, there appears to be a negative correlation between CORT levels and the degree of LTP[113] and PBP.[114] One study demonstrated that the same stressor that impaired learning/memory function also impaired LTP.[112] CORT insufficiency has also been shown to impair LTP.[115] Moreover, a U-shaped relation has been established between PBP induction and circulating CORT levels.[114]

This U-shaped relationship may reflect the dual MR and GR corticosteroid receptor systems. In the CA1 region of the hippocampus, it was shown that a MR agonist mimicked the facilitation of LTP produced by low doses of CORT, and a GR antagonist reversed the impairment of LTP produced by high CORT levels.[115] In the dentate gyrus of the hippocampus, a MR agonist reversed the adrenalectomy-induced LTP suppression and produced even higher LTP than that in nonoperated controls, while LTP was impaired following adrenalectomy and in the presence of a GR agonist.[116] Because of the high binding affinity of CORT to MRs, MRs are almost fully occupied even at basal CORT levels.[14] This maximal binding of CORT to MRs may underlie the optimal induction of LTP. Conversely, because CORT has a lower affinity for GRs than for MRs, GRs are maximally occupied only with high levels of CORT which occur during a stress response.[14] This may underlie the suppressive effects of GRs on LTP. Interestingly, a MR agonist that is known to reverse adrenalectomy-induced impairment of LTP[116] also reversed spatial learning/memory deficits produced by adrenalectomy.[106]

Chronic stress, in which there is elevated CORT levels over an extended period of time, has been shown to decrease cognitive function. The impairment may be mediated, at least partially by, CORT-induced dendritic atrophy, especially in the hippocampus where high concentrations of corticosteroid receptors are located. For example, daily 6 hr restraint stress[117] or daily CORT injections[118] for 21 days decreased dendritic branch points and total dendritic length of apical dendrites in the hippocampal CA3 pyramidal neurons. A functional significance of this dendritic atrophy may be decreased cognitive function, as demonstrated by deficits in spatial learning/memory following this stress regimen.[119] In fact, with this regimen a negative correlation has been established between CORT levels during restraint stress and spatial learning/memory performance.[120] Furthermore, the drugs phenytoin[121] and tianeptine[122] block not only the atrophy of CA3 dendrites, but also the impairments of spatial learning/memory function that are produced by the stress or CORT administration regimens.[119]

The effects of the 21 day CORT exposure regimen, including dendritic atrophy of CA3 hippocampal neurons[123] and spatial learning/memory deficits,[119] appears to be reversible. However, with more extended periods of CORT elevation, permanent neurodegeneration occurs. For example, following 12 wks of daily CORT administration, there was a permanent decrease of CA3 pyramidal cells.[124] The functional significance of this apparent CORT-induced neurodegeneration may be permanent impairment of cognitive function.[125]

Other evidence also supports a relationship between chronic glucocorticoid elevation and cognitive function. Major depression, dementia of the Alzheimer type, and Cushing's disease all have as characteristic features increased cortisol levels as well as decreased cognitive function.[126] With aging, basal levels of CORT are elevated as are CORT levels achieved during the stress response.[11] Accompanying this increased CORT secretion is greater hippocampal pyramidal cell loss, especially in CA3, and impairments on spatial learning/memory tasks.[125] Early handling studies also support the relationship between CORT levels and cognitive function. Early handling involves separation of pups from the dam for several minutes daily during the preweaning period.[127] This procedure produces permanent changes in HPA function. Better modulated CORT feedback in response to stressors, as well as less hippocampal CA1 and CA3 cell loss and better spatial learning/memory task performance are observed in handled compared to nonhandled animals.[128-129] Interestingly, following early handling, LTP has also been shown to be enhanced.[130]

The evidence presented supports a relationship between CORT levels and cognitive function and in its putative physiological correlates, LTP and PBP. Acute elevations of CORT produce impairments on learning/memory tasks and in LTP/PBP induction. Chronic elevations of CORT produce dendritic atrophy and death of hippocampal pyramidal cells, which produces reversible and permanent cognitive impairments, respectively. Prenatal ethanol exposure, which is characterized by hypersecretion of CORT during and following stressors, results in effects that are similar to those that are produced by high CORT exposure. Prenatal ethanol exposure produces cognitive deficits, and it has been shown that there are impairments in LTP in the CA1 region of the hippocampus.[131] Interestingly, prenatal ethanol exposure has also been shown to decrease pyramidal cell density and the number of dendritic spines of neurons in the hippocampus.[132-133] Thus, the decreased cognitive function observed following prenatal ethanol exposure may, in part, result from the hypersecretion of CORT, which also occurs in these animals.

VI. SUMMARY

Prenatal alcohol exposure produces many adverse consequences for the fetus, including hyperresponsiveness to stressors, characterized by increased secretion of HPA axis hormones. The mechanisms underlying this hyperresponsiveness is not fully understood, but may include increased anterior pituitary sensitivity to its secretagogues, alterations in neurotransmitter systems that regulate HPA function, and impairments in negative feedback control of HPA activity. Clearly, more research is required to completely elucidate the mechanisms that underlie this HPA hyperresponsiveness.

Prenatal alcohol exposure also produces many behavioral abnormalities such as hyperactivity and response inhibition, and cognitive impairments. The HPA hyperresponsiveness following prenatal alcohol exposure may play a role in the observed alterations in behavior and cognitive function.

REFERENCES

1. **Lemoine, P., Harousseau, H., Borteyru, J.-P., and Menuet, J.-C.,** Les enfants de parents alcooliques: Anomalies observees a propos de 127 cas, *Quest. Med.*, 21, 476, 1968.

2. **Jones, K.L. and Smith, D.W.,** Recognition of fetal alcohol syndrome in early infancy, *Lancet,* 2, 999, 1973.

3. **Jones, K.L., Smith, D.W., Ulleland, C.N., and Streissguth, A.P.,** Pattern of malformation in offspring of chronic alcoholic mothers, *Lancet,* 1, 1267, 1973.

4. **Sokol, R.J. and Clarren, S.K.,** Guidelines for use of terminology describing the impact of prenatal alcohol on the offspring, *Alc. Clin. Exp. Res.*, 13, 597, 1989.

5. **Streissguth, A.P. and LaDue, R.A.,** Fetal alcohol teratogenic causes of developmental disabilities, in *Toxic Substances and Mental Retardation: Neurobehavioral Toxicology and Teratology*, Schoroeder, S. R., Ed., American Association on Mental Deficiency, Washington, DC, 1987, 1.

6. **Streissguth, A.P., Landesman-Dwyer, S., Martin, J.C., and Smith, D.W.,** Teratogenic effects of alcohol in humans and laboratory animals, *Science*, 209, 353, 1980.

7. **Coles, C.D.,** Prenatal alcohol exposure and human development, in *Development of the Central Nervous System: Effects of Alcohol and Opiates*, Miller, M. W., Ed., Wiley-Liss, New York, 1992, 9.

8. **Schenker, S., Becker, H.C., Randall, C.L., Phillips, D.K., Baskin, G. S., and Henderson, G.I.,** Fetal alcohol syndrome: Current status of pathogenesis, *Alc. Clin. Exp. Res.*, 14, 635, 1990.

9. **Chrousos, G.P. and Gold, P.W.,** The concepts of stress and stress system disorders, *JAMA*, 267, 1244, 1992.

10. **Johnson, E.O., Kamilaris, T.C., Chrousos, G.P., and Gold, P.W.,** Mechanisms of stress: A dynamic overview of hormonal and behavioral homeostasis, *Neurosci. Biobehav. Rev.*, 16, 115, 1992.

11. **Sapolsky, R.M.,** *Stress, the Aging Brain, and the Mechanisms of Neuron Death*, MIT Press, Cambridge, 1992.

12. **Dallman, M.F., Akana, S.F., Cascio, C.S., Darlington, D.N., Jacobson, L., and Levin N.,** Regulation of ACTH secretion: Variations on a theme of B, *Recent Prog. Horm. Res.*, 43, 113, 1987.

13. **Reisine, T., Affolter, H.-U., Rougon, G., and Barbet, J.,** New insights into the molecular mechanisms of stress, *TINS*, 9, 574, 1986.

14. **Reul, J.M.H.M. and De Kloet, E.R.,** Two receptor systems for corticosterone in rat brain: Microdistribution and differential occupation, *Endocrinology*, 117, 2505, 1985.

15. **Reul, J.M.H.M. and De Kloet, E.R.,** Anatomical resolution of two types of corticosterone receptor sites in rat brain with *in vitro* autoradiography and computerized image analysis, *J. Steroid Biochem.*, 24, 269, 1986.

16. **De Kloet, E.R.,** Brain corticosteroid receptor balance and homeostatic control, *Front. Neuroendocrinol.*, 12, 95, 1991.

17. **Herman, J.P., Schafer, M.K.-H., Young, E.A., Thompson, R., Douglass, J., Akil, H., and Watson, S.J.,** Evidence for hippocampal regulation of neuroendocrine neurons of the hypothalamo-pituitary-adrenocortical axis, *J. Neurosci.*, 9, 3072, 1989.

18. **Sapolsky, R.M., Armanini, M.P., Packan, D.R., Sutton, S.W., and Plotsky, P.M.,** Glucocorticoid feedback inhibition of adreno-corticotropic hormone secretagogue release, *Neuroendocrinology*, 51, 328, 1990.

19. **Abou-Samra, A.-B., Catt, K.J., and Aguilera, G.,** Biphasic inhibition of adrenocorticotropin release by corticosterone in cultured anterior pituitary cells, *Endocrinology*, 119, 972, 1986.

20. **Dallman, F.M., Makara, G.B., Roberts, J.L., Levin, N., and Blum, M.,** Corticotrope response to removal of releasing factors and corticosteroids, *Endocrinology*, 117, 2190, 1985.

21. **Diorio, D., Viau, V., and Meaney, M.J.,** The role of the medial prefrontal cortex (cingulate gyrus) in the regulation of hypothalamic-pituitary-adrenal responses to stress, *J. Neurosci.*, 13, 3839, 1993.

22. **Kovacs, K.J., Kiss, Z.J., and Makara, G.B.,** Glucocorticoid implants around the hypothalamic paraventricular nucleus prevent the increase of corticotropin-releasing factor and arginine vasopressin immunostaining induced by adrenalectomy, *Neuroendocrinology*, 44, 229, 1986.

23. **Sawchenko, P.E.,** Evidence for a local site of action for glucocorticoids in inhibiting CRF and vasopressin expression in the paraventricular nucleus, *Brain Res.*, 403, 213, 1987.

24. **Dallman, M.F., Akana, S.F., Levin, N., Walker, C.-D., Bradbury, M.J., Suemaru, S., and Scribner, K.S.,** Corticosteriods and the control of function in the hypothalamo-pituitary-adrenal (HPA) axis, *Ann. N.Y. Acad. Sci.*, 746, 22,1994.

25. **Keller-Wood, M.E. and Dallman, M.F.,** Corticosteroid inhibition of ACTH secretion, *Endocr. Rev.*, 5, 1, 1984.

26. **Ratka, A., Sutanto, W., Bloemers, M., and De Kloet, E.R.,** On the role of brain mineralocorticoid (Type I) and glucocorticoid (Type II) receptors in neuroendocrine regulation, *Neuroendocrinology,* 50, 117, 1989.

27. **Dayanithi, G. and Antoni, F. A.,** Rapid as well as delayed inhibitory effects of glucocorticoid hormones on pituitary adrenocorticotropic hormone release are mediated by type II glucocorticoid receptors and require newly synthesized messenger ribonucleic acid as well as protein, *Endocrinology,* 125, 308, 1989.

28. **De Kloet, E. R., De Kock, S., Schild, V., and Veldhuis, D.,** Antiglucocorticoid RU38486 attenuates retention of a behavior and disinhibits the hypothalamic-pituitary-adrenal axis at different brain sites, *Neuroendocrinology,* 47, 109, 1988.

29. **Root, A.W., Reiter, E.O., Andriola, M., and Duckett, G.,** Hypothalamic-pituitary function in the fetal alcohol syndrome, *J. Pediatr.,* 87, 585, 1975.

30. **Binkiewicz, A., Robinson, M.J., and Senior, B.,** Pseudo-Cushing syndrome caused by alcohol in breast milk, *J. Pediatr.,* 6, 965, 1978.

31. **Jacobson, S.W., Jacobson, J.L., Bihun, J.T., Chiodo, L., and Sokol, R.J.,** Effects of prenatal alcohol exposure on poststress cortisol levels in infants, *Alc. Clin. Exp. Res.,* 17, 456, 1993.

32. **Weinberg, J.,** Prenatal ethanol exposure alters adrenocortical development of offspring, *Alc. Clin. Exp. Res.,* 13, 73, 1989.

33. **Weinberg, J. and Bezio, S.,** Alcohol-induced changes in pituitary-adrenal activity during pregnancy, *Alc. Clin. Exp. Res.,* 11, 274, 1987.

34. **Weinberg, J. and Gallo, P.V.,** Prenatal ethanol exposure: Pituitary-adrenal activity in pregnant dams and offspring, *Neurobehav. Toxicol. Teratol.,* 4, 515, 1982.

35. **Kakihana, R., Butte, J.C., and Moore, J.A.,** Endocrine effects of maternal alcoholization: Plasma and brain testosterone, dihydrotestostersone, estradiol, and corticosterone, *Alc. Clin. Exp. Res.,* 1, 57, 1980.

36. **Taylor, A.N., Branch, B.J., Kokka, N., and Poland, R.E.,** Neonatal and long-term neuroendocrine effects of fetal alcohol exposure, *Monogr. Neural Sci.,* 9, 140, 1983.

37. **Weinberg, J., Nelson, L.R., and Taylor, A.N.,** Hormonal effects of fetal alcohol exposure, in *Alcohol and Brain Development,* West, J. R., Ed., Oxford University Press, New York, 1986, 310.

38. **Angelogianni, P. and Gianoulakis, C.,** Prenatal exposure to ethanol alters the ontogeny of the β-endorphin response to stress, *Alc. Clin. Exp. Res.,* 13, 564, 1989.

39. **Taylor, A.N., Branch, B.J., Nelson, L.R., Lane, L.A., and Poland, R.E.,** Prenatal ethanol and ontogeny of pituitary-adrenal responses to ethanol and morphine, *Alcohol,* 3, 255, 1986.

40. **Taylor, A. N., Branch, B. J., Liu, S. H., and Kokka, N.,** Long-term effects of fetal ethanol exposure on pituitary-adrenal response to stress, *Pharmacol. Biochem. Behav.*, 16, 585, 1982.

41. **Weinberg, J.,** Hyperresponsiveness to stress: Differential effects of prenatal ethanol on males and females, *Alc. Clin. Exp. Res.*, 12, 647, 1988.

42. **Weinberg, J.,** Prenatal ethanol exposure effects: Sex differences in offspring stress responsiveness, *Alcohol,* 9, 219, 1992.

43. **Nelson, L.R., Taylor, A.N., Lewis, J.W., Poland, R.E., Redei, E., and Branch, B.J.,** Pituitary-adrenal responses to morphine and footshock stress are enhanced following prenatal alcohol exposure, *Alc. Clin. Exp. Res.,* 10, 397, 1986.

44. **Nelson, L.R., Taylor, A.N., Redei, E., Branch, B.J., and Lewis, J.W.,** Fetal exposure to ethanol enhances corticosterone release to footshock stress, *Alc. Clin. Exp. Res.*, 8, 109, 1984.

45. **Weinberg, J., Taylor, A.N., and Gianoulakis, C.,** Fetal ethanol exposure: Hypothalamic-pituitary-adrenal and β-endorphin responses to repeated stress, *Alc. Clin. Exp. Res.*, in press.

46. **Taylor, A.N., Branch, B.J., Van Zuylen, J.E., and Redei, E.,** Prenatal ethanol exposure alters ACTH stress response in adult rats, *Alc. Clin. Exp. Res.*, 10, 120, 1986.

47. **Weinberg, J.,** Prenatal ethanol exposure alters adrenocortical response to predictable and unpredictable stressors, *Alcohol,* 9, 427, 1992.

48. **Weinberg, J.,** *In utero* alcohol exposure and hypothalamic-pituitary-adrenal activity: Gender differences in outcome, in *Stress, Gender, and Alcohol-Seeking Behavior*, NIAA Alcohol Research Monograph, in press.

49. **Waltman, R. and Iniquez, E.,** Placental transfer of ethanol and its elimination at term, *Obstet. Gynecol.*, 40, 180, 1972.

50. **Eguchi, Y.,** Interrelationships between the foetal and maternal hypophyseal-adrenal axis in rats and mice, in *Physiology and Pathology of Adaptation Mechanisms*, Bajusz, E., Ed., Pergamon Press, New York, 1969, 3.

51. **Anderson, R.A.,** Endocrine balance as a factor in the etiology of the fetal alcohol syndrome, *Neurobehav. Toxicol. Teratol.*, 3, 89, 1981.

52. **Lee, S., Imaki, T., Vale, W., and Rivier, C.,** Effect of prenatal exposure to ethanol on the activity of the hypothalamic-pituitary-adrenal axis of the offspring: Importance of the time of exposure to ethanol and possible modulating mechanisms, *Mol. Cell Neurosci.*, 1, 168, 1990.

53. **Weichsel, M.E.,** The therapeutic use of glucocorticoid hormones in the perinatal period: Potential neurological hazards, *Ann. Neurol.*, 2, 364, 1977.

54. **Lee, S. and Rivier, C.,** Prenatal alcohol exposure blunts interleukin-1-induced ACTH and β-endorphin secretion by immature rats, *Alc. Clin. Exp. Res.*, 17, 940, 1993.

55. **Taylor, A.N., Branch, B.J.,Van Zuylen, J.E., and Redei, E.,** Maternal alcohol consumption and stress responsiveness in offspring, in *Mechanisms of Physical and Emotional Stress. Advances in Experimental Medicine and Biology,* Vol. 245, Chrousos, G. P., Loriaux, D. L., and Gold, P. W., Eds., Plenum Press, New York, 311, 1988.

56. **Yu, C., Osborn, J.A., and Weinberg, J.,** Increased adreno-corticotropin levels in response to corticotropin-releasing hormone administration following dexamethasone blockade in prenatal ethanol exposed rats, unpublished data.

57. **Lee, S. and Rivier, C.,** Prenatal alcohol exposure alters the hypothalamic-pituitary-adrenal axis response of offspring to interleukin-1: Possible mechanisms, *Alc. Clin. Exp. Res.,* 18, 470, 1994.

58. **Osborn, J.A., Stelzl, G.E., and Weinberg, J.,** Fetal ethanol effects on adrenal sensitivity to adrenocorticotropic hormone (ACTH), *Alc. Clin. Exp. Res.*, 18, 470, 1994.

59. **Palkovits, M.,** Organization of the stress response at the anatomical level, *Prog. Brain Res.,* 72, 47, 1987.

60. **Itoi, K., Suda, T., Tozawa, F., Dobashi, I., Ohmori, N., Sakai, Y., Abe, K., and Demura, H.,** Microinjection of norepinephrine into the paraventricular nucleus of the hypothalamus stimulates corticotropin-releasing factor gene expression in conscious rats, *Endocrinology,* 135, 2177, 1994.

61. **Lavicky, J. and Dunn, A. J.,** Corticotropin-releasing factor stimulates catecholamine release in hypothalamus and prefrontal cortex in freely moving rats as assessed by microdialysis, *J. Neurochem.,* 60, 602, 1993.

62. **Melia, K.R. and Duman, R. S.,** Involvement of corticotropin-releasing factor in chronic stress regulation of the brain noradrenergic system, *Proc. Nat.l Acad. Sci., USA,* 88, 8382, 1991.

63. **Rudeen, P.K. and Weinberg, J.,** Prenatal ethanol exposure: Changes in regional brain catecholamine content following stress, *J. Neurochem.,* 61, 1907, 1993.

64. **Osborn, J.A., Kim, C.K., Yu, W.K., Herbert, L., Zoeller, R.T., and Weinberg, J.,** Fetal ethanol effects on hypothalamic CRF mRNA levels following stress in dexamethasone treated animals, *Soc. Neurosci. Abstr.,* 21, 1390, 1995.

65. **Nelson, L.R., Taylor, A.N., Redei, E., Branch, B.J., and Liebeskind, J.C.,** Corticosterone response to dexamethansone in fetal ethanol-exposed rats, *Proc. West Pharmacol. Soc.,* 28, 299, 1985.

66. **Osborn, J.A., Kim, C.K., Yu, W., Herbert, L., and Weinberg, J.,** Fetal ethanol exposure alters pituitary-adrenal sensitivity to dexamethasone suppression, *Neuroendocrinology*, in press.

67. **Weinberg, J. and Petersen, T.D.,** Effects of prenatal ethanol exposure on glucocorticoid receptors in rat hippocampus, *Alc. Clin. Exp. Res.*, 15, 711, 1991.

68. **Abel, E.L., Jacobson, S., and Sherwin, B.T.,** *In utero* alcohol exposure: Functional and structural brain damage, *Neurobehav. Toxicol. Teratol.*, 5, 363, 1983.

69. **Kim, C.K., Yu, W., Osborn, J.A., and Weinberg, J.,** Prenatal ethanol exposure and glucocorticoid receptors in the hippocampus and hypothalamus, *Alc. Clin. Exp. Res.*, 18, 470, 1994.

70. **Kim, C.K., Yu, W., Edin, G., Herbert, K., Arkinstall, B., Lenger, B., Osborn, J.A., Gorzalka, B., and Weinberg, J.,** Prenatal ethanol exposure and glucocorticoid receptors, *Soc. Neurosci. Abstr.*, 21, 874, 1995.

71. **Lowy, M.T.,** Corticosterone regulation of brain and lymphoid corticosterone receptors, *J. Steroid Biochem. Molec. Biol.*, 39, 147, 1991.

72. **Sapolsky, R.M., Krey, L.C., and McEwen, B.S.,** Stress down-regulates corticosterone receptors in a site-specific manner in the brain, *Endocrinology*, 114, 287, 1984.

73. **Sapolsky, R.M. and McEwen, B.S.,** Down-regulation of neural corticosterone receptors by corticosterone and dexamethasone, *Brain Res.*, 339, 161, 1985.

74. **Streissguth, A.P.,** The behavioral teratology of alcohol: Performance, behavioral, and intellectual deficits in prenatally exposed children, in *Alcohol and Brain Development*, West, J. R., Ed., Oxford University Press, New York, 3, 1986.

75. **Streissguth, A.P., Aase, J.M., Clarren, S.K., Randels, S.P., LaDue, R.A., and Smith, D.F.,** Fetal alcohol syndrome in adolescents and adults, *JAMA*, 265, 1961, 1991.

76. **Bond, N.W.,** Prenatal alcohol exposure in rodents: A review of its effects on offspring activity and learning ability, *Austr. J. Psychol.*, 33, 331, 1981.

77. **Bond, N.W. and DiGiusto, E.L.,** Effects of prenatal alcohol consumption on open-field behavior and alcohol preference in rats, *Psychopharmacology*, 46, 163, 1976.

78. **Martin, J.C., Martin, D.C., Sigman, G., and Radow, B.,** Maternal ethanol consumption and hyperactivity in cross-fostered offspring, *Physiol. Psychol.*, 6, 362, 1978.

79. **Anandam, N., Felegi, W., and Stern, J.M.,** *In utero* alcohol heightens juvenile reactivity, *Pharmacol. Biochem. Behav.*, 13, 531, 1980.

80.   Riley, E.P., Shapiro, N.R., and Lochry, E.A., Nose-poking and head-dipping behaviors in rats prenatally exposed to alcohol, *Pharmacol. Biochem. Behav.*, 11, 513, 1979.
81.   Bond, N.W. and DiGiusto, E.L., Effects of prenatal alcohol consumption on shock avoidance learning in rats, *Psychol. Rep.*, 41, 1269, 1977.
82.   Gallo, P.V. and Weinberg, J., Neuromotor development and response inhibition following prenatal ethanol exposure, *Neurobehav. Toxicol. Teratol.*, 4, 505, 1982.
83.   Riley, E.P., Barron, S., Driscoll, C.D., and Chen, J.-S., Taste aversion learning in preweanling rats exposed to alcohol prenatally, *Teratology*, 29, 325, 1984.
84.   Lochry, E.A. and Riley, E.P., Retention of passive avoidance and T-maze escape in rats exposed to alcohol prenatally, *Neurobehav. Toxicol.*, 2, 107, 1980.
85.   Nelson, L.R., Taylor, A.N., Lewis, J.W., Branch, B.J., and Liebeskind, J.C., Opioid but not nonopioid stress-induced analgesia is enhanced following prenatal exposure to ethanol, *Psychopharmacology*, 85, 92, 1985.
86.   Nelson, L.R., Lewis, J.W., Liebeskind, J.C., Branch, B.J., and Taylor, A.N., Stress induced changes in ethanol consumption in adult rats exposed to ethanol *in utero*, *Proc. West Pharmacol. Soc.*, 26, 205, 1983.
87.   McEwen, B.S., De Kloet, E.R., and Rostene, W., Adrenal steroid receptors and actions in the nervous system, *Physiol. Rev.*, 66, 1121, 1986.
88.   Swanson, L.W., Sawchenko, P.E., Rivier, J., and Vale, W., Organization of ovine corticotropin-releasing factor immunoreactive cells and fibers in the rat brain: An immunohistochemical study, *Neuroendocrinology*, 36, 165, 1983.
89.   Nemeroff, C.B., New Vistas in neuropeptide research in neuropsychiatry: Focus on corticotropin-releasing factor, *Neuropsychopharmacology*, 6, 69, 1992.
90.   Dunn, A.J. and Berridge, C.W., Physiological and behavioral responses to corticotropin-releasing factor administration: Is CRF a mediator of anxiety or stress responses, *Brain Res. Rev.*, 15, 71, 1990.
91.   Valentino, R.J. and Foote, S.L., Corticotropin-releasing hormone disrupts sensory responses of brain noradrenergic neurons, *Neuroendocrinology*, 45, 28, 1987.
92.   Valentino, R.J. and Foote, S.L., Corticotropin-releasing hormone increases tonic but not sensory evoked activity of noradrenergic locus ceruleus neurons in unanesthetized rats, *J. Neurosci.*, 8, 1016, 1988.

233

93. **Arato, M., Banki, C.M., Nemeroff, C.B., and Bissette, G.,** Hypothalamic-pituitary-adrenal axis and suicide, *Ann. N.Y. Acad. Sci.,* 487, 263, 1986.

94. **Nemeroff, C.B., Wilderlov, E., Bissette, G., Walleu, S.H., Karlsson, I., Eklund, K., Kilts, C.D., Loosen, P.T., and Vale, W.,** Elevated concentrations of CSF corticotropin-releasing factor-like immunoreactivity in depressed patients, *Science,* 226, 1342, 1984.

95. **Blanchard, B.A., Riley, E.P., and Hannigan, J.H.,** Deficits on a spatial navigation task following prenatal exposure to ethanol, *Neurotoxicol. Teratol.,* 9, 253, 1987.

96. **Gianoulakis, C.,** Rats exposed prenatally to alcohol exhibit impairment in spatial navigation test, *Behav. Brain Res.,* 36, 217, 1990.

97. **Reyes, E., Wolfe, J., and Savage, D.D.,** The effects of prenatal alcohol exposure on radial arm maze performance in adult rats, *Physiol. Behav.,* 46, 45, 1989.

98. **Abel, E.L.,** Prenatal effects of alcohol on adult learning in rats, *Pharmacol. Biochem. Behav.,* 10, 239, 1979.

99. **Barron, S., Gagnon, W.A., Mattson, S.N., Kotch, L.E., Meyer, L. S., and Riley, E.P.,** The effects of prenatal alcohol exposure on odor associative learning in rats, *Neurotoxicol. Teratol.,* 10, 333, 1988.

100. **Randall, C.L., Becker, H.C., and Middaugh, L.D.,** Effect of prenatal ethanol exposure on activity and shuttle avoidance behavior in adult C57 mice, *Alcohol Drug Res.,* 6, 351, 1986.

101. **Diamond, D.M. and Rose, G.M.,** Stress impairs LTP and hippocampal-dependent memory, *Ann. N.Y. Acad. Sci.,* 743, 411, 1994.

102. **Kant, G.J.,** Effects of psychoactive drugs or stress on learning, memory, and performance as assessed using a novel water maze task, *Pharmacol. Biochem. Behav.,* 44, 287, 1993.

103. **Lambert, R. and Ven Murthy, M.R.,** Memory formation in birds: 2. Effects of stress due to experimental procedures on the conditioning of the budgerigar (melopsittacus undulatus) to sound stimuli, *Prog. Neuropsychopharmacol. Biol. Psychiatry,* 10, 25, 1986.

104. **Sharma, V.M. and Panwar, M.R.,** Variations in mental performance under moderate cold stress, *Int. J. Biometeorol.,* 31, 85, 1987.

105. **De Wied, D. and Croiset, G.,** Stress modulation of learning and memory processes, in *Methods Achieve Exp Pathol,* Vol. 15, Jasmin, G. and Proschek, L., Eds., Karger, Basel, 1991, 167.

106. **Vaher, P., Luine, V., Gould, E., and McEwen, B.S.,** Adrenalectomy impairs spatial memory in rats, *Ann. N.Y. Acad. Sci.,* 743, 405, 1994.

107. **Bliss, T. V. P. and Collingridge, G. L.,** A synaptic model of memory: Long-term potentiation in the hiipocampus, *Nature,* 361, 31, 1993.

108. **Nicoll, R. A. and Malenka, R. C.,** Contrasting properties of two forms of long-term potentiation in the hiipcampus, *Nature,* 377, 115, 1995.

109. **Eichenbaum, H. and Otto, T.,** The hippocampus--what does it do?, *Behav. Neural Biol.,* 57, 2, 1992.

110. **Rose, G.M. and Dunwiddie, T.V.,** Induction of hippocampal long-term potentiation using physiologically patterned stimulation, *Neurosci. Lett.,* 69, 244, 1986.

111. **Shors, T.J. and Dryver, E.,** Effect of stress and long-term potentiation (LTP) on subsequent LTP and the theta burst response in the dentate gyrus, *Brain Res.,* 666, 232, 1994.

112. **Diamond, D.M., Fleshner, M., and Rose, G.M.,** Psychological stress repeatedly blocks hippocampal primed burst potentiation in behaving rats, *Behav. Brain Res.,* 62, 1, 1994.

113. **Foy, M.R., Stanton, M.E., Levine, S., and Thompson, R.F.,** Behavioral stress impairs long-term potentiation in rodent hippocampus, *Behav. Neural Biol.,* 48, 138, 1987.

114. **Diamond, D.M., Bennett, M.C., Fleshner, M., and Rose, G.M.,** Inverted-U relationship between the level of peripheral corticosterone and the magnitude of hippocampal primed burst potentiation, *Hippocampus,* 2, 421, 1992.

115. **Rey, M., Carlier, E., Talmi, M., and Soumireu-Mourat, B.,** Corticosterone effects on long-term potentiation in mouse hippocampal slices, *Neuroendocrinology,* 60, 36, 1994.

116. **Pavlides, C., Watanabe, Y., Magarinos, A.M., and McEwen, B.S.,** Effects of glucocorticoid type I and type II agonists on hippocampal long-term potentiation, *Soc. Neurosci. Abstr.,* 18, 343, 1992.

117. **Watanabe, Y., Gould, E., and McEwen, B.S.,** Stress induces atrophy of apical dendrites of hippocampal CA1 pyramidal neurons, *Brain Res.,* 588, 341, 1992.

118. **Woolley, C.S., Gould, E., and McEwen, B.S.,** Exposure to excess glucocorticoids alters dendritic morphology of adult hippocampal pyramidal neurons, *Brain Res.,* 531, 225, 1990.

119. **Luine, V., Villegas, M., Martinez, C., and McEwen, B.S.,** Repeated stress causes reversible impairments of spatial memory performance, *Brain Res.,* 639, 167, 1994.

120. **Luine, V.N.,** Steroid hormone influences on spatial memory, *Ann. N.Y. Acad. Sci.,* 743, 201, 1994.

121. **Watanabe, Y., Gould, E., Cameron, H., Daniels, D., and McEwen, B. S.,** Phenytion prevents stress- and corticosteroid-induced atrophy of CA3 neurons, *Hippocampus,* 4, 431, 1992.

122. **Watanabe, Y., Gould, E., Daniels, D.C., Cameron, H., and McEwen, B.S.,** Tianeptine attenuates stress-induced morphological changes in the hippocampus, *Eur. J. Pharmacol.,* 222, 157, 1992.

123. **McEwen, B.S.,** Corticosteroids and hippocampal plasticity, *Ann. N.Y. Acad. Sci.,* 746, 134, 1994.

124. **Sapolsky, R.M., Krey, L.C., and McEwen, B.S.,** Prolonged glucocorticoid exposure reduces hippocampal neuron number: Implications for aging, *J. Neurosci.*, 5, 1222, 1985.

125. **Issa, A.M., Rowe, W., Gauthier, S., and Meaney, M.J.,** Hypothalamic-pituitary-adrenal activity in aged, cognitively impaired and cognitively unimpaired rats, *J. Neurosci.*, 10, 3247, 1990.

126. **Martignoni, E., Costa, A., Sinforiani, E., Liuzzi, A., Chiodini, P., Mauri, M., Bono, G., and Nappi, G.,** The brain as a target for adrenocortical steroids: Cognitive implications, *Psychoneuroendocrinology*, 17, 343, 1992.

127. **Meaney, M.J., Bhatnagar, S., Larocque, S., McCormick, C., Shanks, N., Sharma, S., Smythe, J., Viau, V., and Plotsky, P.M.,** Individual differences in the hypothalamic-pituitary-adrenal stress response and the hypothalamic CRF system, *Ann. N.Y. Acad. Sci.*, 697, 70, 1993.

128. **Meaney, M.J., Aitken, D.H., Bhatnagar, S., and Sapolsky, R.M.,** Postnatal handling attenuates certain neuroendocrine, anatomical, and cognitive dysfunctions associated with aging in female rats, *Neurobiol. Aging*, 12, 31, 1991.

129. **Meaney, M.J., Aitken, D.H., Van Berkel, C., Bhatnagar, S., and Sapolsky, R.M.,** Effect of neonatal handling on age-related impairments associated with the hippocampus, *Science*, 239, 766, 1988.

130. **Wilson, D.A., Willner, J., Kurz, E.M., and Nadel, L.,** Early handling increases hippocampal long-term potentiation in young rats, *Behav. Brain Res.*, 21, 223, 1986.

131. **Swartzwelder, H. S., Farr, K. L., Wilson, W. A., and Savage, D. D.,** Prenatal exposure to ethanol decreases physiological plasticity in the hippocampus of the adult rat, *Alcohol*, 5, 121, 1988.

132. **Hammer, R.P.,** Alcohol effects on developing neuronal structure, in *Alcohol and Brain Development*, West, J. R., Ed., Oxford University Press, New York, 1986, 184.

133. **Ward, G.R. and West, J.R.,** Effects of ethanol during development on neuronal survival and plasticity, in *Development of the Central Nervous System: Effects of Alcohol and Opiates*, Miller, M. W., Ed., Wiley-Liss, New York, 1992, 109.

Chapter 11

EFFECTS OF ETHANOL ON LACTATION

Marappa G. Subramanian, Ph.D.

I. INTRODUCTION

Lactation is a major component of reproduction in mammals. Although other animal species may feed their young, only in mammals is this process accomplished by the production of a glandular secretion under endocrine control. Mammary glands are modified cutaneous glands and are found in all mammals including the primitive ones like the duck bill platypus and the spiny anteater. Milk secreted by the mammary glands nourishes the young and colostrum, which has a high antibody titer, protects the young against disease during the initial days after birth. Milk secretion is a complex multistage process which includes the structural development of the mammary gland, the initiation of milk secretion at parturition and the maintenance of postpartum milk production.

Ethanol has multiple and varied effects on reproduction mainly by its effects on the endocrine function. Ethanol-induced changes in maternal endocrine glands could affect the female's ability to have normal lactation. In this chapter, following a brief description of mammary gland development, initiation and maintenance of lactation, studies examining ethanol's effect on lactation will be reviewed.

II. LACTATION

A. MAMMARY GLAND DEVELOPMENT

In humans, mammary gland development begins very early in fetal life, continues during the entire period of gestation and reaches a stage where there is some growth of the lobulo-alveolar system at birth. Additional growth takes place around the pubertal stage. The greatest morphological changes in mammary gland architecture take place during pregnancy. A detailed description of the development and differentiation of the mammary gland before the initiation of lactation is beyond the scope of this chapter and the reader is encouraged to refer to several earlier reviews in this area.[1-6] Mammary gland growth and differentiation is influenced by the pituitary (prolactin, growth hormone), thyroid (thyroxine), adrenal (glucocorticoids), ovarian (estrogen and progesterone) and pancreatic (insulin) hormones. In addition, the fetoplacental unit also functions as an endocrine organ influencing mammary development during late pregnancy by serving as a major source of steroids (estrogen and progesterone) and placental lactogen.

0-8493-7685-8/96/$0.00+$.50

The relative contribution of various hormones and the sequence of events in mammogenesis is difficult to assess. An additional factor in this complex process is the variation among species in the role played by different hormones in mammogenesis. Detailed studies in rodents have established that estrogen is essential for mammary gland duct growth, and estrogen and progesterone treatment results in both duct growth and lobulo-alveolar development. The full mammogenic response is accomplished by the presence of the pituitary hormones (prolactin or growth hormone) in addition to estrogen and progesterone. Other hormones that are listed above are required for providing optimal metabolic factors.[6-7]

B.   INITIATION OF LACTATION

During pregnancy increased secretion of prolactin, placental lactogen, cortisol, estrogens and progesterone completes the development of the mammary gland secretory apparatus. Although prolactin continues to rise throughout pregnancy, the full expression of prolactin action and the initiation of lactation during pregnancy is prevented by the presence of high levels of estrogen and progesterone, antagonizing prolactin's effects.   Following delivery, the levels of progesterone and estrogens decline, prolactin receptors in the mammary tissue increase, and milk secretion is initiated.

C.   MAINTENANCE OF LACTATION

Prolactin is not only essential for the development of the mammary gland during pregnancy, it is also needed for the initiation and maintenance of lactation after delivery. During lactation, prolactin level in the nonsuckled state is not elevated. Lactation is maintained by the surges of bioactive prolactin (molecular weight = 23,000) which occur in response to suckling.[8] It has long been known that the magnitude and the pattern of the rise in serum prolactin is affected by suckling.[9-10] This suckling-induced prolactin release maintains lactation and is essential for the mammary gland to produce adequate milk prior to the next feeding. It has also been suggested that optimal lactation is dependent on the frequency but not the duration of suckling.[11-12]

For normal milk ejection and emptying of the breast, oxytocin is necessary. This hormone is synthesized within the paraventricular and supraoptic nuclei of the hypothalamus. Bundles of long axons, the hypothalamo-hypophysial nerve tracts, connect the nuclei with the neural lobe of the pituitary gland. Oxytocin is synthesized within the above hypothalamic nuclei and packaged along with a specific protein called neurophysin into large granules that travel down the long axons. Oxytocin is released into the blood as part of a neuroendocrine reflex initiated by the suckling stimulus. Oxytocin causes the myoepithelial cells surrounding the alveoli and alveolar ducts to contract and expel the secreted milk.

III. ETHANOL AND LACTATION

Ethanol is a widely available and abused social drug. Many have expressed an opinion that ethanol consumed in moderation by lactating mothers would not have any discernible adverse effects. In a study done with eight nursing mothers given ethanol, it was reported that because of the large dilution of the ethanol contained in the milk by the baby's body water, the baby's resultant blood ethanol level was very low.[13] Although studies such as the above imply that occasional moderate intake of ethanol might not have any harmful effects on the infant, other studies detailed below indicate that lactating mothers should avoid ethanol consumption. It is of interest that the Committee on Drugs, established by the American Academy of Pediatrics[14-15] to study the transfer of drugs and other chemicals, classified ethanol as a drug compatible with breast feeding, although it is recognized that adverse effects may occur. These adverse effects include a decrease in linear growth, abnormal weight gain and decrease in the milk ejection reflex.

As noted previously, alcoholic beverages are believed to have a beneficial effect on lactation by promoting the milk "let down" reflex. Contrasting this belief, recent studies have shown that breast-fed infants consumed less milk during a 3-hour test session after their nursing mothers drank a small dose of ethanol in orange juice.[16] These same investigators have also reported that beer intake by lactating women adversely affected the sensory qualities of the milk and the nursing behavior of their infants. The infants consumed less milk during a 4-hour test session.[17]

A.   ETHANOL EXCRETION IN MILK

Ethanol is easily absorbed from the gastrointestinal tract. It is metabolized by oxidative pathways in the liver and the metabolized products are eliminated in the breath and urine. Ethanol freely passes into breast milk.[18] Wilson et al.[19] have reported that the amount of ethanol received by the infant in a single feeding from the mother with a blood ethanol level of 100% mg would be 164 mg, which is an insignificant amount.

It has been known for a long time that ethanol reaches human milk almost in the same concentration as it is in the blood and the elimination of ethanol in blood and milk is closely correlated.[13,20-21] In contrast, following ethanol intake, no acetaldehyde was found in milk, even though significant amounts were measured in the blood.[20] This observation is important because acetaldehyde, the major metabolite of ethanol, has been suggested to be the toxicity factor responsible for ethanol induced damage. Contrary to this report, Guerri and Sanchis[22] demonstrated that in rats administered ethanol via a liquid diet or gavage, acetaldehyde was present in milk and the concentration was about 35-50% that of blood.

B.   EXAGGERATED   ETHANOL   CLEARANCE   DURING LACTATION

In a series of studies, Abel and co-workers reported that ethanol clearance is faster in lactating rats compared to non-lactating rats. Further, the rate of ethanol disappearance was related to the intensity of suckling.[23-24] Our laboratory has reported a higher ethanol clearance rate for lactating rats[25] compared to ovariectomized rats.[26] A 40-50% hypertrophy of the liver is one of the many physiological changes that occur during lactation[27] and would explain the increased ethanol clearance rate during lactation. The faster ethanol clearance in lactating rats compared to non-lactators was not evident when the clearance rates were expressed per gram of liver.[28]

C.   ETHANOL EFFECTS ON THE MAMMARY GLAND AND MILK CONSTITUENTS

When rats were given ethanol in their drinking water (5%) from day 11 of gestation (term = day 22), the mammary gland weighed less and there was an indication of a reduced efficiency of milk secretion. When ethanol was given from parturition throughout lactation, no effects on the mammary gland were observed.[29] Ethanol administration in a liquid diet for 25 days prior to mating and then throughout pregnancy to lactation (day 2 or 10), altered the mammary gland structure during the early stages of lactation. A shorter duration of ethanol administration from day 1 of pregnancy through lactation day 2 or 10 did not result in any mammary tissue changes.[30] By employing a chronic ethanol administration regimen which started 4 weeks before mating and continued throughout pregnancy and into the latter part of lactation, Vilaro et al.[31] observed that, as measured by arterio-venous differences, the efficiency of acetaldehyde extraction by the lactating mammary gland was higher than that of ethanol. A histological examination of the mammary gland revealed that chronic ethanol administration resulted in a loss of mammary cell polarization, a reduction of the Golgi dictyosomal elements and abnormalities at the level of casein maturation and secretion; however, lipid secretion was not affected. Chronic ethanol administration also seems to affect mammary gland amino acid uptake. The effect appears to be selective and different according to the amino acid studied.[32]

When milk composition was examined following chronic ethanol administration starting from 4 to 5 weeks before mating, Sanchis and Guerri[33] noted that in the milk of alcoholic rats, the pH, protein and lipids were increased and lactose was decreased compared to controls. Ethanol administration in drinking water for 4 weeks before mating, during pregnancy and lactation, impaired mammary gland function as shown by the decline in milk production and other adverse effects. These effects include increases in dry weight and lipoprotein lipase activity of the mammary gland, and decreases in both absolute and relative mammary gland weight and protein content. The triacylglycerol concentration of milk from ethanol treated dams was increased whereas lactose concentration was decreased.[34] By employing a liquid diet paradigm for chronic ethanol administration to weanling rats (21-22 days old), it was observed that the density of carcinogen-sensitive terminal end bud structures of the developing mammary gland were increased and carcinogen-insensitive alveolar bud structures were decreased in ethanol fed rats compared to ad-lib and pair-fed controls. Ethanol feeding also adversely affected progesterone levels measured on the afternoon of proestrus and the adverse effect on the mammary gland development could be related to a decreased progesterone secretion in the ethanol fed group.[35] From the observations it is apparent that ethanol, especially when consumed over a longer duration, can affect the lactational process by influencing mammary gland development and physiology as well as milk constituents.

IV. ETHANOL'S EFFECT ON THE ENDOCRINE FUNCTIONS INFLUENCING LACTATION

As stated earlier, mammary gland development and the initiation and maintenance of lactation is influenced by a number of endocrine factors from the pituitary, ovarian, adrenal and thyroid glands. The act of suckling results in the release of oxytocin from the posterior pituitary which causes the contraction of myoepithelial cells surrounding the alveoli, resulting in milk ejection. Suckling also causes a sustained release of prolactin from the anterior pituitary which is essential for the maintenance of lactation. As Short[12] stated, "oxytocin serves today's meal and prolactin prepares tomorrow's." The effects of ethanol on these two major hormones involved in lactation will be reviewed here.

A.   ETHANOL'S EFFECT ON PROLACTIN SECRETION

Although a multitude of hormones are involved in the lactational process, prolactin is the key hormone controlling milk synthesis. Prolactin release from the anterior pituitary is stimulated by suckling-induced neural signals, transmitted by sensory nerves and transduced by the maternal hypothalamus to the anterior pituitary gland. This suckling-induced release of prolactin maintains lactation and is essential for the mammary gland to produce adequate quantities of milk prior to the next feeding.[12] Suckling is a powerful stimulus for the release of prolactin into the circulation during lactation. This suckling-induced prolactin has been well studied and characterized.[10,36-37]

For obvious ethical reasons, no studies have examined prolactin release in lactating women given ethanol. During the past decade we have studied the effects of acute and chronic ethanol administration on prolactin secretion and other lactational parameters in lactating rats. These studies have shown that acute and chronic (for 8 days) ethanol administration do not affect basal prolactin in the lactating rat when separated from pups; however, suckling-induced prolactin was inhibited.[25,38-41] Ethanol, when administered after the establishment of a suckling-induced prolactin surge, inhibited prolactin release; however, continued nursing pups for 120 minutes over-comes the inhibitory effect.[42] Our studies have established that ethanol does not act at the pituitary level to inhibit suckling-induced prolactin release. This was examined by the administration of prolactin secretagogues to lactating rats given ethanol[43-45] and *in vitro* studies.[43] The other mechanisms by which ethanol could inhibit suckling-induced prolactin release are by either acting at the hypothalamic and higher central nervous system or by disrupting the neural impulse transmission, engendered at the nipples in response to suckling.

In a study examining ethanol's effect on prolactin secretion in non-lactating normal women, ethanol diminished prolactin secretion following breast stimulation.[46]

B.   ETHANOL'S EFFECT ON OXYTOCIN SECRETION

In earlier studies, utilizing uterine contraction as the end point, it was implied that ethanol inhibited oxytocin release in the lactating rabbit,[47-49] rat[50] and woman.[51] In women given ethanol at doses up to 2.0 g/kg body weight, milk ejection was inhibited in a dose-dependent manner.[52] Similar to its effect on prolactin secretion,[46] ethanol inhibited oxytocin response to breast stimulation.[53]

V. PRENATAL ETHANOL EXPOSURE AND SUCKLING DEFICITS IN THE OFFSPRING

Infants born to mothers abusing ethanol exhibited severe feeding dysfunctions characterized by poor suck patterns. They also tired quickly while feeding and were distracted.[54-56] Similarly, rat pups prenatally exposed to ethanol take a longer time to attach to the nipple,[57] exert a lower maximum suckling pressure, spend less time suckling, and have a reduced number of rapid rhythmic sucks per unit amount of suckling time.[58] Prolactin released in foster dams in response to suckling by prenatally ethanol-exposed pups showed an interesting pattern. Although there was no difference between the control and the ethanol-exposed pups on day 6, suckling-induced prolactin was amplified in dams suckled by prenatally ethanol-exposed pups on day 10 of lactation. This paradoxical response was attributed to either a compensatory neuroendocrine mechanism in the foster dams for adequate milk secretion in response to the poor suckling or to the shorter but more frequent suckling episodes by prenatally ethanol-exposed pups. Increased time taken by the pups to attach to the nipple, a decreased milk consumption and a decreased growth rate were also observed in the group exposed to ethanol prenatally.[59] From these studies, it is obvious that prenatal ethanol exposure adversely affects suckling, which in turn may contribute to postnatal growth retardation

From these studies, it is obvious that prenatal ethanol exposure adversely affects suckling, which in turn may contribute to postnatal growth retardation and behavioral problems.[57-58,60-61]

VI. SUMMARY

The information presented above clearly indicates that ethanol has adverse effects on various aspects of lactation. It is safe to assume that ethanol has a disruptive effect at the hypothalamic, pituitary and mammary gland levels. This would result in the modulation of various endocrine and other factors directly involved in mammary gland growth, initiation and maintenance of lactation, and suckling behavior resulting in both the qualitative and quantitative changes in milk production. With the availability of a number of newer and more sensitive investigative tools, future investigations should delineate the mechanisms and sites of action of ethanol on endocrine, nutritional and other factors controlling lactation.

ACKNOWLEDGMENTS

The author is grateful to Dr. Michael W. Church for his valuable suggestions and comments in preparation of this review. This work was supported by National Institute on Alcohol Abuse and Alcoholism Grant No. AA07670.

REFERENCES

1. **Meites, J.,** Control of mammary growth and lactation, in Neuroendocrinology, Martini L. and Ganong W., Eds., Academic Press, New York, 1966, p. 669.
2. **Cowie, A.T. and Tindal, J.S.,** *The Physiology of Lactation*, Williams and Wilkins, Baltimore, 1971.
3. **Cowie, A.T.,** Overview of the mammary gland, *J. Invest. Dermatol.* 63, 2, 1974.
4. **Tucker, H.N.,** Endocrinology of lactation, *Semin. Perinatol.*, 3, 199, 1979.
5. **Topper, Y.J. and Freeman, C.S.,** Multiple hormone interactions in the developmental biology of mammary glands, *Physiol. Rev.*, 60, 1049, 1980.
6. **Whitworth, N.S.,** Lactation in Humans, *Psychoneuro-endocrinology*, 13, 171, 1988.

7. **Philip, J.,** Milk production and the effects of drugs, in *Drugs and Human Lactation,* Bennett, P.N., Ed., Elsevier, New York, 1988, p. 9.

8. **Liu, J.H., Lee, D.W., and Markoff, E.,** Differential release of prolactin variants in postpartum and early follicular phase women, *J. Clin. Endocrinol. Metab.*, 71, 605, 1990.

9. **Grosvenor, C.E. and Whitworth, N.S.,** Evidence for a steady rate of secretion of prolactin following suckling in the rat, *J. Dairy Sci.*, 57, 900, 1974.

10. **Subramanian, M.G. and Reece, R.P.,** Anterior pituitary and plasma prolactin in rats after 2 to 90 minutes of suckling, *Proc. Soc. Exp. Biol. Med.*, 149, 754, 1975.

11. **Konner, M. and Worthman, C.,** Nursing frequency, gonadal function, and birth spacing among Kung hunter-gatherers, *Science*, 207, 788, 1980.

12. **Short, R.V.,** Breast-feeding, *Sci. Am.*, 250, 35, 1984.

13. **Lawton, M.E.,** Alcohol in breast milk, *Aust. N.Z. J. Obstet. Gynaec.*, 25, 71, 1983.

14. **Committee on Drugs, American Academy of Pediatrics,** Transfer of drugs and other chemicals into human milk, *Pediatrics,* 84, 924, 1989.

15. **Committee on Drugs, American Academy of Pediatrics,** Transfer of drugs and other chemicals into human milk, *Pediatrics*, 93, 137, 1994.

16. **Mennella, J.A. and Beauchamp, G.K.,** The transfer of alcohol to human milk: Effects on flavor and infant's behavior, *N. Engl. J. Med.*, 325, 981, 1991.

17. **Mennella, J.A. and Beauchamp, G.K.,** Beer, Breastfeeding and Folklore, *Dev. Psychobiol.*, 26(8), 454, 1993.

18. **Vorheer, H.,** Drug excretion in breast milk, *Post-graduate Med.*, 56, 97, 1974.

19. **Wilson, J.T., Brown, R.D., Cherek, D.R., Dailey, J.W., Hilman, B., Jobe, P.C., Manno, B.R., Manno, J.E., Redetzki, H.M., and Stewart, J.J.,** Drug excretion in breast milk: Principles, pharmacokinetics and projected consequences, *Clin. Pharmacokinet.*, 5, 1, 1980.

20. **Kesaniemi, Y.A.,** Ethanol and acetaldehyde in the milk and peripheral blood of lactating women after ethanol administration, *J. Obstet. Gynaecol. Br. Common Wealth*, 81, 84, 1974.

21. **Flores-Hureta, S., Hernandez-Montes, H., Argote, R.M., and Villalpando, S.,** Effects of ethanol consumption during pregnancy and lactation on the outcome and postnatal growth of its offspring, *Ann. Nutr. Metab.*, 36, 121, 1992.

22. **Guerri, C. and Sanchis, R.,** Alcohol and acetaldehyde in rat's milk following ethanol administration, *Life Sci.*, 38, 1543, 1986.

23. **Abel, E.L.**, Effects of lactation on rate of blood ethanol disappearance, ethanol consumption, and serum electrolytes in the rat, *Bull. Psychonomic Soc.*, 14, 365, 1979.

24. **Abel, E.L., Greizerstein, H.B., and Siemens, A.J.**, Influence of lactation on rate of disappearance of ethanol in the rat, *Neurobehav. Toxicol.*, 1, 185, 1979.

25. **Subramanian, M.G., Chen, X.G., and Bergeski, B.A.**, Pattern and duration of the inhibitory effect of alcohol administered acutely on suckling-induced prolactin in lactating rats, *Alc. Clin. Exp. Res.*, 14, 771, 1990.

26. **Subramanian, M.G., Savoy-Moore, R.T., Bergeski, B.A., Kruger, M.L., and Abel, E.L.**, Acute alcohol infusion does not alter plasma gonadotropins or prolactin in ovariectomized rats. *Alc. Clin. Exp. Res.*, 14, 191, 1990.

27. **Williamson, D.H.**, Regulation of metabolism during lactation in the rat, *Reprod. Nutr. Dev.*, 26, 597, 1986.

28. **Gordon, B.H.J., Baraona, E., Miyakawa, H., Finkelman, F., and Lieber, C.S.**, Exaggerated acetaldehyde response after ethanol administration during pregnancy and lactation, *Alc. Clin. Exp. Res.*, 9, 17, 1985.

29. **Jones, W.L. and Stewart, D.B.**, Effects of orally-administered ethanol on mammary gland morphology and functional efficacy in lactating rats, *Exp. Pathol.*, 25, 205, 1984.

30. **Steven, W.M., Bulloch, B., and Seelig, Jr., L.L.**, A morphometric study of the effects of ethanol consumption on lactating mammary glands of rats, *Alc. Clin. Exp. Res.*, 13, 209, 1989.

31. **Vilaro, S., Vinas, O., and Remesar, X.**, Altered ultrastructure of lactating rat mammary epithelial cells induced by chronic ethanol ingestion, *Alc. Clin. Exp. Res.*, 13, 128, 1989.

32. **Vinas, O., Vilaro, S., Herrera, E., and Remesar, X.**, Effects of chronic ethanol treatment on amino acid uptake and enzyme activities in the lactating rat mammary gland, *Life Sci.*, 40, 1745, 1989.

33. **Sanchis, R. and Guerri, C.**, Chronic ethanol intake in lactating rats: Milk analysis, *Comp. Biochem. Physiol.*, 85, 107, 1986.

34. **Vilaro, S., Vinas, O., Remesar, X., and Herrera, E.**, Effects of chronic ethanol consumption on lactational performance in rat: Mammary gland and milk composition and pups' growth on metabolism, *Pharmacol. Biochem. Behav.*, 27, 333, 1987.

35. **Singletary, K.W. and McNary, M.Q.**, Effect of moderate ethanol consumption on mammary gland structural development and DNA synthesis in the female rat, *Alcohol*, 9, 95, 1992.

36.   Grosvenor, C.E., Mena, F., and Whitworth, N.S., The secretion rate of prolactin in the rat during suckling and its metabolic clearance rate after increasing intervals of non-suckling, *Endocrinology,* 104, 372, 1979.

37.   Mattheij, J.A.M., Guisen, E.F.M., and Swarts, J.J.M., The suckling-induced rise of prolactin in lactating rats: Its dependence on stage of lactation and litter size, *Hormone Res.*, 11, 325, 1979.

38.   Subramanian, M.G. and Abel, E.L., Alcohol inhibits suckling-induced prolactin release and milk yield, *Alcohol*, 5, 95, 1988.

39.   Subramanian, M.G., Chen, X.G., Bergeski, B.A., and Savoy-Moore, R.T., Alcohol inhibition of suckling-induced prolactin release in lactating rats: Threshold evaluation, *Alcohol*, 8, 203, 1991.

40.   Subramanian, M.G. and Savoy-Moore, R.T., Alcohol and Endocrine Function: Effects on Prolactin Release, in *Advances in Endocrinology, Metabolism and Diabetes*, Vol. 1, Kochupillai, Ed., McMillan India Ltd., New Delhi, 1992, 191.

41.   Subramanian, M.G., Effects of chronic alcohol administration on lactational performance in the rat, *Alcohol*, 12, 137, 1995.

42.   Subramanian, M.G., Inhibitory effect of alcohol on the established suckling-induced prolactin surge in lactating rats, *Proc. Soc. Exp. Biol. Med.*, 198, 579, 1991.

43.   Subramanian, M.G. and Savoy-Moore, R.T., Alcohol effects on TRH-induced prolactin response in lactating rats: *In vivo* and *in vitro* studies, *Alcohol*, 10, 11, 1993.

44.   Subramanian, M.G., ß-endorphin stimulated prolactin release in lactating rats following alcohol administration, *Alcohol*, 11, 269, 1994.

45.   Subramanian, M.G., Prolactin secretion in lactating rats following chronic alcohol exposure: Provocative tests with secretagogues, *Life Sci.*, 57, 533, 1995.

46.   Volpi, R., Chiodera, P., Gramellini, D., Cigarini, C., Papadia, C., Caffarri, G., Rossi, G., and Coiro, V., Endogenous opioid mediation of the inhibitory effect of ethanol on the prolactin response to breast stimulation in normal women, *Life Sci.*, 54, 739, 1994.

47.   Fuchs, A.R. and Wagner, G., Effect of alcohol and release of oxytocin, *Nature*, 198, 92, 1963.

48.   Fuchs, A.R. and Wagner, G., Quantitative aspects of release of oxytocin by suckling in unanesthetized rabbits, *Acta Endocrinol.*, 44, 581, 1963.

49.   Fuchs, A.R. and Wagner, G., The effect of ethyl alcohol on the release of oxytocin in rabbits, *Acta Endocrinol.*, 44, 593, 1963.

50.   Fuchs, A.R., Ethanol and the inhibition of oxytocin release in lactating rats, *Acta Endocrinol.*, 62, 546, 1969.

51. **Wagner, G. and Fuchs, A.R.**, Effect of ethanol on uterine activity during suckling in post-partum women, *Acta Endocrinol.*, 58, 133, 1968.

52. **Cobo, E.**, Effect of different doses of ethanol on the milk-ejecting reflex in lactating women, *Am. J. Obstet. Gynecol.*, 15, 817, 1973.

53. **Coiro, V., Alboni, A., Gramellini, D., Cigarini, C., Bianconi, L., Pignatti, D., Volpi, R., and Chiodera, P.**, Inhibition by ethanol of the oxytocin response to breast stimulation in normal women and the role of endogenous opioids, *Acta Endocrinol.*, 126, 213, 1992.

54. **Ouelette, E.M., Rosett, H.L., Rosman, N.P., and Weiner, L.**, Adverse effects on offspring of maternal alcohol abuse during pregnancy, *N. Engl. J. Med.*, 297, 528, 1977.

55. **Martin, D.C., Martin, J.C., Streissguth, A.P., and Lund, C.A.**, Suckling frequency and amplitude in newborns as a function of maternal drinking and smoking, in *Currents in Alcoholism*, Vol. 5, Galanter, M., Ed., Grune and Stratton, New York, 1979, 359.

56. **Van Dyke, D.C., Mackay, L., and Zriaglek, E.N.**, Management of severe feeding dysfunction in children with fetal alcohol syndrome, *Clin. Pediatr.*, 21, 336, 1982.

57. **Chen, J., Driscoll, C.D., and Riley, E.P.**, Ontogeny of suckling behavior in rats prenatally exposed to alcohol, *Teratology*, 26, 145, 1982.

58. **Rockwood, G.A. and Riley, E.P.**, Suckling deficits in rat pups exposed to alcohol *in utero*, *Teratology*, 33, 145, 1986.

59. **Subramanian, M.G.**, Lactation and prolactin release in foster dams suckling prenatally exposed pups, *Alc. Clin. Exp. Res.*, 16, 891, 1992.

60. **Abel, E.L.**, *In utero* alcohol exposure and developmental delay of response inhibition, *Alc. Clin. Exp. Res.*, 6, 369, 1982.

61. **Lochry, E.A., Shapiro, N.R., and Riley, E.P.**, Growth deficits in rats exposed to alcohol *in utero*, *J. Stud. Alcohol*, 4, 1031, 1980.

Chapter 12

INVOLVEMENT OF PROSTAGLANDINS
IN FETAL ALCOHOL SYNDROME

Jocelynn L. Saulnier and Carrie L. Randall

I. GENERAL OVERVIEW

It is generally well established that alcohol is a teratogen, producing classical behavioral and physical anomalies in exposed offspring. Although there has been much progress since the fetal alcohol syndrome was first described and recognized in 1973,[1-2] the underlying biochemical mechanism remains to be elucidated. Many mechanisms have been proposed to describe at least some of ethanol's teratogenic effects. One suggested mechanism is ethanol-induced changes in physiological mediators called *prostaglandins*.

The rationale for studying prostaglandin involvement in the fetal alcohol syndrome is based on experimental evidence in a number of areas. It has been well documented that prostaglandins play roles in fetal development and that the administration of exogenous prostaglandins is associated with fetal anomalies. Also, it is known that ethanol influences prostaglandin production and that prenatal exposure to ethanol induces fetal abnormalities in growth and development. These concepts have led to theories implicating a role for prostaglandins in alcohol-induced fetal anomalies. Based on these findings, it has been postulated that prostaglandins, either directly or indirectly, may contribute to the teratogenic actions of alcohol.[3-4]

II. PROSTAGLANDINS

As a result of their ubiquitous nature, interest in prostaglandins has been generated in many scientific fields, including biochemistry, physiology, pharmacology, neuroscience, and obstetrics and gynecology. As stated above, prostaglandins have been implicated to play roles in the induction of alcohol-induced birth defects. However, before further examination of this issue, it is necessary to discuss briefly the biochemistry of prostaglandins.

Prostaglandins are 20-carbon chain fatty acids that act as local hormones to regulate physiological functions of almost all cells of the body. Prostaglandins may be of the 2-series type, derived from arachidonic acid, or of the 1-series type, derived from related fatty acid precursors. This chapter will focus on the 2-series prostaglandins because of the roles they play in pregnancy[5] and because of their implications in alcohol research.[6]

Prostaglandins of the 2-series are formed by the liberation of arachidonic acid from the plasma membrane by the enzyme phospholipase A_2. The enzyme cyclooxygenase converts arachidonic acid to the 2-series prostaglandins, including thromboxane (TXA_2), prostacyclin (PGI_2), prostaglandin E_2 (PGE_2), and prostaglandin F_{2a} (Figure 1). Non-steroidal anti-inflammatory agents (NSAIA), such as aspirin, indomethacin, and ibuprofen prevent the production of prostaglandins by inhibiting cyclooxygenase. These drugs have been used experimentally, as well as clinically, to reduce prostaglandin levels in conditions characterized by excess prostaglandin production.[7-10]

The Arachidonic Acid Cascade

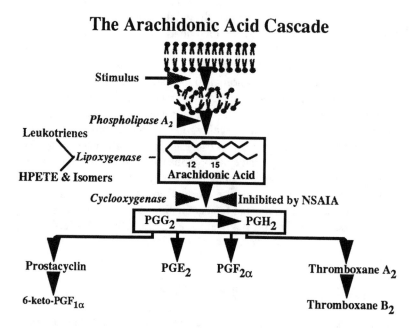

Figure 1. The generation of prostaglandins through the arachidonic acid cascade involves the liberation of arachidonic acid from the plasma membrane by phospholipase A_2. Cyclooxygenase converts arachidonic acid to PGG_2, which then converts to PGH_2. From PGH_2, specific prostaglandins, including prostacyclin, prostaglandins E_1 and E_2, prostaglandin F_{2a}, and thromboxane, are generated through the action of specific prostaglandin synthetase enzymes. Cyclooxygenase is inhibited by non-steroidal anti-inflammatory agents (NSAIA), such as ibuprofen, indomethacin, and aspirin.

Prostaglandins are sensitive to alcohol in many model systems, and exposure of human and animal tissues to ethanol, *in vivo* and *in vitro*, has been shown to alter prostaglandin levels.[11-17] The prostaglandins influenced by ethanol and their direction of change seem to differ in a dose- and tissue-specific manner. The step that ethanol influences in the arachidonic acid cascade remains to be clarified, an issue that will be discussed in the following sections of this chapter.

A.   ROLES OF PROSTAGLANDINS IN PREGNANCY

The roles that prostaglandins play in pregnancy and in fetal development are important to recognize when evaluating the involvement of prostaglandins in the fetal alcohol syndrome. Since prostaglandins play roles in almost all stages of pregnancy as well as in fetal development itself, disruptions in these mediators may result in abnormal *in utero* development.

There is abundant evidence that prostaglandins play important regulatory roles in various aspects of human pregnancy and parturition, including in implantation,[18] in labor,[5,19] and in fetal growth and development.[20-21] On a clinical level, these compounds have been used in pregnancy since 1967 for induction of labor,[22] for the termination of pregnancy,[23] and for preparation of the cervix for the induction of labor.[24]

Clinical studies have found high concentrations of prostaglandins in decidua, in amniotic fluid, and in blood of women in labor.[25-28] These data provide strong evidence that prostaglandins play important physiological roles in human labor. Additionally, prostaglandins have also been shown, *in situ*, to exhibit marked contractile effects on the pregnant human uterus,[29-30] lending further support to their importance in parturition.

Because of the involvement of prostaglandins in many stages of pregnancy, there is promising potential for pharmacological intervention in obstetrics. Drugs, such as aspirin, that inhibit the cyclooxygenase enzyme reduce prostaglandin production and have been used clinically to arrest premature labor and to delay the progress of induced abortion.[31] Aspirin is also used to treat pre-eclampsia, a condition characterized by abnormal prostaglandins levels where perinatal outcome is at risk.[10,32] In cases of induced abortion and situations of pre-eclampsia, the importance of pharmacological intervention and of the resulting therapeutic benefits of prostaglandins and prostaglandin inhibitors is apparent.

B.   ROLES OF PROSTAGLANDINS IN FETAL DEVELOPMENT

Perhaps related to their roles in fetal development is the fact that elevated prostaglandin levels, especially PGE, often lead to abnormal fetal development. *In utero* exposure to exogenous prostaglandins has been shown to result invariably in maternal and fetal complications, including termination of pregnancy,[33] degeneration of corpora lutea,[34-35] and either embryonic death[36] or the induction of fetal malformations.[37-38] In this way, the elevation of prostaglandin levels may be considered to influence fetal development *directly*.

In general, the induction of fetal malformations as a result of direct *in utero* exposure to prostaglandins suggests that prostaglandins may exert teratogenic effects. There are, in fact, data supporting evidence that the elevation of prostaglandin levels in response to ethanol may play roles in alcohol-induced teratogenesis in animals.[39-41]

1. PGE

Persaud showed that intra-amniotic administration of prostaglandin E_2 to rat fetuses resulted in either fetal death or in resorptions in 100% of the fetuses.[42] Similar embryopathic evidence was found when developing chick eggs[37] and pregnant rabbits[43] were treated with prostaglandin E_2. In another study, treatment of pregnant mice with a single dose of prostaglandin E_2 did not significantly increase the incidence of embryonic deaths and of fetal resorptions compared to the corresponding controls but did increase the incidence of abnormal fetuses.[38] These studies provide evidence that PGE_2 administration to pregnant animals results in abnormal pregnancy outcome, including fetal malformations in surviving pups.

2. PGF_{2a}

The teratogenic role of PGF_{2a} is less clear, although it does play a potential role in fetal development. For instance, it is known that $PGF2_a$ promotes implantation[44] and that the F-series prostaglandins act as extremely powerful growth factors for neonatal rat hepatocytes.[45] In fact, administration of prostaglandin F_{2a} to pregnant mice resulted in a high incidence of intrauterine deaths and fetal resorptions but did not, however, induce developmental defects.[46] This suggests that PGF_{2a} may interfere with fetal survival by compromising maternal ability to maintain pregnancy or by inducing fetal malformations extreme enough to result in resorption or to result in *in utero* death.

3. Thromboxane

Like PGE and $PGF2_a$, elevated fetal thromboxane levels have also been suggested to influence normal fetal growth and development. However, there are few studies where this relationship has been examined. Direct exposure to exogenous thromboxane B_2 was found to be embryopathic in the chick, with administration provoking a high incidence of anomalies, including growth retardation and everted viscera.[36] Since thromboxane is a potent vasoconstrictor, it is tempting to speculate that these effects are a result of vascular changes within the fetus or within the umbilical vessels. It is less likely that thromboxane itself has direct teratogenic effects.

4. Prostaglandin Precursors

Results from a study using arachidonic acid, a prostaglandin precursor, also provide evidence that elevated prostaglandins play a role in the induction of fetal complications. Reproductive outcomes in pregnant mice who received an injection of exogenous arachidonic acid were worse than those in mice receiving only vehicle injections.[47] Exogenous administration of a prostaglandin precursor, such as arachidonic acid, will increase prostaglandin production by target tissues. Once again, data indicate that elevated prostaglandin levels may play a role in adverse pregnancy outcomes.

5. Prostaglandin Inhibitors

Studies involving prostaglandin inhibitors have provided evidence for the possible involvement of prostaglandins in alcohol-induced teratogenesis. Data have been published by researchers using chicks,[39] mice,[48-49] and sheep,[50-52] indicating that the cyclooxygenase inhibitors ibuprofen and indomethacin antagonize alcohol's effects on fetal growth and development. One study, on the other hand, did not find evidence that aspirin antagonized the effects of prenatal alcohol exposure.[53]

In general, however, aspirin seemed to be a powerful protectant against alcohol-induced birth defects.[49] Pretreatment with aspirin prior to alcohol exposure caused an attenuation of alcohol-induced birth defects in mice.[54] On the other hand, aspirin did not block the teratogenic actions of ethanol if it was administered following intragastric alcohol treatment.[54] This indicates that the inhibition of the prostaglandin-synthesizing enzyme cyclooxygenase must be completed before introduction of alcohol for there to be any protective effect. Presumably, inhibition after alcohol introduction is too late to prevent alcohol-induced increases in prostaglandins, especially in PGE. More recently, the magnitude of prostaglandin E inhibition in mouse uterine/embryo tissue has been positively correlated with the extent to which aspirin protects against alcohol-induced fetal malformations.[55]

Aspirin has been shown to cross the placenta easily,[56] and this may account for aspirin's powerful protective effect. By crossing the placenta, the drug administered to the maternal circulation is able to reach the fetal circulation quickly. In this way, aspirin may be acting to inhibit prostaglandin production in fetal tissues, thus offering its protective effect against alcohol. On the other hand, indomethacin crosses the placenta of rodents during the period of organogenesis with difficulty,[49] if at all.[57] The inability of indomethacin to cross the placenta readily and to reach the fetal circulation at the time of alcohol exposure may explain its less effective protective effect in rodents.

6. Prostaglandins and the Neurobehavioral Effects of Ethanol

In addition to mediating the physical teratogenic effects of ethanol discussed above, increased prostaglandin levels have also been proposed as a potential mechanism for some of alcohol's *neurobehavioral* teratogenic effects. This theory stems from the fact that ethanol increases prostaglandin levels in the brains of mice. In one study, data indicate that ethanol administration increased brain prostaglandin levels in a dose-, sex-, and genotype-dependent manner,[15] and results are consistent with the theory that ethanol stimulates prostaglandin production. These data suggest that ethanol-induced stimulation of prostaglandin production may explain some of ethanol's behavioral effects.

Prostaglandin inhibitors have been successful, in some cases, in antagonizing some ethanol-induced behaviors in adult mice not exposed prenatally to ethanol.[15,58-61] However, prostaglandin inhibitors given to pregnant rats fed a liquid diet containing alcohol failed to antagonize alcohol-induced behavioral anomalies in the offspring.[62] Also, Bonthius and West [63] did not show any benefit of concomitant alcohol and aspirin administration to neonatal rat pups on brain weight. Whether these negative findings are a result of species differences, of methodological differences, or of differential protective capacity (e.g., aspirin can protect against ethanol-induced physical malformations, but not against behavioral anomalies or brain weight) remains to be clarified. The differential effects of the prostaglandin inhibitors on alcohol-induced morphological and behavioral teratogenesis may have important implications, for they suggest that prostaglandins may be involved in only *some* of the features of the fetal alcohol syndrome.

C. THE VASOACTIVE EFFECTS OF PROSTAGLANDINS

In addition to their possible teratogenic actions, prostaglandins also exert potent vasoactive effects on uterine, placental, and umbilical vessels. The indirect role that prostaglandins have been implicated to play in the mechanism of ethanol-induced fetal malformations centers around the disruption of blood flow in these tissues. This indirect role of prostaglandins is important because reduced blood flow in the uterine, placental, or umbilical vessels may decrease vitamin, amino acid, glucose, and nutrient availability to the fetus by impairing placental transport of these compounds. Fetal oxygen supply may also be limited by decreased blood flow. These reductions in substrate availability may adversely affect the developing fetus.

It has been documented that as little as 5% to 10% reduction in placental volume may be associated with poor perinatal outcomes including growth retardation, fetal hypoxia, and perinatal death.[64] Since prenatal ethanol exposure to animals has been associated with all of these problems, it is possible, then, that ethanol may be inducing abnormal perinatal outcome by decreasing blood flow in uterine, in placental, and/or in umbilical vessels. An ethanol-induced reduction of blood flow in these tissues has been proposed as a potential mechanism for the pathophysiology of alcohol.[4,65-66] Vasoactive prostaglandins that regulate blood flow in these tissues may mediate this indirect effect of alcohol.

Vasoactive prostaglandins include PGE, PGF_{2a}, PGI_2, and TXA_2. Neither PGE nor PGF_{2a} exerts strong vasoactive effects on uterine, on placental, nor on umbilical vessels, and for that reason, this chapter will focus on the more potent prostaglandins, PGI_2 and TXA_2. The specific roles that TXA_2 and pro-stacyclin PGI_2 play in the normal physiology of human pregnancy remain to be established, although these vasoactive prostaglandins have been implicated as major regulators of umbilical/placental blood flow.[8,67-68] Prostacyclin is a potent platelet anti-aggregator and vasodilator produced mainly by endothelial cells. Thromboxane, the biological antagonist to prostacyclin, is produced in large amounts by platelets and to a lesser degree by vascular endothelium and by smooth muscle. Thromboxane functions as a platelet aggregator and as a powerful vasoconstrictor.

A shift in the normal ratio of TXA_2 to PGI_2 characterizes a condition in pregnancy called pre-eclampsia. Pre-eclampsia and other chronic placental insufficiency syndromes are accompanied by a reduction in PGI_2 levels in the mother and in fetomaternal tissues as well as by an overproduction of TXA_2 in the placenta.[10,32] In pre-eclamptic patients there is decreased uteroplacental blood flow and often uteroplacental ischemia. The consequences of placental vascular insufficiency, such as the vascular insufficiency characteristic of pre-eclampsia, on perinatal outcome are mentioned above, and it is possible that ethanol might influence fetal growth and development through shifting the TXA_2 to PGI_2 ratio.

1. Prostaglandins and Uterine Blood Flow

Adequate maintenance of uterine blood flow during pregnancy is crucial for normal fetal growth as fetal growth has been shown to be directly related to incremental increases in uterine blood flow.[69] Thus, a significant decrease in uterine blood flow during pregnancy may be associated with both maternal and fetal complications.[70] For example, temporary clamping of the uterine blood vessels during late pregnancy in rats resulted in hemorrhage and in tissue necrosis in the extremities of the fetuses.[71] This study was done to mimic uterine trauma, but the significant reduction in blood flow due to clamping may resemble a consequence of maternal exposure to high levels of ethanol. Consequently, long term alterations in the normal incremental increase of this flow could disrupt oxygen and nutrient supply to the fetus,[69] thus leading to abnormal growth of the fetus and of the placenta.

The utero-placental unit has been shown to produce significant amounts of prostaglandins E and F[72-73] during pregnancy. These prostaglandins have been purported to play important roles in the regulation of uterine blood flow throughout pregnancy. Consequently, alterations in prostaglandin levels may impair uterine blood flow. If ethanol influences prostaglandin production in the uterus, disrupting normal blood flow, this may be a mechanism by which ethanol interferes with fetal growth and development. Indeed, prostaglandins are influenced by alcohol in both human and animal uterine tissue. Alcohol increased uterine PGE_2 and PGF_{2a} levels both when given in a liquid diet[74] and when given as a single injection to rats.[75]

Prostaglandins play a regulatory role in uterine contractility [76] as well as in the regulatory role in uterine blood flow discussed above. Interestingly, PGE_2 and PGF_{2a} both induce contraction, to some degree, of the uterus.[77-79] This may explain the usefulness of prostaglandins as abortifacients.

However, although PGE_2 and PGF_{2a} are increased by ethanol and induce uterine contractions, alcohol has traditionally been used to inhibit uterine contractions in both humans and animals. The ability of ethanol to induce contractions or to induce relation of the myometrium may be dependent upon concentration of ethanol and duration of exposure (e.g., chronic ethanol may influence uterine contraction differently that acute ethanol exposure). Alcohol infusions have been used to attenuate uterine contractions and to prevent threatened premature labor[80] in obstetrical patients. Similarly, increased gestation length associated with administration of ethanol to rodents[81] may also be attributable to alcohol's inhibitory effects on uterine contractions. The ability of ethanol to relax the uterine myometrium, however, is the result of the anti-oxytocic actions of ethanol[82-84] and does not seem to involve ethanol-induced changes in prostaglandins.

Results from human and from animal studies reveal that there is a definite relationship between alcohol, prostaglandins, and uterine contraction. Data also indicate that the regulation of uterine blood flow may be altered by ethanol and by prostaglandins. However, these are yet other areas where further study is needed to define the interactions.

2. Prostaglandins and Blood Flow in the Umbilical/Placental System

Adequate placental and umbilical vessel perfusion ensures that substrates necessary for fetal growth and development become available to the growing fetus. The umbilical vein is the sole vessel carrying substances, via the placenta, from the mother to the fetus. Two umbilical arteries return fetal waste to the placenta, where it is transferred to the maternal circulation for removal. The maintenance of blood flow in these vessels dictates fetal substrate availability. Hence, alterations in either placental or umbilical blood flow could restrict compounds available to the fetus, many of which may be necessary for normal *in utero* growth and development. Decreased umbilical artery flow could affect the ability of the fetus to remove waste metabolites and could impair fetal oxygenation. Decreased blood flow in the umbilical vein could impair oxygen and other substrates from reaching the fetal circulation.

Ethanol is known to interfere with umbilical/placental blood flow,[85] although the mechanisms are not well understood. Ethanol diffuses freely across the placenta,[86-89] rendering the fetal tissues susceptible to the effects of ethanol as a result of maternal ingestion. By crossing the placenta and entering the fetal circulation, ethanol may affect prostaglandins in fetal as well as in maternal tissues.

It is of importance to note that the vessels of the umbilical/placental system lack nervous innervation,[90] and blood flow regulation in this system is entirely dependent upon the local production of humoral factors, including prostaglandins. In fact, it is the *balance* between vasoactive prostaglandins that has been proposed as a major factor in the regulation of blood flow in the umbilical/placental system.[32,67]

a. Umbilical Vessels

The prostaglandins PGE_2, $PGF_{2\alpha}$,[91] and TXA_2[92] have all been shown to constrict umbilical vessels, while PGI_2 acts to vasodilate them. The production of these vasoactive prostaglandins has demonstrated an ethanol influence.[93-95] Ethanol may differentially affect the vasoactive prostaglandins. Ethanol may increase[13,96] or decrease[7] the levels of vasoconstrictive prostaglandins, and, in other cases, ethanol may affect the production of the vasodilatory prostaglandins.[97-98] Whether ethanol acts to contract or to relax umbilical vessels seems dependent upon the dose of ethanol and the duration of exposure.

Ethanol exerts vasoactive effects in umbilical arteries and in veins, both of which have been shown to constrict in response to ethanol exposure.[99-100] Umbilical vessels, however, under normal circumstances are maximally dilated with very little resistance and with high blood flow, which may be a result of the high levels of prostacyclin produced in these vessels. This may be a feto-protective mechanism, especially given the fact that umbilical veins are less sensitive to the vasoconstrictive effects of ethanol than are umbilical arteries.[101]

Our laboratory has shown that perfusion of human umbilical veins with an ethanol solution results in prostaglandin levels that differ from control levels. These ethanol-induced differences in prostaglandins may be the way that ethanol compromises blood flow in the umbilical-placental unit. For example, PGI_2 levels were decreased by about 50% after 60 minutes of perfusion with 100 mM ethanol, and the ratio between thromboxane and PGI_2 was significantly increased after just five minutes of perfusion with the 100 mM ethanol solution.[98] The shift towards vasoconstriction through reduction of PGI_2, the major vasodilator present in this tissue, and the lack of PGI_2 to oppose other vasoconstrictive agents such as endothelins, angiotensin II, and catecholamines indicate that the umbilical vein may have increased tension and resistance during exposure to ethanol.[102] This may cause the fetus to be particularly vulnerable to the possible consequences of disrupted blood flow discussed above.

The maintenance of blood flow in the umbilical vessels is important for adequate oxygenation of fetal vessels. A study that involved direct occlusion of an umbilical artery in lambs was shown to limit placental oxygen diffusion capacity and transport.[103] Hence, results from studies involving umbilical vein perfusion with a vasoconstrictor and from studies where umbilical arteries were occluded effectively illustrate some possible consequences of blood flow reduction in umbilical vessels.

b. The Placenta

The possibility that placental prostaglandin production is a target for ethanol's actions has become evident. In sheep, PGE_2 concentrations in maternal and fetal plasma[14] and in fetal cerebrospinal fluid[51] have been shown to increase after maternal ethanol infusion. Similar data from our laboratory have shown that perfusion of an isolated cotyledon of the human placenta with ethanol increases PGE concentration when compared to placentas perfused with buffer alone.[104]

In addition to increasing prostaglandin production, ethanol has also been shown to affect blood flow in the placenta. In pregnant rats exposed to alcohol, placental blood flow decreased by a third.[85] In pregnant women, however, alcohol did not influence placental blood flow.[105] Whether these discrepant findings can be attributed to species differences or to dosage differences is not certain.

A recent study[102] illustrated that ethanol perfusion of the fetal circulation in isolated human placental lobules resulted in a concentration-related rise in fetal arterial pressure. This rapid pressor response could be inhibited by indomethacin, a prostaglandin inhibitor. The inhibition of ethanol's pressor effect indicates a role for prostaglandins in this effect. This pressor action of ethanol in the fetal circulation is thought to contribute to the pathogenesis of the fetal alcohol syndrome and may represent an underlying mechanism for ethanol-induced hypertension.[102]

Another study[106] illustrated additional consequences of ethanol-induced reductions in placental blood flow. Intravenous infusion of ethanol over a one-hour period to catheterized pregnant ewes decreased blood flow on both sides of the placenta. These reductions, interestingly, were maintained for at least two hours after the cessation of ethanol perfusion. Consequently, fetal glucose supply and consumption were both decreased,[106] and it is probable that fetal utilization of other substrates, including oxygen, might have been affected.

Whether or not prenatal ethanol exposure compromises oxygen availability to the fetus, rendering it hypoxic, is a controversial area. Some studies have indicated that maternal exposure to ethanol results in the transient collapse of umbilical vessels, rendering the fetus hypoxic.[65] Other studies indicate either that fetal hypoxia does not occur[17] or that fetal oxygenation is increased[107] as a result of prenatal ethanol exposure. Clearly, whether or not ethanol exposure results in fetal hypoxia is an important issue, especially given the fact that the developing brain is particularly vulnerable to hypoxic conditions. If fetal use of oxygen and glucose is decreased by maternal ethanol ingestion, this may be an important contributing factor underlying some of the neurological problems associated with fetal alcohol syndrome. Perhaps chronic ethanol consumption, for these reasons, may result in changes that contribute to growth defects typical in the fetal alcohol syndrome.

In summary, the vasoactive prostaglandins are differentially sensitive to ethanol. Since ethanol has been shown to influence vascular tone and resistance[100] as well as blood flow[85] in the umbilical/placental system, these effects may be a result of ethanol-induced fluctuations in prostaglandin levels. Hence, vasoactive prostaglandins may play an indirect role in ethanol-induced teratogenesis by disrupting uterine, umbilical, or placental blood flow, which could result in potential pathological consequences for the fetus.

III. PROSTAGLANDINS AND FETAL ALCOHOL SYNDROME: A SUMMARY

It has been established here that prostaglandins appear to play a role in fetal growth and development and that ethanol affects prostaglandin levels in both maternal and fetal tissues. Together, these findings lead to the probability that ethanol may mediate at least some of its teratogenic effects through interference with prostaglandin metabolism in maternal tissues[40-41,108-109] and through prostaglandin synthesis in the embryo-fetus.[110]

Generally, data provide evidence that prostaglandins appear to mediate at least some of ethanol's teratogenic effects through direct actions on the fetus and/or through fluctuations in blood flow in the maternal-fetal utero-placental unit (i.e., ethanol may influence prostaglandins that play roles in fetal morphological development, or ethanol may influence vasoactive postaglandins that regulate blood flow in uterine, placental, and umbilical vessels). The maintenance of blood flow in the uterus, placenta, and umbilical vessels is important for normal fetal growth and development. Ethanol can be exerting an effect at any, or all, of these sites to alter vasoactiove prostaglandins and, hence, blood flow. It will be important to determine the biochemical mechanism through which ethanol interferes with prostaglandin production and with metabolism in order that pharmacological intervention be made possible. Data indicate that ethanol affects almost all aspects of the arachidonic acid cascade. Ethanol may liberate arachidonic acid from the membrane's lipid bilayer through actions on phospholipase A_2,[111] it may alter the amount of constitutive cyclooxygenase present,[112] and/or ethanol may interact selectively with the specific prostaglandin synthetase enzymes[98] to result in differential effects on prostaglandin expression. The mechanism whereby ethanol interferes with prostaglandin production, on a biochemical level, may differ in a concentration-dependent and tissue- and/or cell-specific manner and is beyond the scope of this chapter.

IV. SUMMARY

In vivo and *in vitro* data from animal as well as human studies indicate that prostaglandins play integral roles in pregnancy and in reproduction. There is also strong evidence that indicates a definite interaction between ethanol and prostaglandin levels in many tissues, including placental, uterine, and umbilical vessels. These effects may be mediated through changes in synthesis, through changes in degradation, or through altering compounds that regulate prostaglandin production and release. The specific prostaglandins that are sensitive to ethanol and the directions in which their levels change are unknowns that elude us. The interaction between ethanol and prostaglandins is complicated and remains to be clarified.

Perhaps the most important issue is a recurrent one. Although prostaglandins have been implicated in teratogenesis, their roles in ethanol-induced birth defects and in the fetal alcohol syndrome remain unclear. It is generally understood that alcohol alters prostaglandin levels, but it is not understood how, or where, alcohol acts to do so. It is known that altered prostaglandin levels may influence fetal development or influence blood flow in the maternal-fetal unit.

It is tempting to speculate that the prostaglandins affecting fetal growth are different prostaglandins from those affecting fetal morphological development. For instance, prostaglandins of the E and F series seem to be directly involved in embryonic morphological *development*, while the potent vasoactive prostaglandins prostacyclin and thromboxane may influence fetal *growth* through compromising blood flow in the uterine/placental/umbilical unit. Thus, ethanol may *differentially* influence fetal growth and development by exerting differential effects on prostaglandins involved either directly or indirectly in these processes.

Studies tend to differ in terms of which prostaglandins are affected, in the concentrations of alcohol used to produce an effect, in the duration of ethanol exposure, and in animal species used as model systems. Still, there is ample evidence for a relationship between alcohol, prostaglandins, and pregnancy. Their specific involvement in the fetal alcohol syndrome, however, remains to be defined.

REFERENCES

1. **Jones, K.L. and Smith, D.W.**, Recognition of the fetal alcohol syndrome in early infancy, *Lancet*, 2, 999, 1973.
2. **Jones, K.L., Smith, D.W., Ulleland, C.N., and Streissguth, P.**, Pattern of malformation in offspring of chronic alcoholic mothers, *Lancet*, 1, 1267, 1973.
3. **Schenker, S., Becker, H.C., Randall, C.L., Phillips, D.K., Baskin, G.S., and Henderson, G.I.**, Fetal alcohol syndrome: Current status of pathogenesis, *Alc. Clin. Exp. Res.*, 14, 635, 1990.
4. **Randall, C.L., Ekblad, U., and Anton, R.F.**, Perspectives on the pathophysiology of fetal alcohol syndrome, *Alc. Clin. Exp. Res.*, 14, 807, 1990.
5. **Keirse, M.J.**, Biosynthesis and metabolism of prostaglandins in the pregnant human uterus, *Adv. Prostaglandin Thromb. Res.*, 4, 87, 1978.
6. **Anggard, E.**, Ethanol, essential fatty acids and prostaglandins, *Pharmacol. Biochem. Behav.*, 18, 401, 1983.
7. **Thorp, J.A., Walsh, S.W., and Brath, P.C.**, Low-dose aspirin inhibits thromboxane, but not prostacyclin, production by human placental arteries, *Am. J. Obstet. Gynecol.*, 159, 1381, 1988.

8. **Mak, K.K., Gude, N.M., Walters, W.A. and Boura, A.L.**, Effects of vasoactive autacoids on the human umbilical-fetal placental vasculature, *Br. J. Obstet. Gynaecol.*, 91, 99, 1984.

9. **Ylikorkala, O. and Viinikka,L.**, The role of prostaglandins in obstetrical disorders, *Baillieres. Clin. Obstet. Gynaecol.*, 6, 809, 1992.

10. **Walsh, S.W.**, Low-dose aspirin: Treatment for the imbalance of increased thromboxane and decreased prostacyclin in preeclampsia, *Am. J. Perinatol.*, 6, 124, 1989.

11. **Ylikorkala, O., Halmesmaki, E., and Viinikka, L.**, Urinary prostacyclin and thromboxane metabolites in drinking pregnant women and in their infants: Relations to the fetal alcohol effects, *Obstet. Gynecol.*, 71, 61, 1988.

12. **Dubin, N.H., Wolff, M.C., Thomas, C.L., and Di Blasi, M.C.**, Prostaglandin production by rat vaginal tissue, *in vitro*, in response to ethanol, a mild mucosal irritant, *Toxicol. Appl. Pharmacol.*, 78, 458, 1985.

13. **Anton, R.F., Becker, H.C., and Randall, C.L.**, Ethanol increases PGE and thromboxane production in mouse pregnant uterine tissue, *Life Sci.*, 46, 1145, 1990.

14. **Smith, G.N., Brien, J.F., Homan, J., Carmichael, L., Treissman, D., and Patrick, J.**, Effect of ethanol on ovine fetal and maternal plasma prostaglandin E2 concentrations and fetal breathing movements, *J. Dev. Physiol.*, 14, 23, 1990.

15. **George, F.R. and Collins, A.C.**, Ethanol's behavioral effects may be partly due to increases in brain prostaglandin production, *Alc. Clin. Exp. Res.*, 9, 143, 1985.

16. **Landolfi, R. and Steiner, M.**, Ethanol raises prostacyclin *in vivo* and *in vitro*, *Blood*, 64, 679, 1984.

17. **Bocking, A.D., Sinervo, K.R., Smith, G.N., Carmichael, L., Challis, J.R., Olson, D.M., and Brien, J.F.**, Increased uteroplacental production of prostaglandin E2 during ethanol infusion, *Am. J. Physiol.*, 265, R640, 1993.

18. **Labhsetwar, A.P.**, Effects of prostaglandins E1, E2 and F2 on zygote transport in rats: Induction of delayed implantation, *Prostaglandins*, 4, 115, 1973.

19. **Goldberg, V.J. and Ramwell, P.W.**, Role of prostaglandins in reproduction, *Physiol. Rev.*, 55, 325, 1975.

20. **Challis, J.R. and Patrick, J.E.**, The production of prostaglandins and thromboxanes in the feto-placental unit and their effects on the developing fetus, *Semin. Perinatol.*, 4, 23, 1980.

21. **Persaud, T.V.**, Prostaglandins and organogenesis, *Adv. Prostaglandin Thromboxane Res.*, 4, 139, 1978.

22. **Karim, S. M. and Sharma, S. D.,** Oral administration of prostaglandin E2 for the induction and acceleration of labor, *J. Reprod. Med.,* 9, 346, 1972.

23. **Karim, S.M., Sharma, S.D., Filshie, G.M., Salmon, J.A., and Ganesan, P.A.,** Termination of pregnancy with prostaglandin analogs, *Adv. Biosci.,* 9, 811, 1973.

24. **Mac Kenzie, I.Z. and Embrey, M.P.,** Intravaginal PGE2 gel prior to labor induction, *Adv. Prostaglandin Thromboxane Res.,* 8, 1477, 1980.

25. **Karim, S.M. and Devlin, J.,** Prostaglandin content of amniotic fluid during pregnancy and labour, *J. Obstet. Gynaecol. Br. Commonw.,* 74, 230, 1967.

26. **Karim, S.M.,** Physiological role of prostaglandins in the control of parturition and menstruation, *J. Reprod. Fertil. Suppl.,* 16, 105, 1972.

27. **Karim, S.M. and Sharma, S.D.,** Oral administration of prostaglandins for the induction of labour, *Br. Med. J.,* 1, 260, 1971.

28. **Curbelo, V., Bejar, R., Benirschke, K., and Gluck, L.,** Premature labor. I. Prostaglandin precursors in human placental membranes, *Obstet. Gynecol.,* 57, 473, 1981.

29. **Bygdeman, M. and Hamberg, M.,** The effect of eight new prostaglandins on human myometrium, *Acta. Physiol. Scand.,* 69, 320, 1967.

30. **Wiqvist, N., Bygdeman, M.,Kwon, S. U., Mukherjee, T., and Roth-Brandel, U.,** Effect of prostaglandin E1 on the midpregnant human uterus. Intravenous, intramuscular, intra-amniotic, and vaginal administration, *Am. J. Obstet. Gynecol.,* 102, 327, 1968.

31. **Waltman, R., Tricomi, V., Shabanah, E. H., and Arenas, R.,** The effect of anti-inflammatory drugs on parturition parameters in the rat, *Prostaglandins,* 4, 93, 1973.

32. **Ylikorkala, O. and Makila, U.M.,** Prostacyclin and thromboxane in gynecology and obstetrics, *Am. J. Obstet. Gynecol.,* 152, 318, 1985.

33. **Labhsetwar, A.P.,** Prostaglandin E1: Studies on antifertility and luteolytic effects in hamsters and rats, *Biol. Reprod.,* 8, 103, 1973.

34. **Labhsetwar, A.P.,** Prostaglandin E2: Analysis of effects on pregnancy and corpus luteum in hamsters and rats, *Acta. Endocrinol. Suppl.,* 170, 3, 1972.

35. **Labhsetwar, A.P.,** Prostaglandin E2: Evidence for luteolytic effects, *Prostaglandins,* 2, 23, 1972.

36. **Gilani, S.H. and Persaud, T.V.,** Embryopathic effects of thromboxane B2 in the chick, *Prostaglandins Med.,* 6, 627, 1981.

37. **Persaud, T.V., Mann, R.A., and Moore, K.L.,** Teratological studies with prostaglandin E2 in chick embryos, *Prostaglandins,* 4, 343, 1973.

38. **Persaud, T.V.,** The effects of prostaglandin E2 on pregnancy and embryonic development in mice, *Toxicology,* 5, 97, 1975.

39. **Pennington, S., Allen, Z., Runion, J., Farmer, P., Rowland, L., and Kalmus, G.,** Prostaglandin synthesis inhibitors block alcohol-induced fetal hypoplasia, *Alc. Clin. Exp. Res.*, 9, 433, 1985.

40. **Randall, C.L., Anton, R.F., and Becker, H.C.,** Alcohol, pregnancy, and prostaglandins, *Alc. Clin. Exp. Res.*, 11, 32, 1987.

41. **Randall, C.L., Anton, R.F., Becker, H.C., and White, N.M.,** Role of prostaglandins in alcohol teratogenesis, *Ann. N.Y. Acad. Sci.,* 562, 178, 1989.

42. **Persaud, T.V.,** Pregnancy and progeny in rats treated with prostaglandin E2, *Prostaglandins*, 3, 299, 1973.

43. **Persaud, T. V.,** Fetal development in rabbits following intra-amniotic administration of prostaglandin E2, *Exp. Pathol.*, 9, 336, 1974.

44. **Chida, S. and Mettler, L.,** Effects of indomethacin, prostaglandin E2 and prostaglandin F2 alpha on mouse blastocyst attachment and trophoblastic outgrowth *in vitro, Prostaglandins*, 37, 411, 1989.

45. **Armato, U. and Andreis, P. G.,** Prostaglandins of the F series are extremely powerful growth factors for primary neonatal rat hepatocytes, *Life Sci.*, 33, 1745, 1983.

46. **Persaud, T.V.,** The effects of prostaglandin F2a on pregnancy and fetal development in mice, *Toxicology*, 2, 25, 1974.

47. **Wainwright, P., Ward, G.R., and Molnar, J.D.,** g-Linolenic acid fails to prevent the effects of prenatal ethanol exposure on brain and behavioral development in B6DF$_2$ mice, *Alc. Clin. Exp. Res.*, 1985.

48. **Randall, C.L., Becker, H.C., and Anton, R.F.,** Effect of ibuprofen on alcohol-induced teratogenesis in mice, *Alc. Clin. Exp. Res.*, 15, 673, 1991.

49. **Randall, C.L., Anton, R.F., and Becker, H.C.,** Effect of indomethacin on alcohol-induced morphological anomalies in mice, *Life Sci.*, 41, 361, 1987.

50. **Smith, G.N., Brien, J.F., Homan, J., Carmichael, L,. and Patrick, J.,** Indomethacin antagonizes the ethanol-induced suppression of breath activity but not the suppression of brain activity in the near-term fetal sheep, *J. Dev. Physiol.*, 12, 69, 1989.

51. **Smith, G.N., Brien, J.F., Homan, J., Carmichael, L., and Patrick, J.,** Indomethacin reversal of ethanol-induced suppression of ovine fetal breathing movements and relationship to prostaglandin E2, *J. Dev. Physiol.*, 14, 29, 1990.

52. **Smith, G.N., Sinervo, K.R., Carmichael, L., Patrick, J., Bocking, A.D., and Brien, J.F.,** The effects of indomethacin and prostaglandin E$_2$ on the ethanol-induced supression of ovine fetal breathing movements, *J. Dev. Physiol.*, 16, 239, 1991.

53. **Guy, J.F. and Sucheston, M.E.,** Teratogenic effects on the CD-1 mouse embryo exposed to concurrent doses of ethanol and aspirin, *Teratology*, 34, 249, 1986.

54. **Randall, C.L. and Anton, R.F.,** Aspirin reduces alcohol-induced prenatal mortality and malformations in mice, *Alc. Clin. Exp. Res.*, 8, 513, 1984.

55. **Randall, C.L., Anton, R.F., Becker, H.C., Hale, R.L., and Ekblad, U.,** Aspirin dose-dependently reduces alcohol-induced birth defects and prostaglandin E levels in mice, *Teratology*, 44, 521, 1991.

56. **Jacobson, R.L., Brewer, A., Eis, A., Siddiqi, T.A., and Myatt, L.,** Transfer of aspirin across the perfused human placental cotyledon, *Am. J. Obstet. Gynecol.*, 165, 939, 1991.

57. **Klein, K.L., Scott, W.J., Clark, K.E., and Wilson, J.G.,** Indomethacin--placental transfer, cytotoxicity, and teratology in the rat, *Am. J. Obstet. Gynecol.*, 141, 448, 1981.

58. **George, F.R. and Collins, A.C.,** Prostaglandin synthetase inhibitors antagonize the depressant effects of ethanol, *Pharmacol. Biochem. Behav.*, 10, 865, 1979.

59. **George, F.R., Jackson, S.J., and Collins, A.C.,** Prostaglandin synthetase inhibitors antagonize hypothermia induced by sedative hypnotics, *Psychopharmacology*, 74, 241, 1981.

60. **George, F.R., Elmer, G.I., and Collins, A.C.,** Indomethacin significantly reduces mortality due to acute ethanol overexposure, *Subst. Alcohol. Actions Misuse*, 3, 267, 1982.

61. **George, F. R., Howerton, T. C., Elmer, G. I., and Collins, A. C.,** Antagonism of alcohol hypnosis by blockade of prostaglandin synthesis and activity: Genotype and time course effects, *Pharmacol. Biochem. Behav.*, 19, 131, 1983.

62. **Mattson, S.N., Carlos, R., and Riley, E.P.,** The behavioral teratogenicity of alcohol is not affected by pretreatment with aspirin, *Alcohol*, 10, 51, 1993.

63. **Bonthius, D.J. and West, J.R.,** Aspirin augments alcohol in restricting brain growth in the neonatal rat, *Neurotoxicol. Teratol.*, 11, 135, 1989.

64. **Macpherson, T.,** Fact and fancy. What can we really tell from the placenta?, *Arch. Pathol. Lab. Med.*, 115, 672, 1991.

65. **Mukherjee, A.B. and Hodgen, G.D.,** Maternal ethanol exposure induced transient impairment of umbilical circulation and fetal hypoxia in monkeys, *Science*, 218, 700, 1982.

66. **Altura, B.M. and Altura, B.T.,** Microvascular and vascular smooth muscle actions of ethanol, acetaldehyde, and acetate, *Fed. Proc.*, 41, 2447, 1982.

67. **Makila, U.M., Jouppila, P., Kirkinen, P., Viinikka, L., and Ylikorkala, O.,** Placental thromboxane and prostacyclin in the regulation of placental blood flow, *Obstet. Gynecol.*, 68, 537, 1986.

68. **Howard, R.B., Hosokawa, T., and Maguire, M.H.,** Pressor and depressor actions of prostanoids in the intact human fetoplacental vascular bed, *Prostaglandins. Leukot. Med.*, 21, 323, 1986.

69. Clapp, J.F., McLaughlin, M.K., Larrow, R., Farnham, J., and Mann, L.I., The uterine hemodynamic response to repetitive unilateral vascular embolization in the pregnant ewe, *Am. J. Obstet. Gynecol.*, 144, 309, 1982.

70. Whitney, E.A., Ducsay, C.A., and Valenzuela, G.J., Is uterine blood flow controlled locally or systemically in the pregnant rabbit?, *Am. J. Obstet. Gynecol.*, 169, 1507, 1993.

71. Webster, W.S., Lipson, A.H., and Brown-Woodman, P.D., Uterine trauma and limb defects, *Teratology*, 35, 253, 1987.

72. Walsh, S.W., Thromboxane production in placentas of women with preeclampsia [letter], *Am. J. Obstet. Gynecol.*, 160, 1535, 1989.

73. Venuto, R.C., O'Dorisio, T., Stein, J.H., and Ferris, T.F., Uterine prostaglandin E secretion and uterine blood flow in the pregnant rabbit, *J. Clin. Invest.*, 55, 193, 1975.

74. Franchi, A.M., Faletti, A., Fernandez-Pardal, J., Gimeno, M.F., and Gimeno, A.L., The output of uterine prostaglandins and the activity of 15-hydroxy-prostaglandin dehydrogenase are enhanced in chronic ethanol fed rats, *Prostaglandins. Leukot. Essent. Fatty. Acids.*, 33, 69, 1988.

75. Jaerbaum, A., Chaud, M., Gonzalez, E.T., Gimeno, A.L., and Gimeno, M.A., Acute effects of a single ethanol injection on *in vitro* rat uterine spontaneous motility, on uteri prostaglandin production and on tissue metabolism of triglycerides, *Prostaglandins. Leukot. Essent. Fatty. Acids.*, 47, 219, 1992.

76. Bygdeman, M., Gemzell, K., and Swahn, M.L., The role of prostaglandins and ovarian hormones in the regulation of human uterine contractility, *Adv. Prostaglandin Thromboxane Leukot. Res.*, 1, 799, 1991.

77. Bygdeman, M., Gemzell, K., Gottlieb, C., and Swahn, M.L., Uterine contractility and interaction between prostaglandins and antiprogestins. Clinical implications, *Ann. N.Y. Acad. Sci.*, 626, 561, 1991.

78. Martin, J.N. and Bygdeman, M., The effect of locally administered PGF2alpha on the contractility of the nonpregnant human uterus, *Prostaglandins*, 9, 245, 1975.

79. Herabutya, Y. and O-Prasertsawat, P., Control of uterine hyperactivity caused by prostaglandin with intravenous terbutaline: A case report, *J. Med. Assoc. Thai.*, 1, 100, 1993.

80. Zervoudakis, I.A., Krauss, A., and Wilson, K.H., Infants of mothers treated with ethanol for premature labor, *Am. J. Obstet. Gynecol.*, 137, 713, 1980.

81. Bond, N.W., Prenatal exposure to ethanol: Association between increased gestational length and offspring mortality, *Neurobehav. Toxicol. Teratol.*, 4, 501, 1982.

82. **Dumont, M., Thoulon, J.M., Guibaud, S., Broussard, P., and Glehen, D.,** Ethanol perfusions during threatened premature labor. Special study of oxytocinase activity, *J. Gynecol. Obstet. Biol. Reprod.,* 6, 107, 1977.

83. **Fuchs, A.R.,** The inhibitory effect of ethanol on the release of oxytocin during parturition in the rabbit, *J. Endocrinol,* 35, 125, 1966.

84. **Lauersen, N.H., Wilson, K.H., and Fuchs, F.F.,** The inhibitory effect of ethanol on oxytocin-induced labor at term, *J. Reprod. Med.,* 26, 547, 1981.

85. **Jones, P.J.H., Leichter, J., and Lee, M.,** Placental blood flow in rats fed alcohol before and during gestation, *Life Sci.,* 29, 1153, 1981.

86. **Idanpaan-Heikkila, J.E., Fritchie, G.E., Ho, B.T., and McIsaac, W. M.,** Placental transfer of C14-ethanol, *Am. J. Obstet. Gynecol.,* 110, 426, 1971.

87. **Ho, B.T., Fritchie, G.E., Idanpaan-Heikkila, J.E., and McIsaac, W.M.,** Placental transfer and tissue distribution of ethanol-1- 14 C. A radioautographic study in monkeys and hamsters, *Q. J. Stud. Alcohol,* 33, 485, 1972.

88. **Dilts, P., Jr.,** Placental transfer of ethanol, *Am. J. Obstet. Gynecol.,* 107, 1195, 1970.

89. **Waltman, R. and Iniquez, E.S.,** Placental transfer of ethanol and its elimination at term, *Obstet. Gynecol.,* 40, 180, 1972.

90. **Spivack, M.,** On the presence or absence of nerves in the umbilical blood vessels of man and guinea pig, *Anat. Rec.,* 85, 85, 1943.

91. **Haugen, G., Bjoro, K., and Stray-Pedersen, S.,** The influence of extra-umbilical serotonin, PGE2 and PGF2 alpha on prostanoid production in human umbilical arteries, *Scand. J. Clin. Lab. Invest.,* 51, 131, 1991.

92. **Di Grande, A., Malatino, L.S., Boura, A.L., Read, M.A., and Walters, W.A.,** Modulation by adenosine of thromboxane A2 receptor-mediated constriction in the human umbilical artery, *Int. J. Clin. Pharmacol. Ther.,* 32, 344, 1994.

93. **Kontula, K., Viinikka, L., Ylikorkala, O., and Ylikahri, R.,** Effect of acute ethanol intake on thromboxane and prostacyclin in human, *Life Sci.,* 31, 261, 1982.

94. **Mikhailidis, D.P., Jeremy, J.Y., Barradas, M.A., Green, N., and Dandona, P.,** Effect of ethanol on vascular prostacyclin (prostaglandin I2) synthesis, platelet aggregation, and platelet thromboxane release, *Br. Med. J.,* 287, 1495, 1983.

95. **Toivanen, J., Ylikorkala, O., and Viinikka, L.,** Ethanol inhibits platelet thromboxane A_2 production but has no effect on lung prostacyclin synthesis in humans, *Thromb. Res.,* 33, 1, 1983.

96. **Ouwendijk, R.J.T., Zijlstra, F.J., Wilson, J.H.P., Bonta, I.L., and Vincent, J.E.,** Raised plasma thromboxane B2 levels in alcoholic liver disease, *Prostaglandins Leukotrienes Med.,* 10, 115, 1983.

97. **Greenberg, S.S., Xie, J., Wang, Y., Kolls, J., Shellito, J., Nelson, S., and Summer, W.R.,** Ethanol relaxes pulmonary artery by release of prostaglandin and nitric oxide, *Alcohol,* 10, 21, 1993.

98. **Randall, C.L. and Saulnier, J.L.,** The effect of ethanol on prostacyclin, thromboxane, and prostaglandin E production in human umbilical veins, *Alc. Clin. Exp. Res.,* 19, 741, 1995.

99. **Altura, B.M., Malaviya, D., Reich, C.F., and Orkin, L.R.,** Effects of vasoactive agents on isolated human umbilical arteries and veins, *Am. J. Physiol.,* 222, 345, 1972.

100. **Savoy-Moore, R.T., Dombrowski, M.P., Cheng, A., Abel, E.A., and Sokol, R. J.,** Low dose alcohol contracts the human umbilical artery *in vitro, Alc. Clin. Exp. Res.,* 13, 40, 1989.

101. **Yang, H.Y., Shum, A.Y., Ng, H.T., and Chen, C.F.,** Effect of ethanol on human umbilical artery and vein *in vitro, Gynecol. Obstet. Invest.,* 21, 131, 1986.

102. **Taylor, S.M., Heron, A.E., Cannell, G.R., and Florin, T.H.,** Pressor effect of ethanol in the isolated perfused human placental lobule, *Eur. J. Pharmacol.,* 270, 371, 1994.

103. **Wilkening, R.B. and Meschia,G.,** Effect of occluding one umbilical artery on placental oxygen transport, *Am. J. Physiol.,* 260, H1319, 1991.

104. **Randall, C.L., White, N.M., Becker, H.C., and Ekblad,U.,** Ethanol perfusion of human placenta increases PGE levels over time, *Alc. Clin. Exp. Res.,* 16, 383, 1992.

105. **Erskine, R.L. and Ritchie, J.W.,** The effect of maternal consumption of alcohol on human umbilical artery blood flow, *Am. J. Obstet. Gynecol.,* 154, 318, 1986.

106. **Falconer, J.,** The effect of maternal ethanol infusion on placental blood flow and fetal glucose metabolism in sheep, *Alc. Alcohol.,* 25, 413, 1990.

107. **Reynolds, J.D., Penning, D.H., Atkins, B., Dexter, F., Hardy, J., Poduska, D., and Brien, J. F.,** Effect of maternal administration of ethanol or cocaine, or maternal hemorrhage on uterine blood flow and fetal oxygen status in the near-term pregnant ewe, *Alc. Clin. Exp. Res.,* 19, 21, 1995.

108. **Pennington, S.N., Smith, C.P., Jr., and Strider, J.B., Jr.,** Alterations in prostaglandin catabolism in rats chronically dosed with ethanol, *Biochem. Med.,* 21, 246, 1979.

109. **Brien, J.F. and Smith, G.N.,** Effects of alcohol (ethanol) on the fetus, *J. Dev. Physiol.,* 15, 21, 1991.

110. **Horrobin, D.F.,** A biochemical basis for alcoholism and alcohol-induced damage including the fetal alcohol syndrome and cirrhosis: Interference with essential fatty acid and prostaglandin metabolism, *Med. Hypotheses*, 6, 929, 1980.

111. **Spach, P.I., Parce, J.W., and Cunningham, C.C.,** Effect of chronic ethanol administration on energy metabolism and phospholipase A_2 activity in rat liver, *Biochem. J.*, 178, 23, 1979.

112. **Bondy, S.C. and Orozco, J.,** Effects of ethanol treatment upon sources of reactive oxygen species in brain and liver, *Alc. Alcohol.*, 29, 375, 1994.

Chapter 13

ETHANOL-NUTRIENT INTERACTION AND THE FETUS

Stanley E. Fisher and Peter I. Karl

I. INTRODUCTION

Good maternal and fetal nutrition have long been recognized as important aspects of a successful pregnancy. General maternal health, genetics and environmental exposure also contribute to the success of every pregnancy. Among environmental factors, alcohol exposure stands out as a major human embryotoxin and teratogen. The fetal alcohol syndrome (FAS) is the most serious manifestation of fetal alcohol exposure. This almost invariably involves mental retardation, as well as low birthweight and a series of specific and non-specific congenital anomalies.[1-2] The FAS is one of the major causes of severe mental retardation in Western society. Moreover, there are more subtle and isolated clinical deficits caused by fetal alcohol exposure, without full manifestation of the FAS.

While ethanol (and probably its metabolic products, as well) undoubtedly has direct toxic effects upon the fetus, there may be indirect effects as well. Ethanol use has the potential to adversely affect maternal nutritional health and may be toxic to the placenta, an important organ for fetal nutrition. This might be reflected in altered maternal nutritional status, as well as impaired placental nutrient transport or placental metabolic function. In addition, the mechanisms by which ethanol has direct fetal toxicity may include nutrient interaction. These aspects of ethanol-nutrient interaction and the potential for altering fetal health will be addressed in the following review.

II. ALCOHOL AND MATERNAL NUTRITION

During pregnancy, the fetal/placental unit functions as a sort of "parasite" deriving oxygen, essential nutrients and many growth factors from its host. It depends upon maternal nutrient stores and maternal general well being to provide an environment suitable for optimal growth. More than 70% of brain growth occurs during pregnancy, with a large percentage of brain differentiation and some growth occurring early, before the placenta is fully developed. In general, maternal nutritional status influences birthweight, with a strong relationship between birthweight and maternal preconceptual nutrition.[3-4]

Maternal nutritional deficiencies before or during pregnancy can obviously result in fetal nutrient deprivation and, when particularly severe, even fetal wastage. More commonly, the clinical manifestation would be fetal growth retardation. Maternal nutrient intake during pregnancy correlates with birthweight, even after controlling for smoking or alcohol intake.[3] Hence, the mother's diet and general nutritional status are important to fetal growth. Maternal nutritional status can easily be influenced by ethanol. Interaction between alcohol and maternal nutritional status may be viewed at a global level or at the level of individual nutrients, such as essential vitamins. Specifically, chronic alcoholics are notorious for being poorly nourished. Yet, recent studies would indicate that this generalization may be more applicable to those alcoholics who are in the lower socioeconomic classes.[5] Hence, the habitual use of alcohol may be associated with generally poor maternal nutrition; which would be expected to be present at the time of conception, when good maternal nutrition may be particularly critical to brain development.[3] Moreover, continued poor general nutrition throughout pregnancy would be expected to compound any specific interactions between ethanol and particular nutrients.

Interaction between ethanol and nutrients could affect fetal development in any habitual user, regardless of preconceptual nutritional status or nutritional intake during pregnancy. Certain micronutrients, such as vitamins and zinc, are essential to normal fetal development. Even without diminished maternal vitamin intake, alcohol use during pregnancy may contribute to vitamin deficiency via altered vitamin metabolism. Metabolism of four vitamins has been shown to be altered in alcoholics: thiamine, folate, pyridoxal (B_6) and vitamin A (retinoic acid). These will be discussed in terms of the potential for affecting the fetus.

1. Thiamine

This vitamin is essential to normal fetal growth.[6] Severe thiamine deficiency is neurotoxic. Ethanol abuse might reduce maternal thiamine stores through decreased intestinal absorption.[7] The net result would be a potentially decreased thiamine supply for the fetus. However, this interaction remains speculative, as no studies have evaluated the effect of maternal ethanol exposure on fetal thiamine status.

2. Folate

A co-factor for DNA/RNA synthesis, folate is essential to cell growth and differentiation. Pregnancy appears to increase maternal requirements for intake of folate, presumably because of increased demands by the fetus. With heavy ethanol use, maternal folate stores may be decreased by impaired intestinal absorption, as well as increased renal losses.[8-9] More importantly, hepatic metabolism of folate may be impaired by ethanol,[10] including increased catabolism due to superoxide generation from oxidation of ethanol to acetaldehyde.[11] The ultimate consequences would be a diminished supply for the fetus. A relatively diminished supply of folate may be manifest in neural tube defects, which have been described in the FAS.[12-14] Ethanol and folate metabolism may also interact in the presence of iron deficiency, common in pregnancy, and expected to be present in those with poor nutritional intake, such as alcoholics. In the mouse, it has been suggested that reproduction is adversely affected by the combination of iron deficiency and chronic ethanol intake, apparently by way of alterations in maternal folate metabolism.[15] Despite the potential for ethanol induced maternal folate deficiency, studies have failed to conclusively show that the effect of ethanol on the fetus is related to diminished maternal folate status.[16-19] Indeed, the effect of ethanol appears to be independent of maternal folate; Larroque *et al.* found lowered birth weight to be related to ethanol intake in the first trimester, which occurred in the face of enhanced maternal folate status.[19]

3. Vitamin B₆

B_6 is also an essential vitamin for fetal growth. Ethanol might be expected to reduce maternal vitamin B_6 levels by increased hepatic catabolism (reviewed in Mezey[20]). With regard to the FAS, the potential role of B_6 deficiency in the pathophysiology has received little attention, despite the observation that maternal B_6 deficiency exacerbates the effect of ethanol on fetal growth in experimental animals.[21]

4. Vitamin A

The effects of ethanol on hepatic vitamin A levels and subsequent tissue distribution have the potential to alter the fetal supply of vitamin A. However, it is more likely that the ethanol-vitamin A interaction at the fetal level has greater impact, which will be discussed later in this review.

The pathways for ethanol-vitamin A interaction in the drinking adult have been reviewed recently.[20-22] Briefly, ethanol ingestion causes a reduction in vitamin A stores within the liver. This is due in part to increased metabolism via the cytochrome P450 system. It is also secondary to a decrease in binding proteins and redistribution of vitamin A to peripheral tissues. The serum levels of vitamin A may remain normal until hepatic vitamin A stores are depleted. Depending on the circumstances, a chronic alcoholic could eventually become vitamin A deficient. This could have consequences for the fetus, in the form of vitamin deprivation. On the other hand, especially during the early phases of altered vitamin A metabolism, an opposite effect might occur: increased transfer of Vitamin A to the fetus as the result of hepatic mobilization and tissue redistribution. Both deficiency and excess vitamin A have been associated with teratogenic effects, many of which mimic the findings in the FAS (reviewed in Keir,[23] Duester,[24] and Pullarkat[25]). Hence, there is the theoretical potential for double jeopardy. At one stage or another, the mother may become Vitamin A deficient through the action of ethanol plus poor diet and deprive the fetus; or she may eat well but cause excess Vitamin A to reach the fetus.

5. Zinc

Zinc deficiency may occur in alcoholics[23] and ethanol lowers serum zinc levels in pregnant women.[27] In the latter study, the authors concluded that zinc deficiency contributes to the teratogenesis in FAS. Experimentally, maternal zinc deficiency leads to low birthweight and developmental anomalies seen in the FAS.[28-29] One study in mice indicates that maternal zinc deficiency may be a cofactor in ethanol toxicity.[30] However, supplementation of the diet with zinc failed to alter the effect of ethanol.[31] Moreover, most other experimental studies have failed to demonstrate a direct relationship between ethanol-induced teratogenesis and maternal/fetal zinc deficiency.[32-35] Hence, while maternal zinc deficiency, presumably with resultant fetal zinc deficiency, may sometimes be a co-teratogen in man, the evidence is conflicting and there appears to be no consistent interaction between ethanol, overall zinc nutrition and the FAS.

III. ALCOHOL AND THE PLACENTA

During the last two trimesters, the human placenta is the virtually exclusive conduit for transport of essential nutrients, such as glucose, amino acids or vitamins, from the maternal to the fetal compartment. Therefore, any compromise in placental transport activity may contribute to the fetal malnutrition seen in the FAS. Deficient placental transport may result from diminished blood flow to the placenta, hypoxia and/or interference with placental transport mechanisms. This section will discuss the latter. With regard to all the placental studies cited below, an important caveat is that the effect of ethanol may not be identical for placentas from humans versus non-human animals.

1. Glucose

Glucose is a primary energy substrate for the fetus. During the third trimester, it is the major energy source for fetal growth. In experimental animals, chronic maternal alcohol exposure decreases glucose uptake and transfer by the placenta.[36] This study suggested that ethanol-induced intrauterine growth retardation correlated best with impairment of glucose transfer. In contrast, brief ethanol exposure does not appear to affect transplacental transfer of glucose, as studied in the perfused human placental cotyledon.[37]

2. Amino acids

The human fetus, like postnatal man, is dependent on certain essential amino acids for protein synthesis. In addition, fetal growth increases the need for many nonessential amino acids. A special case is the increased need for taurine, important primarily for central nervous system growth. Coupled with marginal fetal synthetic capacity, taurine is considered to be a conditionally essential amino acid for the fetus. Also, the growing fetus utilizes large amounts of gluconeogenic amino acids, such as alanine, requiring an external source. Accordingly, the human placenta transports both essential and nonessential amino acids from the maternal to the fetal circulation (with the exception of glutamine/glutamate, see below). Ethanol-induced interference with placental amino acid uptake (maternal side) or release (fetal side) could contribute to the intrauterine growth retardation associated with the FAS.

In rodents and sheep, both acute and chronic ethanol treatment decrease transplacental transport of certain amino acids[38-42] (reviewed in Fisher and Karl[43]). This has been associated with reduced activity of placental Na^+/K^+-ATPase.[44] In placentas from chronically treated nonhuman primates, amino acid uptake is also inhibited.[45]

In human placentas, clinically relevant concentrations (≤ 65 mM) do not acutely alter transplacental transfer in the perfused human placental cotyledon.[37,46] Similarly, in cultured placental trophoblasts, chronic treatment with clinically relevant concentrations of ethanol does not affect basal amino acid uptake. However, when the experimental system includes trophic factors which normally circulate or are locally produced, namely insulin or IGF-1, chronic ethanol exposure impairs amino acid uptake.[47] This suggests that the human, unlike the experimental animals, is at risk for impaired placental amino acid transport only when exposed chronically. In keeping with the Na^+/K^+-ATPase findings in rodents, inhibition of human placental amino acid transport is limited to Na^+-dependent active transport systems. This might provide insight into at least one mechanism of ethanol toxicity, since *in vivo* active transport of amino acids (both in the placenta and other tissues) is partially regulated by hormones and growth factors, including insulin and IGF-1.

3. Glutamine/Glutamate

A unique aspect of placental amino acid transport and metabolism is the handling of glutamine and glutamate. In excess quantities, glutamate is potentially neurotoxic. During fetal growth, glutamate is generated in the fetal tissue. Since the neonatal blood/brain barrier is immature and permeable to glutamate throughout most of pregnancy, an accumulation of glutamate in the fetal circulation would be potentially dangerous. To help prevent such a situation, net movement of glutamate is normally from the fetus to the placenta. There, glutamate is used as a placental fuel. Most of the remainder is released back into the fetal circulation as glutamate, to be utilized by the fetus as a metabolic fuel.[48] In rats exposed to ethanol throughout pregnancy, fetal serum glutamate is elevated.[49] This suggests increased fetal glutamate production and/or impaired placental glutamate uptake and/or decreased capacity for placental conversion to glutamine. In preliminary experiments in rats, ethanol does not alter the message level for the placental glutamate transporter proteins.[50] On the other hand, preliminary work in cultured human placental trophoblasts suggests that ethanol impairs conversion of glutamate to glutamine.[50] Altered placental handling of glutamate and glutamine represents another ethanol-nutrient interaction which may contribute to neurotoxicity in the developing fetus.

4. Thiamine

Thiamine is actively transported to the fetus by the human placenta.[51-53] The effect of chronic ethanol exposure on placental thiamine transport has not been studied in animals or *in vitro* human models. However, Schenker and colleagues have utilized the perfused human cotyledon to study acute ethanol exposure and found no alteration in thiamine transport.[53]

5. Folate

Folate is thought to be actively transported across the placenta to the fetus.[54] Chronic ethanol treatment reduces folate receptor levels in rat placenta.[55] However, chronic ethanol treatment in rats does not appear to reduce net folate transfer to fetal tissue; more importantly, tissue folate deficiency was not observed in newborn growth retarded rats from dams treated with ethanol throughout gestation.[18] Acutely, ethanol does not impair folate transport in the perfused human placental cotyledon.[54] At this point, the evidence would indicate that placental transport of folate is not a likely pathway for ethanol toxicity.

6. Vitamin B_6

B_6 is selectively transported across the placenta to the fetus. Some of the vitamin is phosphorylated in the placenta and released into the fetus circulation.[56] The effect of chronic ethanol exposure on transport or phosphorylation has not been evaluated. However, in the *in vitro* perfused human cotyledon, acute exposure to ethanol inhibits the transport of B_6 from the maternal to fetal compartments.[56] Inhibition of this placental transport system may, therefore, contribute to the fetal toxicity of ethanol.

7. Vitamin A

While this vitamin is the subject of hypotheses regarding ethanol and the FAS (see below), there have been no reports of placental studies. This may due to the technical difficulty in studying transport of lipid soluble substrates.

8. Zinc

Although overall maternal zinc deficiency is not a consistent accompaniment to chronic ethanol ingestion, the possibility exists that placental transfer of zinc might be impaired. In rats, one study demonstrated diminished placental transfer of zinc in the face of short or long term ethanol exposure.[57] Zinc supplementation did not correct this placental deficit.[58] In human tissue, short term ethanol exposure failed to alter zinc transfer by the isolated perfused placental cotyledon.[59] This discrepancy may be related to species differences, although several other studies have failed to demonstrate generalized deficits in fetal tissue zinc levels, in the face of long-term maternal ethanol exposure.[32-35] Moreover, placental zinc levels were unaltered by ethanol.[35] Hence, any impairment of placental zinc transport which might be induced by ethanol is insufficient to alter fetal stores; this would argue against an important role for ethanol-zinc interaction at the placental level.

IV. ETHANOL-NUTRIENT INTERACTION IN THE FETUS

In the foregoing sections, we examined ethanol-nutrient interactions in the mother and the placenta, with attention to how they might influence growth and development of the fetus. In this section, we will discuss the potential effects of ethanol-nutrient interaction at the level of the fetal tissue per se. Some of the physiologic alterations which occur in the maternal or placental tissue may be applicable to fetal tissue as well. Plus, there are interactions which may be uniquely harmful to the fetus.

1. Glucose

The mechanism by which ethanol impairs glucose uptake and transport in the human placenta is not well defined; but progress has been made in identifying ethanol-induced abnormalities in glucose metabolism in fetal tissue. These observations are particularly important in that glucose is virtually the sole fuel for neuronal tissue. Chronic ethanol exposure during pregnancy decreases fetal tissue uptake of glucose and lowers liver glycogen content in rats.[60-62] In the brain, chronic ethanol consumption inhibits expression of glucose transporter I.[63] All of these findings correlate with altered fetal growth.

2. Glutamine/Glutamate

The potential for accumulation of glutamate in the fetal circulation, which may be neurotoxic, was discussed in the previous section. In addition to the placental mechanisms presented above, there is recent evidence for derangement of glutamate production at the fetal level. Studies in pregnant sheep indicate that ethanol exposure increases extracellular glutamate in the cerebral cortex.[64] The source of the increased extracellular CNS glutamate, whether blood (i.e., extraneural tissue), neuronal tissue or both, is not clear.

3. Vitamin A

As initially indicated in this review, fetal abnormalities similar to some of those found in the FAS have been observed with both vitamin A deficiency and exposure to excess vitamin A. These teratogenic effects include the type of neural crest abnormalities seen in some cases of FAS. At the fetal level, ethanol may induce intracellular "deficiency" by competitive inhibition of the oxidative pathway for retinal formation, or "excess" via displacement of the vitamin from fetal hepatic stores (similar to what may be occurring in the mother). Recent publications on these two concepts are discussed below.

Vitamin A (retinol) is bound to carrier proteins in the serum and in the cytosol. Within the cell, retinol is reversibly oxidized by retinol dehydrogenase. This enzyme appears to be identical to class I alcohol dehydrogenase found in the human liver. The product of oxidation, retinal, is further oxidized to retinoic acid by the enzyme aldehyde dehyrogenase. The first step, i.e. catalyzed by retinol dehydrogenase, is felt to be the rate limiting step in retinoic acid synthesis. Since ethanol may compete with retinol for oxidation by retinol dehydrogenase in peripheral tissues[65-66] as well as in the liver,[65,67] it has been proposed that such inhibition of retinoic acid formation may cause a "deficiency" state within fetal tissue.[24-25] This intriguing hypothesis has yet to be confirmed experimentally, but many of the findings of the FAS could be explained in part by ethanol induced inhibition of retinoic acid formation.

On the other hand, ethanol interaction with fetal vitamin A metabolism may be fetotoxic by an opposite mechanism: tissue excess. This could be via mechanisms similar to those which probably occur in the mother (described above). In the fetus, ethanol may induce a shift in vitamin A from fetal liver, with resultant deposit in peripheral tissue and peripheral "excess." Zachman and colleagues have begun to address this alternate hypothesis. They point out that only 54% of retinol oxidation is inhibited by ethanol, even at extremely high concentrations, such as 100 mM.[68-69] In rats, they have shown depletion of vitamin A in the fetal liver and an increase in the lung and kidney, similar to what is found in adult, nonpregnant animals.[70] In a more recent study, they looked at binding proteins and vitamin A levels in the whole embryo, head and brain tissue of animals exposed to ethanol *in vivo*. They found that ethanol exposure caused increased levels of <u>retinol,</u> including the brain.[71] While this might be the result of a shift in vitamin A from fetal liver to the peripheral tissue, the possibility remains that this is the result of inhibition of retinol oxidation. Hence, it is not certain whether the peripheral tissue is actually being exposed to increased or decreased levels of <u>retinoic acid</u>. Nonetheless, the findings do indicate that ethanol induced alterations in fetal vitamin A metabolism may contribute to the pathophysiology of the FAS.

4. Zinc

While most studies fail to show a decrease in fetal tissue zinc following intrauterine ethanol exposure, one study indicates that there may be regional effects at the level of the fetal tissue. Savage and colleagues looked at rat pups at postnatal day 45. The pups which had been exposed to intrauterine ethanol had decreased zinc levels in the hippocampal mossy fibers, but not in other tissues.[72] Unfortunately, data are not available at birth and postnatal factors might have influenced these findings. Nonetheless, this study raises the possibility that there is ethanol-zinc interaction in certain fetal neuronal tissues.

V. SUMMARY

This review has examined the role of ethanol-nutrient interaction in the pathophysiology of the FAS. Ethanol effects on nutrient supply and metabolism are probably more important than "nutrition" (i.e., diet) alone in the decreased birthweight seen with intrauterine ethanol exposure. Indeed, in evaluating a large number of rat studies, Hannigan and Abel have concluded that ethanol exposure, *per se*, or the interaction between alcohol and caloric restriction as opposed to restricted caloric intake alone, is most responsible for decreased birthweight; the latter being a consistent effect of intrauterine ethanol exposure.[73] Ethanol-nutrient interaction may occur at the maternal, placental or fetal level. Since none are mutually exclusive, there is a strong possibility that ethanol-induced alterations are occurring at all levels. Figure 1 provides a graphical overview of potential ethanol-nutrient interactions.

Ethanol-Nutrient Interaction and the FAS

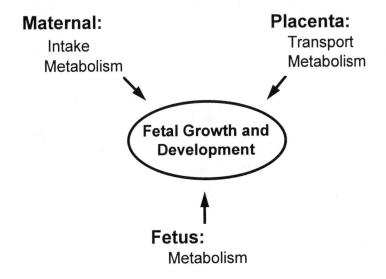

Figure 1: Summary of different levels of ethanol-nutrient interaction in the pathophysiology of the FAS

REFERENCES

1. **Jones, K.L., Smith, D.W., Ulleland, C.N., and Streissguth, A.P.,** Patterns of malformation in offspring of chronic alcoholic mothers, *Lancet*, i, 1076, 1973.
2. **Lemoine, P., Harroussean, H., Borteyru, J.P., and Menuet, J.C.,** Les enfants de parents alcooliques. Anomalies observees. A propos de 127 cas, *Questions de Medicine*, 25, 476, 1968.
3. **Crawford, M.A., Doyle, W., Leaf, A., Laigfield, M., Ghebremeskel, K., and Phylactos, A.,** Nutrition and Neurodevelopmental Disorders, *Nutr. Health,* 9, 81, 1993.
4. **Luke, B.,** Nutritional influences on fetal growth, *Clin. Obstet. Gynecol.,* 37, 538, 1994.
5. **Salaspuro, M.,** Nutrient intake and nutritional status in alcoholics, *Alcohol Alcohol.,* 28, 85, 1993.
6. **Roecklein, B., Levin, S.W., Comly, M., and Mukherjee, A.B.,** Intrauterine growth retardation induced by thiamine deficiency and pyrithiamine during pregnancy in the rat, *Am. J. Obstet. Gynecol,* 151, 455, 1985.
7. **Hoyumpa, A.M. Jr., Breen, K.J., Schenker, S., and Wilson, F.A.,** Thiamine transport across the rat intestine. Effect of ethanol, *J. Lab. Clin. Med.,* 86, 803, 1975.
8. **Mezey, E.,** Intestinal function in chronic alcoholism, *Ann. N.Y. Acad. Sci.,* 252, 215 1975.
9. **Muldoon, R.T. and McMartin, K.E.,** Ethanol acutely impairs the renal conservation of 5-methyltetrahydrofolate in the isolated perfused rat kidney, *Alc. Clin. Exp. Res.,* 18, 233, 1994.
10. **Hidiroglou, N., Camilo, M.E., Beckenhauer, H.C., and Tuma, D.J.,** Effect of chronic alcohol ingestion on hepatic folate distribution in the rat, *Biochem. Pharmacol.,* 47, 1561-6, 1994
11. **Shaw, S., Jayatilleke, E., Herbert, V., and Colman, N.,** Cleavage of folates during ethanol metabolism. Role of acetaldehyde/xanthine oxidase-generated superoxide, *Biochem. J.,* 257, 277-80, 1989.
12. **de Cornulier, M., de Lacour, F., Avet-Loiseau, H., Passuti N; *et al.,*** Vertebral involvement and fetal alcohol syndrome, *Pediatrie (Bucur),* 46, 685, 1991
13. **Goldstein, G. and Arulanantham, K.,** Neural tube defect and renal anomalies in a child with fetal alcohol syndrome, *J. Pediatr.,* 93, 636, 1978.
14. **Kovetski, N.S.,** Neural tube dysraphia at the level of the midbrain in alcoholic embryopathy, *Zh Nevropatol Psikhiatr. Im. S. S. Korsakova,* 91, 79, 1991.

15. **El Banna, N., Picciano, M.F., and Simon, J.,** Effect of chronic alcohol consumption and iron deficiency on maternal folate status and reproduction outcome in mice, *J. Nutr.,* 115, 2059, 1983.

16. **Leichter, J. and Lee, M.,** Intestinal folate conjugase activity and folate absorption in the ethanol-fed pregnant rat, *Drug Nutr. Interact,* 3, 53, 1984.

17. **Switzer, B.R., Anderson, J.J., and Pick, J.R.,** Effects of dietary protein and ethanol intake on pregnant beagles fed purified diets, *J. Nutr.,* 116, 689, 1986.

18. **Lin, G.W.,** Maternal-fetal folate transfer: Effect of ethanol and dietary folate deficiency, *Alcohol,* 8, 169, 1991.

19. **Larroque, B., Kaminski, M., Lelong, N., d'Herbomez, M.** *et al.,* Folate status during pregnancy: Relationship with alcohol consumption, other maternal risk factors and pregnancy outcome, *Eur. J. Obstet. Gynecol. Reprod. Biol.,* 43, 19, 1992.

20. **Mezey, E.,** Interaction between alcohol and nutrition in the Pathogenesis of alcoholic liver disease, *Semin. Liver Dis.,* 11, 340, 1991.

21. **Lin, G.W.,** Effect of ethanol and vitamin B_6 deficiency on pyridoxal 5-phosphate levels and fetal growth in rats, *Alc. Clin. Exp. Res.,* 13, 236, 1989.

22. **Lieber, C.S.,** Biochemical factors in alcoholic liver disease, *Semin. Liver Dis.,* 13, 136, 1993.

23. **Keir, W.J.,** Inhibition of retinoic acid synthesis and its implications in fetal alcohol syndrome, *Alc. Clin. Exp. Res.,* 15, 560, 1991.

24. **Duester, G.,** A hypothetical mechanism for fetal alcohol syndrome involving ethanol inhibition of retinoic acid synthesis at the alcohol dehydrogenase step, *Alc. Clin. Exp. Res.,* 15, 568, 1991.

25. **Pullarkat, R.K.,** Hypothesis: Prenatal ethanol-iduced birth defects and retinoic acid, *Alc. Clin. Exp. Res.,* 15, 565, 1991.

26. **McClain, C.J. and Su, L.C.,** Zinc deficiency in the alcoholic: A review, *Alc. Clin. Exp. Res.,* 7, 5, 1983.

27. **Flynn, A., Miller, S.I., Martier, S.S., Golden, N.L.** *et al.,* Zinc status of pregnant alcoholic women: A determinant of fetal outcome, *Lancet,* i, 551, 1981.

28. **Hurley, L.S.,** The fetal alcohol syndrome: Possible implications of nutrient deficiencies, in *NIAAA Monograph 2: Alcohol and Nutrition,* Li, T.K., Schenker, S., and Lumeng, L., Eds. DHEW Publications 79-780, US Government Printing Office, Washington, D.C., 1979.

29. **Rosso, P. and Cramoy, C.,** Nutrition and pregnancy, in *Nutrition, Pre- and Postnatal Development,* Winick, M., Ed., Plenum Press, New York, 1979, pp. 133-228.

30. **Keppen, L.D., Pysher, T., and Rennert, O.M.,** Zinc deficiency acts as a co-teratogen with alcohol in fetal alcohol syndrome, *Pediatr. Res.,* 19, 944, 1985.

31. **Keppen, L.D., Moore, D.J., and Cannon, D.J.,** Zinc nutrition in fetal alcohol syndrome, *Neurotoxicology,* 11, 375, 1990.

32. **Fisher, S.E., Alcock, N.W., Amirian, J., and Altshuler, H.L.,** Neonatal and maternal hair zinc levels in a nonhuman primate model of the fetal alcohol syndrome, *Alc. Clin. Exp. Res.,* 12, 417, 1988.

33. **Zeidenberg-Cherr, S., Benak, P.A., Hurley, L.S., and Keen, C.L.,** Altered mineral metabolism: A mechanism underlying the fetal alcohol syndrome in rats, *Drug Nutr. Interact.,* 5, 257, 1988.

34. **Harris, J.E.,** Hepatic glutathione, metallothionein and zinc in the rat on gestational day 19 during chronic ethanol administration, *J. Nutr.,* 120, 1080, 1990.

35. **Greeley, S., Johnson, W.T., Schafer, D., and Johnson, P.E.,** Gestational alcoholism and fetal zinc accretion in Long-Evans rats, *J. Am. Coll. Nutr.,* 9, 265, 1990.

36. **Snyder, A.K., Singh, S.P., and Pullen, G.L.,** Ethanol-induced intrauterine growth retardation: Correlation with placental glucose transfer, *Alc. Clin. Exp. Res.,* 10, 167, 1986.

37. **Schenker, S., Dicke, J.M., Johnson, R.F., Hays, S.E., and Henderson, G.I.,** Effect of ethanol on human placental transport of model amino acids and glucose, *Alc. Clin. Exp. Res.,* 13, 112, 1989.

38. **Lin, G.W.,** Effect of ethanol feeding during pregnancy on placental transfer of alpha-amino isobutyric acid in the rat, *Life Sci.* 28, 595, 1981.

39. **Fisher, S.E., Atkinson, M., Holzman, I., David, R., and Van Thiel, D.H.,** Effect of ethanol upon placental uptake of amino acids, in *Endocrinological Aspects of Alcoholism, Progress in Biochemical Pharmacology Series,* Messiha, F.S. and Tyner, B.D., Eds., Karger Verlag Publisher, Basel, Switzerland, 18, 216, 1981.

40. **Henderson, G.I., Turner, D., Patwardhan, R.V., Lumeng, L, Hoyumpa, A.M., and Schenker, S.,** Inhibition of placental valine uptake after acute and chronic maternal ethanol consumption, *J. Pharmacol. Exp. Ther.,* 216, 465, 1981.

41. **Henderson, G.I., Patwardhan, R.V., McLeroy, S., and Schenker, S.,** Inhibition of placental amino acid uptake in rats following acute and chronic ethanol exposure, *Alc. Clin. Exp. Res.,* 6, 495, 1982.

42. **Patwardhan, R.V., Schenker, S., Henderson, G.I., Abou-Mourad, N.N., and Hoyumpa, A.M.,** Short-term and long-term ethanol administration inhibits the placental uptake and transport of valine in rats, *J. Lab. Clin. Med.,* 98, 251, 1981.

43. **Fisher, S.E. and Karl, P.I.**, Alcohol and the Foetus, in *The Molecular Pathology of Alcoholism*, Palmer, T.N., Ed., Oxford University Press, New York, 1991, 254-279.

44. **Fisher, S.E., Duffy, L., and Atkinson, M.,** Selective fetal malnutrition: Effect of acute and chronic ethanol exposure upon rat placental Na,K-ATPase activity, *Alc. Clin. Exp. Res.,* 10, 150, 1986.

45. **Fisher, S.E., Atkinson, M., Jacobson, S., Sehgal, P., Burnap, J., Holmes, E., Teichberg, S., Kahn, E., Jaffe, R., and Van Thiel, D.H.,** Selective fetal malnutrition: The effect of *in vivo* ethanol exposure upon *in vitro* placental uptake of alpha amino isobutyric acid in the non-human primate, *Pediatr. Res.,* 17, 704, 1983.

46. **Fisher, S.E. and Karl, P.I.,** Histidine transfer across the human placenta: Characteristics in the isolated perfused human placenta and the effect of ethanol, *Placenta*, 11, 157, 1990.

47. **Karl, P.I. and Fisher, S.E.,** Chronic ethanol exposure inhibits insulin and IGF-1 stimulated amino acid uptake in cultured human placental trophoblasts, *Alc. Clin. Exp. Res.,* 18, 942, 1994.

48. **Vaughn, P.R., Lobo, C., Battaglia, F.C., Fennessey, P.V., Wilkening, R.B., and Meschia, G.,** Glutamine-glutamate exchange between placenta and fetal liver, *Am. J. Physiol.,* 268, 705, 1995.

49. **Karl, P.I., Kwun, R., Slonim, A., and Fisher, S.E.,** Ethanol elevates fetal serum glutamate levels in the rat, *Alc. Clin. Exp. Res.,* 19, 177, 1995.

50. **Karl, P.I. and Fisher, S.E.,** unpublished material.

51. **Baker, H., Frank, D., DeAngelis, B., Feingold, S., and Kaminetzky, H.E.,** Role of placenta in maternal-fetal vitamin transfer in humans, *Am. J. Obstet. Gynecol.,* 141, 792, 1981.

52. **Dancis J., Wilson D., Hoskins I.A., and Levitz M.,** Placental transfer of thiamine in the human subject: *In vitro* perfusion studies and maternal-cord plasma concentrations, *Am. J. Obstet. Gynecol.,* 159, 1435, 1988.

53. **Schenker, S., Johnson, R.F., Hoyumpa, A.M., and Henderson, G.I.,** Thiamine transfer by human placenta: Normal transport and effects of ethanol, *J. Lab. Clin. Med.,* 116, 106, 1990.

54. **Henderson, G.I., Perez, T., Schenker, S., Mackins, J., and Antony, A.C.,** Maternal-to-fetal transfer of 5-methyltetrahydrofolate by the perfused human placental cotyledon: Evidence for a concentrative role by placental folate receptors in fetal folate delivery, *J. Lab. Clin. Med.,* 126, 184, 1995.

55. **Fisher, S.E., Inselman, L.S., Duffy, L., Atkinson, M., Spencer, H., and Chang, B.,** Ethanol and fetal nutrition: Effect of chronic ethanol exposure on rat placental growth and membrane associated folic acid receptor binding activity, *J. Pediatr. Gastroenterol. Nutr.,* 4, 645, 1985.

56. **Schenker, S., Johnson, R.F., Mahuren, J.D., Henderson, G.I., and Coburn, S,P.,** Human placental vitamin B_6 (pyridoxal) transport: Normal characteristics and effects of ethanol, *Am. J. Physiol.,* 262, 966, 1992.

57. **Ghishan, F.K., Patwardhan, R., and Greene H.L.,** Fetal alcohol syndrome: Inhibition of placental zinc transport as a potential mechanism for fetal growth retardation in the rat, *J. Lab. Clin. Med.,* 100, 45, 1982.

58. **Ghishan, F.K. and Greene, H.L.,** Fetal alcohol syndrome: Failure of zinc supplementation to reverse the effect of ethanol on placental transport of zinc, *Pediatr. Res.,* 17, 529, 1983.

59. **Beer, W.H., Johnson, R.F., Guentzel, M.N., Lozano, J., Henderson, G.I., and Schenker, S.,** Human placental transfer of zinc: Normal characteristics and role of ethanol, *Alc. Clin. Exp. Res.,* 16, 98, 1992.

60. **Singh, S.P., Snyder, A.K., and Singh, S.K.,** Effects of ethanol ingestion on maternal and fetal glucose homeostasis, *J. Lab. Clin. Med.,* 104, 176, 1984.

61. **Singh, S.P., Snyder, A.K., and Pullen, G.L.,** Fetal alcohol syndrome: Glucose and liver metabolism in term rat fetus and neonate, *Alc. Clin. Exp. Res.,* 10, 54, 1986.

62. **Singh, S.P., Snyder, A.K, and Pullen, G.L.,** Maternal alcohol ingestion inhibits fetal glucose uptake and growth, *Neurotoxicol. Teratol.,* 11, 215, 1989.

63. **Singh, S.P., Pullen, G.L., Srivenugopal, K.S., Yuan, X.H., Snyder, A.K.,** Decreased glucose transporter 1 gene expression and glucose uptake in fetal brain exposed to ethanol, *Life Sci.,* 51, 527, 1992.

64. **Reynolds, J.D., Penning, D.H., Dexter, F., Atkins, B., Hrdy, J., Poduska, D., Chestnut, D.H., and Brien, J.F.,** Dose-dependent effects of acute *in vivo* ethanol exposure on extracellular glutamate concentration in the cerebral cortex of the near-term fetal sheep, *Alc. Clin. Exp. Res.,* in press.

65. **Mezey, E. and Holt, P.R.,** The inhibitory effect of ethanol on retinol oxidation by human liver and cattle retina, *Exp. Mol. Pathol.,* 15, 148, 1971.

66. **Van Thiel, D.H., Gavaler, J., and Lester, R.,** Ethanol inhibition of vitamin A metabolism in the testes: Possible mechanism of sterility in alcoholics, *Science,* 186, 941, 1974.

67. **Leo, M.A., Kim, C., and Lieber, C.S.,** NAD+ dependent retinol dehydrogenase in liver microsomes, *Arch. Biochem. Biophys.,* 259, 241, 1987.

68. **Zachman, R.D. and Grummer, M.A.,** [Letter], *Alc. Clin. Exp. Res.,* 16, 141, 1992.

69. **Napoli, J.L. and Race, K.R.,** The biosynthesis of retinoic acid from retinol in rat tissues *in vitro, Arch. Biochem. Biophys.,* 255, 95, 1987.

70. **Grummer, M.A. and Zachman, R.D.,** The effect of maternal ethanol ingestion on fetal vitamin A in the rat, *Pediatr. Res.,* 28, 1867, 1990.

71. **Grummer, M.A., Langhough, R.E., and Zachman, R.D.,** Maternal ethanol ingestion effects on fetal rat brain vitamin A as a model for fetal alcohol syndrome, *Alc. Clin. Exp. Res.,* 17, 592, 1993.

72. **Savage, D.D., Montano, C.Y., Paxton, L.L., and Kasarskis, E.J.,** Prenatal ethanol exposure decreases hippocampal mossy fiber zinc in 45-day-old rats, *Alc. Clin. Exp. Res.,* 13, 588, 1989.

73. **Hannigan, J.H., Abel, E.L., Kruger, M.L.,** Population characteristics of birthweight in an animal model of alcohol-related developmental effects, *Neurotoxicol. Teratol.,* 15, 97, 1993.

Chapter 14

BROWN ADIPOSE TISSUE: A MODEL SYSTEM TO INVESTIGATE FETAL ALCOHOL EFFECTS ON THERMOREGULATION

Betty Zimmerberg

I. INTRODUCTION

Despite increased educational efforts to curtail alcohol intake in pregnant women, exposure to alcohol *in utero* persists as a major medical problem in this country. The effects of prenatal alcohol exposure are now known to be dose-related: Fetal Alcohol Syndrome only describes the extreme end of numerous fetal alcohol effects (FAE). At birth, the alcohol-exposed neonate is likely to be hyperactive, hypotonic, tremulous, less easily aroused, slower to habituate, and irritable.[1-2] Spontaneous seizure activity and increased respiratory rate are viewed as signs of alcohol withdrawal.[3] In 23 FAS cases, 17% of the newborns died by one week of age; one infant died of respiratory distress.[4] Among full-term infants, the incidence of respiratory distress syndrome was greater among infants born to binge drinkers and alcoholic women compared to more moderate drinkers.[5] Neonatal state regulation also is disrupted - FAS infants take longer to fall asleep and spend less total time in REM sleep and quiet sleep,[6-7] and their EEG's are hypersynchronous during all stages of sleep.[8]

One aspect of neonatal state regulation that has not been examined in FAS infants is thermoregulation. Although full-term human neonates show the same average body temperature as adults, they are less resistant to high and low temperatures. Low birth weight infants may be particularly sensitive to ambient temperatures below thermoneutrality.[9] Indeed, survival rates of low birth weight infants are lower when the environmental temperature is decreased by only a few degrees. Since low birth weight and growth retardation are consistently observed in FAS[10-12] and chronic maternal alcoholism,[13] any alcohol-induced altered development of temperature regulation in newborns would have negative consequences for growth and neural development. An alcohol-exposed infant with body temperature dysregulation is an infant at greater risk for respiratory distress, sudden infant death, and delayed neural and body growth. Normal processes subserving recovery from neuronal damage (e.g., resealing of lesioned fibers, removal of damaged debris, protein synthesis and distribution of structural components through axonal transport) are temperature-dependent[14] and thus an FAS newborn with an immature thermoregulatory system might be less able to recover from alcohol-induced neural damage sustained *in utero*. In addition, an infant with a lower body temperature may be lethargic and fail to elicit care, which would exacerbate a postnatal growth retardation.[15]

In addition to its potential clinical importance, a study of the mechanisms subserving thermoregulation provides a model system to understand more broadly how prenatal alcohol exposure may be affecting neural function, both peripherally and centrally. To maintain an adequate body temperature, immature mammals rely principally on the activation by the sympathetic nervous system of non-shivering thermogenesis in brown adipose tissue (discussed in Section III). Thermoregulation thus has several levels at which to examine the effects of prenatal alcohol exposure. Prenatal alcohol exposure may alter the growth of brown adipose tissue, impair its functional capacity, or affect the development of peripheral or central neural control of non-shivering thermogenesis in brown adipose tissue. This chapter will first describe the initial studies demonstrating that prenatal alcohol exposure impairs thermoregulation in animal models of FAE, and then relate the more mechanistically-oriented studies attempting to elucidate the bases of alcohol-related dysfunctions.

II. FETAL ALCOHOL-RELATED THERMOREGULATORY DISTURBANCES

A. ANIMAL MODEL OF FETAL ALCOHOL EXPOSURE

In all of the studies in this laboratory, subjects were bred from Long Evans hooded male and female rats. Pregnant dams were assigned to one of the three treatment groups: LC, 0% EDC and 35% EDC. Females in the Lab Chow (LC) control group had continuous access to standard lab chow and water throughout their pregnancies. Pregnant dams in the other two treatment groups were treated identically to LC dams from Gestational Day (GD) 1 - GD 5 but then received liquid diets beginning on GD 6. In the alcohol treatment condition, the pregnant dams were given a liquid diet consisting of 6.7% v/v ethanol (Liquid Diet F1265, Bioserv Inc, Frenchtown, NJ). This diet provided 35% of the total caloric content as ethanol (35% ethanol derived calories, 35% EDC). In the nutritional pair-fed control group, the pregnant dams on GD6 received a similar liquid diet (Liquid Diet F1264) except that the ethanol was replaced isocalorically with maltose-dextrin (0% ethanol-derived calories, 0% EDC). Dams in the 0% EDC group were provided the mean amount consumed by 35% EDC dams, corrected for body weight on a ml/kg basis, for each specific day of pregnancy. Thus, each yoked pair received the same relative volume of diet and hence the same number of calories on a body weight basis; the only difference will be the presence or absence of alcohol. On GD 20, liquid diets were replaced by continuous access to lab chow and water. Following parturition, pups were weighed and culled randomly to 10 pups per litter, maintaining 5 of each sex whenever possible. In all of the experiments described in this chapter, only one male and female subject from any one litter were tested to avoid litter confounds.

B. FETAL ALCOHOL EXPOSURE AND NEONATAL THERMOREGULATION

The body temperature of the neonatal rat is regulated by both its own physiological status and the presence of the mother and siblings in the nest. To determine whether prenatal alcohol exposure would affect the ability to thermoregulate, subjects were removed from their home cage and placed individually in small compartments for four hours.[16] Rectal temperatures were recorded hourly. Pups from the three prenatal treatment groups were tested at four ages. With increasing age, all pups developed the ability to maintain thermoneutrality, However, prenatal alcohol-exposed pups were not able to maintain as high a body temperature as control pups at five and ten days of age. Since the 35% EDC pups weighed less than control pups, an additional study demonstrated that reduced body weight was not itself responsible for the thermoregulatory deficit. This effect was also found to be largely independent of any maternal factors; a replication of the previous study using a cross-fostering paradigm had identical results.[17] There was a significant interaction between Prenatal Treatment, Age and Time on body temperature (see Figure 1). Non-fostered prenatal alcohol-exposed pups at both 5 and 10 days of age had significantly greater decreases in body temperature over time compared to all three control groups. Fostered prenatal alcohol-exposed pups at some time points did not differ from pair-fed control pups, but at all time points after leaving the nest they did differ significantly from both fostered and non-fostered lab chow groups.

Although in this initial study thermoregulation appeared normative in 20-day-old alcohol-exposed offspring, studies from other laboratories suggested underlying deficits might remain since thermoregulatory deficits could be unmasked after pharmacological challenge in older offspring.[18-22] Thermoregulatory deficits can be detected in 20-day-old prenatal alcohol-exposed offspring under more stressful testing conditions. If pups are placed in a 10°C environment, alcohol-exposed pups lose body temperature at a faster rate and drop to a lower set-point compared to control pups.[23] Thermoregulatory deficits can also be detected at 20 days of age by directly measuring brown adipose tissue temperature. When pups at this age are removed from the home nest and placed individually in small compartments with an indwelling guide cannula in their interscapular brown adipose tissue, the baseline temperature of alcohol offspring is significantly lower than that of both control groups during a 20 minute test.[24]

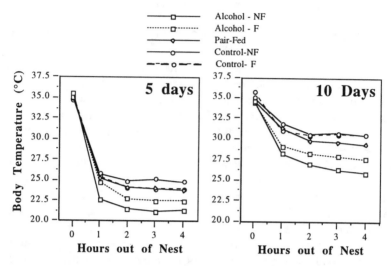

Figure 1. Mean body temperatures (°C) in Long-Evans rats at five and ten days of age individually removed from the home nest for four hours. Subjects (n's = 8 - 11/sex/ group/age) represent offspring from one of three prenatal treatment groups (Alcohol, Pair-fed or Control) who were either fostered at birth to control dams (F, fostered groups - dotted lines) or remained with their birth dams (NF, non-fostered groups - solid lines).

In order to determine whether prenatal alcohol exposure affects neonatal thermoregulation in the home nest, body temperatures of rat pups were assessed using telemetry techniques (Mini-Mitter Inc., Sun River OR). This system consisted of implantable AM transmitters (Mini-Mitter Inc., Model XM), receiver platforms placed under each home cage, two consolidation matrices (BCM-100), and a computer (Zenith Data Systems Model XT) for data acquisition. At 12 days of age, one female or one male subject was randomly chosen from each of sixteen litters from the three prenatal treatment groups and implanted interperitoneally with a transmitter. After recovery from surgery, the subject was replaced in the home nest with its mother and siblings. The subject's body temperature could then be continuously recorded during its normal activities without any disturbance from experimenters. The results for the first week of this study are shown in Figure 2. There was a main effect of Prenatal Condition on the daily mean body temperature from postnatal days 13 through 20. All three groups differed significantly from each other. There was not a significant interaction between Day and Prenatal Condition, indicating that although the rate of improvement in thermoregulatory mechanisms does develop over time in parallel with controls, prenatal alcohol exposure results in a lower basal body temperature in rat pups despite the presence of the dam and siblings. This lower body temperature appears to normalize after the third week of life, however. When mean body temperatures of these subjects was analyzed by week for the next six weeks, no significant differences by prenatal treatment were obtained (see Figure 3).

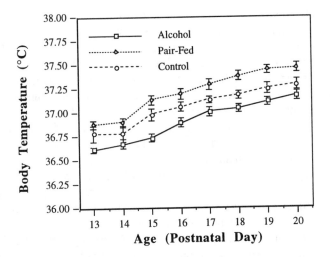

Figure 2. Mean daily body temperatures (°C) + S.E.M. measured telemetrically in subjects (n's = 8/sex/group) representing litters from each of three prenatal treatment groups (Alcohol, Pair-fed or Control) from 13 to 20 days of age.

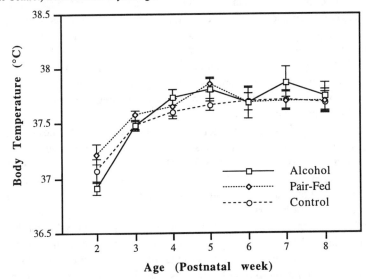

Figure 3. Mean daily body temperatures (°C) ± S.E.M. measured telemetrically in subjects (n's = 8/sex/group) representing litters from each of three prenatal treatment groups (Alcohol, Pair-fed or Control) averaged over each week from 2-8 weeks of age.

Pups rely on a combination of self-initiated non-shivering thermogenesis, maternal heat, and huddling behavior to maintain an adequate body temperature.[25-26] The results of this telemetry study supports the hypothesis that thermoregulatory deficits observed in studies in which the pup was removed from the home nest were not due to the stress of removal but were indeed a reflection of a physiological dysfunction. Studies to determine whether the deficit is due to inadequate non-shivering thermogenesis are described later in this chapter. Prenatal alcohol-related thermoregulatory deficits do not appear to be due to a difference in maternal body temperature, since telemetry studies conducted in this laboratory on body temperatures of dams during lactation did not reveal any differences between dams who had consumed alcohol during pregnancy compared to pair-fed or lab chow control dams. Another hypothesis is that alcohol-exposed pups are deficient in their ability to engage in behavioral thermoregulation (e.g, huddling behavior); studies to explore this hypothesis are described in section E.

Studies in other laboratories have replicated our observation of prenatal alcohol related-thermoregulatory deficits in both neonatal rats[27] and mice.[28] Both Long Sleep and Short Sleep mice exposed to alcohol prenatally were found to have lower body temperatures at one and two hours after removal from the home nest compared to controls. This thermoregulatory deficit was apparent from postnatal days 7 through 21. Interestingly, although prenatal alcohol exposed Short Sleep mice had similar thermoregulatory dysfunction, they did not have body weight deficits; this observation confirms that an unfavorable body surface to mass ratio is not responsible for the results seen in both species. In another study looking at offspring of dams fed beer both before, during and after pregnancy, offspring at 29 days of age had lower baseline body temperatures.[22] The deficit was not seen when subjects were retested at 85 days of age. In our laboratory, we did not find any evidence of body temperature differences among prenatal treatment groups in either sex at 28 days of age using either the rectal probe or telemetry procedures under standard laboratory housing conditions.

The presence of thermoregulatory deficits in the first few weeks of life might have significant implications for both body growth and neural development in offspring exposed to alcohol prenatally. One easily measured index of temperature-dependent growth in rodents is the length of their tails. In mammals whose habitats spread across from varying climates, peripheral body parts (e.g., tails, ears, paws, antlers) reach shorter final lengths as you move further north in colder climate's. This naturalistic observation has been confirmed in the laboratory - mice reared in lower temperatures have shorter ears and tails than controls reared at room temperature.[29] Since neonatal rats exposed to alcohol in utero have lower body temperatures, one demonstration of a functional consequence might be seen in tail length. Indeed, tails of rat pups exposed to alcohol prenatally grew at a slower rate than tails of control pups, although their body lengths grew at parallel rates.[30] This disproportionate reduction in tail growth was an indirect indication that alcohol-exposed neonatal rats were experiencing periods of lower ambient nest temperature than controls.

C. FETAL ALCOHOL EXPOSURE AND ADULT THERMOREGULATION: CIRCADIAN RHYTHMS

One important aspect of thermoregulation is its circadian rhythm, so we have also examined the effects of prenatal alcohol exposure on body temperature rhythms in adult offspring.[31-32] Adult male and female offspring were monitored for body temperature and activity using the telemetry system described above under various light-dark (LD) schedule conditions. Baseline measures were unaffected by prenatal treatment under standard housing conditions (12:12 LD). There were, however, main effects of sex: females were more active, had higher mean body temperatures, and had higher maximal temperatures that peaked earlier in the evening than males regardless of prenatal condition.

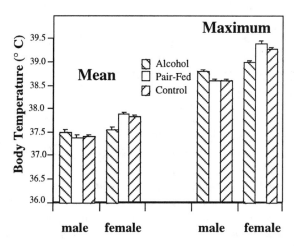

Figure 4. Mean and maximum body temperatures (°C) ± S.E.M. measured telemetrically in male and female adult offspring (n's ≐ 8/sex/group) from each of three prenatal treatment groups (Alcohol, Pair-fed or Control) during the second week of a constant light (LL) schedule.

Although thermoregulatory deficits do not appear to be detectable in adult offspring under standard laboratory conditions, environmental stress might reveal underlying deficits. A mild shift to 14:10 LD schedule did not detect any thermoregulatory differences between prenatal treatment groups. We did see some persistent effects of prenatal alcohol exposure on body temperature, however, when we switched the animals to an all light schedule (LL), which is a greater environmental stressor. Mean and maximal daily body temperatures during the second week of the LL schedule were significantly higher in alcohol-exposed males and significantly lower in alcohol-exposed females than same sex controls. Thus, alcohol-exposed offspring no longer displayed the typical sex-dependent pattern of body temperature under constant light stress, as seen in Figure 4. There was also one interesting effect of prenatal alcohol exposure of switching to an all light schedule on circadian rhythms of body temperature in males (but not females). Although all subjects demonstrated phase advancement when placed in a "free-running" all-light environment, alcohol-exposed male subjects lagged significantly behind male controls, as measured by the period length and the "acrophase" (time before midnight when the body temperature reaches its peak).

D.   FETAL ALCOHOL EXPOSURE AND THERMIC RESPONSE TO ETHANOL

These results suggested that the stress of the constant light schedule revealed underlying thermoregulatory dysfunction in alcohol-exposed adult offspring. Similarly, although studies of drug challenges with alcohol and other hypothermic agents in adult rats prenatally exposed to alcohol have been inconsistent, they all suggest a persistent underlying alteration in thermoregulatory mechanisms. In the first study, alcohol-exposed male offspring had a decreased hypothermic response to 2 g/kg ethanol, and alcohol-exposed females had a decreased hypothermic response to 2 or 3 g/kg of ethanol compared to controls.[18] In contrast, two subsequent studies, using a different strain and a different prenatal alcohol administration model, found that both male and female alcohol-exposed offspring demonstrated an augmented hypothermic response to 0.75, 1.5 and 3 g/kg of ethanol compared to controls.[19-20] Male offspring of beer-drinking dams were less hypothermic than controls in response to 3 g/kg ethanol.[22] Interestingly, rats exposed to alcohol only on gestational day 8 were less hypothermic in response to 2.82 g/kg alcohol than controls at 60-63 days of age.[21] Finally, a recent study looking at the effects of postnatal handling on subsequent thermic response to 2 g/kg of ethanol reported that non-handled prenatal alcohol exposed males had no differential response to ethanol, but that handled prenatal alcohol exposed and pair-fed control males had an augmented hyperthermic response.[33] There were no effects of prenatal treatment on thermic response to this dose of ethanol in females, regardless of the handling condition.

None of these studies, however, used a biotelemetry system. Using the telemetry system, we compared thermic responses to saline, 1.5 g/kg and 3.0 g/kg ethanol (20% w/v in saline) in adult male and female rats from the three prenatal treatment groups implanted with telemetry transmitters.[32] Injections (i.p.) were spaced four to five days apart and counter-balanced. There were no prenatal treatment differences in response to saline or the lower dose of ethanol. There was a sex-dependent response to the higher dose of ethanol: prenatal alcohol-exposed females were less hypothermic than controls. Male offspring did not differ in their response to ethanol by prenatal treatment group. Results from these studies are seen in Figure 5. To determine whether circulating gonadal hormones were responsible for the sex difference in outcome, we included a group of ovariectomized females. Ovariectomized females from the alcohol prenatal treatment group were also less hypothermic in response to alcohol compared to controls, suggesting a non-hormonal mediation of the sex difference in thermic response between male and female prenatal alcohol exposed adult offspring.

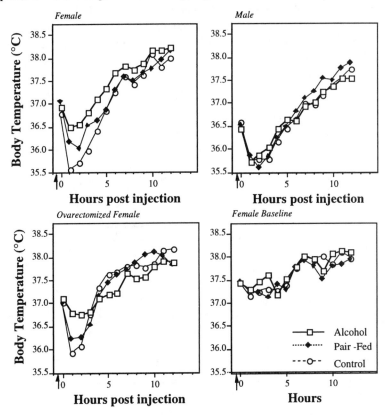

Figure 5. Mean body temperatures (°C) measured telemetrically in female, male and ovariectomized female subjects (n's = 8/sex/group) from each of three prenatal treatment groups (Alcohol, Pair-fed or Control) after administration of 3.0 g/kg ethanol. The lower right graph represents body temperatures in intact females during the same time period but without any injections.

Most studies of thermoregulatory response after pharmacological challenge use rectal probes, and measure body temperature by inserting probes hourly. Many factors, including rectal probes and handling, can alter thermic response to alcohol via "stress hyperthermia."[34-35] Since there have been discrepancies between various laboratories in their results, as discussed above, the next experiment was designed to determine whether the stress response to the probe alone might be affected by prenatal treatment.[32] In this experiment, male and female subjects from the three prenatal treatment groups with telemetry transmitters implanted previously were individually removed from their home cages, and had a standard thermistor (RT-3, Physiotemp Instruments, Clifton,

NJ) inserted rectally once every hour for six hours. After this "fake" temperature measurement replicating the procedure in previous studies, the subjects were placed back in their cages on top of the receivers, and their body temperature monitored telemetrically every 15 minutes. The results of this study are shown in Figure 6. All subjects showed a "stress" hyperthermia immediately after the rectal probe, and this hyperthermic response habituated over the six hours.

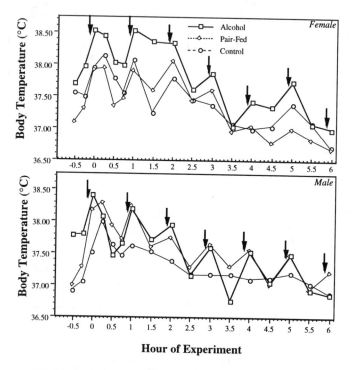

Figure 6. Mean body temperatures (°C) measured telemetrically in female and male subjects (n's = 8/sex/group) from each of three prenatal treatment groups (Alcohol, Pair-fed or Control) after insertion of a standard rectal thermistor every hour for six hours.

However, females exposed to alcohol prenatally had a greater hyperthermic response than female controls. Among the male subjects, both the prenatal alcohol exposure group and the pair-fed control group had greater hyperthermic responses than standard lab chow controls. Sex differences in stress response in prenatal alcohol exposed subjects and pair-fed effects have also been demonstrated in other studies.[36-37] The results of this experiment suggest that interpretations of the thermic response to a pharmacological challenge using a standard rectal temperature paradigm may be subject to a confounding stress response variable.

E.   FETAL ALCOHOL EXPOSURE AND BEHAVIORAL THERMOREGULATION

Thermoregulation may be impaired in young rodents because of a prenatal alcohol-related impairment of behavioral thermoregulation. The investigation of behavioral thermoregulation in small mammals has employed a variety of apparati, each designed to offer the subject either a choice of environments with different ambient temperatures or the opportunity to change the ambient temperature of an otherwise constant environment.   Infants of several mammalian species can seek heat and can move along a thermal gradient (thermocline) from cold to warm positions.[38] The consistent ability to choose a warm environment has been reported to develop in neonatal rats at about 6 days of age.[39] Even younger pups have demonstrated some limited ability to regulate their temperature behaviorally by selecting an appropriate position on a thermal gradient, given suitable testing conditions.[40-41]

In an initial study of the effects of prenatal alcohol exposure on behavioral thermoregulation, alcohol-exposed rat pups were found to be slower to reach a wall to huddle compared to controls.[16] In a subsequent experiment, behavior in a thermocline was assessed.[42] Alcohol-exposed pups at 5 days of age were found to move further along a temperature gradient than controls when tested repeatedly for 5 ten-min. trials. These results suggested that alcohol-exposed offspring are not impaired in learning a behavioral thermoregulatory response. Similar results have been reported in three day old mice prenatally exposed to alcohol.[43] Although 5 day old pups from all prenatal treatment groups moved towards the hot end of the thermocline, none of the pups chose a position that would maintain their body temperature at thermoneutrality.

Since this age was too young to determine the effects of prenatal alcohol exposure on body temperature "set-point," older offspring were tested in a larger thermocline for a longer observational period in order to better assess the effects of prenatal alcohol on behavioral thermoregulation.[44] In this study, the temperature preference behaviors of 10, 15 and 125 day old male and female offspring from the three prenatal treatment conditions were observed. Subjects were placed in the thermocline in the cold (20° C), hot (45° C) or middle start positions and observed for 60 minutes. Ten and fifteen day old rats exposed to alcohol prenatally preferred warmer temperatures when started at the hot end of the thermocline, and colder temperatures when started at the cold end, compared to control subjects. Adult subjects did not differ by prenatal treatment. From these three studies, we can thus conclude that alcohol-exposed offspring are not impaired in behavioral thermoregulation. However, our study does indicate that thermoregulatory set-point is affected by prenatal alcohol exposure. The thermoregulatory set-point has been defined as a reference body temperature that is defended physiologically and behaviorally.[45] Within this set-point are body temperatures considered to constitute a thermoneutral zone, in which the basal rate of heat production is equivalent to the rate of heat loss, thus conserving energy by requiring very little thermoregulatory effort.[46]

During the first two weeks of life, alcohol-exposed neonatal rats have lower body temperatures than controls when placed in an experimental situation of low ambient temperature,[16,27] and have higher body temperatures than controls when placed in an experimental situation of high ambient temperature.[42] This inability to retain heat during cold exposure coupled with an inability to dissipate heat during heat exposure may lead to a "widening" of the thermoneutral zone in young rats prenatally exposed to alcohol. A wider thermoneutral zone might allow the alcohol-exposed animal to adapt to naturally occurring alternating experiences of heat and cold stress. If a neonatal rat is constantly challenged by thermal stress, food energy is diverted from normal growth processes. For example, neonatal rats separated from their dams at room temperature grew more slowly and did not show normal developmental increases in brain weight, brain protein, RNA or DNA content compared to similarly separated rats maintained at nest temperature.[47-48] In summary, these results (a) ruled out behavioral thermoregulation as an important factor in thermoregulatory deficits in alcohol-exposed offspring, and (b) established that these alcohol-related thermoregulatory deficits have functional consequences in terms of thermoregulatory set-point. The next series of studies were designed to determine the mechanism of these thermoregulatory deficits.

III. BROWN ADIPOSE TISSUE AND NON-SHIVERING THERMOGENESIS

Newborns use a combination of physiological and behavioral mechanisms to maintain thermoneutrality. The major physiological mechanism is the activation of non-shivering thermogenesis in a specialized "thermogenic" organ - brown adipose tissue - located around vital organs and the interscapular area. Figure 7A presents an electronmicrograph of brown adipose tissue from an adult rat bred in our laboratory. Brown adipose tissue is characterized by an abundance of mitochondria, sympathetic nerve terminals, capillary networks and multiple vacuoles.[49] The importance of non-shivering thermogenesis for maintaining body temperature appears to lessen with age, except in conditions of cold-acclimation.[50] Figure 7B presents an electronmicrograph from a cold-acclimated rat in our laboratory; the increase in the number of mitochondria is indeed striking. Although there are over a dozen locations in the body where brown adipose tissue is located, the samples shown in these figures, and used in all of the following experiments, comes from one particular site located between the shoulder blades on the dorsal surface. This interscapular area allows an easy dissection and an adequate sample size.

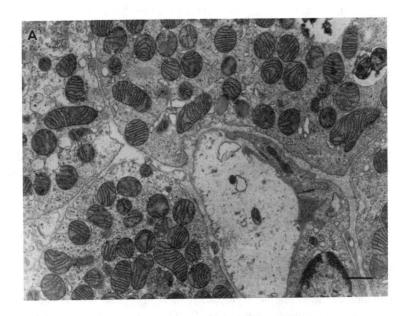

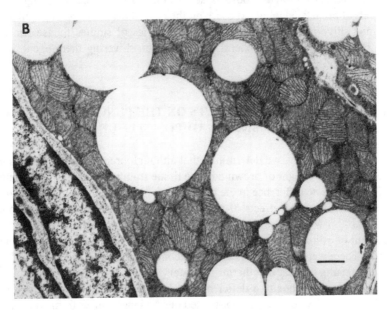

Figure 7. Electron micrographs of brown adipose tissue from adult Long-Evans rats housed either (A) under standard laboratory conditions (23°C) or (B) for four weeks at 5°C in a cold room. Brown adipose tissue differs from white adipose tissue in that there are many sympathetic nerve endings and capillaries, numerous mitochondira, and multiple small triglyceride droplets.[49] (Magnification X 8,840; bar = 1 micron. N. P. Piatczyc)

In non-shivering thermogenesis, heat is generated by lipolysis via a proton conductance pathway across the inner membrane of the mitochondria leading to a controlled uncoupling of respiration from the synthesis of ATP.[51] Proton conductance is regulated by a protein unique to brown adipose tissue called uncoupling protein or "thermogenin."[52]   Non-shivering thermogenesis is regulated by the sympathetic nervous system, which, in turn, is regulated by the hypothalamus.[53] For example, electrical stimulation of the ventromedial hypothalamus in rats increases temperature, norepinephrine turnover and lipid metabolism in brown adipose tissue; this effect is mediated by the sympathetic nervous system.[54-55] The preoptic anterior hypothalamus is also implicated in the control of sympathetic innervation of brown adipose tissue[56-57] although its effects may be mediated through the ventromedial hypothalamus.[58] Local application of glutamate in several hypothalamic nuclei also activates brown adipose tissue, also mediated via the sympathetic nervous system.[59] Prenatal alcohol exposure has been found to alter the functioning of dopamine, norepinephrine and serotonin neurochemical systems in the hypothalamus.[60-61] These three hypothalamic neurotransmitter systems are all involved in thermoregulation, and could be sites for alcohol's teratological effects on regulation of the developing sympathetic nervous system and its control of thermogenesis in brown adipose tissue (BAT). However, before turning to the effects of prenatal alcohol exposure on the central nervous system regulation of non-shivering thermogenesis, the next series of studies focuses on the functional status and peripheral control of non-shivering thermogenesis in brown adipose tissue.

IV. FETAL ALCOHOL EFFECTS ON THE FUNCTIONAL STATUS OF BROWN ADIPOSE TISSUE

In the first study, we determined that although prenatal alcohol exposure decreased the weight of brown adipose tissue from postnatal days 1 through 20, there was no difference in the proportion of brown adipose tissue to body weight.[30] Next, the effects of prenatal alcohol exposure on the functional status of brown adipose tissue were assessed by immunoblot analysis of the content of mitochondrial uncoupling protein (UCP) on postnatal days 1 and 20.[62] There were no effects of prenatal alcohol exposure on the UCP content. These results suggest that thermoregulatory deficits seen in alcohol-exposed offspring are not due to a deficiency in the concentration of mitochondrial UCP. At 20 days of age, alcohol-treated rats no longer differ from controls in their ability to maintain thermoneutrality when removed from the home nest. It seems likely that alcohol-treated offspring compensate for their delayed development in thermoregulation by increasing sympathetic activation of brown adipose tissue as opposed to synthesizing additional UCP. The results of this study were corroborated by our subsequent finding that protein concentration in brown adipose tissue was not affected by prenatal treatment.

In another laboratory, the ratio of brown adipose tissue weight to body weight was found to be greater in two week old alcohol-exposed pups compared to controls.[63] They also found that there was a greater protein content, and higher activities of cytochrome oxidase and succinate dehydrogenase, two mitochondrial oxidative enzymes in BAT, compared to controls. It is difficult to compare our results to those of this study because a different alcohol administration paradigm was employed - alcohol was the sole source of fluids for dams for several weeks prior to pregnancy, during gestation, and during lactation, and there was no nutritional control group.

V. FETAL ALCOHOL EFFECTS ON THE SYMPATHETIC INNERVATION OF BROWN ADIPOSE TISSUE

There are few previous studies on the effects of prenatal alcohol exposure on the developing sympathetic nervous system (SNS). Prenatal alcohol exposure altered SNS development in the heart,[64-66] thymus and spleen.[67] Alcohol added to cultured rat sympathetic neurons changes axonal growth and Schwann cell number.[68] Gastric intubation on GD 10-16, however, did not affect beta-adrenergic receptor binding in the heart, although the alcohol administration procedure as well as the tissue differed from our methods.[69] The following studies were conducted to determine the effects of prenatal alcohol exposure on the developmental pattern of sympathetic innervation to BAT in an attempt to elucidate the nature of alcohol-related thermoregulatory dysfunction and how the SNS might attempt to compensate for prenatal insult by alcohol.

A. FETAL ALCOHOL EXPOSURE AND NOREPINEPHRINE CONCENTRATIONS

To determine whether prenatal alcohol exposure alters the normal developmental course of norepinephrine concentration in brown adipose tissue, the concentrations of norepinephrine in interscapular brown adipose tissue in 5, 10, and 20 day old male and female offspring from the three prenatal treatment groups were assessed.[70] Norepinephrine was measured by reverse-phase high performance liquid chromatography, using electrochemical detection. There was a significant interaction between prenatal treatment and age (see Figure 8). At five days of age, the mean norepinephrine concentration was significantly lower in the alcohol group than in the pair-fed and control groups, which did not differ from each other. At twenty days of age, the mean norepinephrine concentration in the alcohol group was significantly higher than the pair-fed and control groups, which did not differ from each other. There was also a significant effect of age; the norepinephrine concentrations were lower at five days of age than at ten or twenty days of age, but norepinephrine concentrations did not differ at the two older ages. These results suggested a delay in the development of the sympathetic activation thermogenesis, followed by a compensatory overactivation. The early deficiency may have been due to the late arrival of sympathetic neurons. At 20 days of age, the increased norepinephrine concentration may reflect neuronal sprouting by the sympathetic fibers.

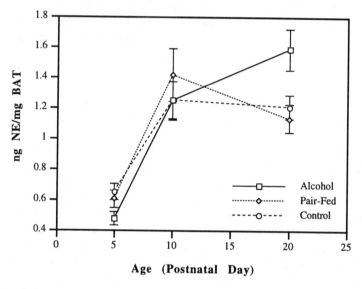

Figure 8. Mean concentration of norepinephrone (NE) in brown adipose tissue (ng/mg tissue) (± SEM) for three prenatal treatment groups at 5, 10 and 20 days of age. (From Zimmerberg, B. *et al.*, Alc. Clin. Exp. Res. 17, 418, 1993. With permission.)

B.   FETAL ALCOHOL EXPOSURE AND NOREPINEPHRINE TRANSPORTER

One measure of terminal density is the concentration of transporter protein sites.[71-72] To determine, indirectly, whether prenatal alcohol exposure was associated with increased norepinephrine concentration because of an increased number of terminal boutons, we assessed the density and sensitivity of norepinephrine transporter protein in 10 and 20 days old male and female subjects from the three prenatal treatment groups. All assays were performed in triplicate in a final volume of 1.0 ml containing 50 µl of ^{3}H-nisoxetine (Dupont New England Nuclear (NEN), Boston, MA), 500 µl tissue homogenate and 450 µl incubation buffer for total binding. To define non-specific binding, 400 µl of incubation buffer and 50 µl of 1 µM mazindol (Sigma Chemical Co., St. Louis, MO) was added to the radioactive ligand and tissue. Saturation analyses were performed over three log units of radioligand concentration (0.01-10 nM). Tubes were incubated for 2 hours at 0° C.[71,73] The incubation was terminated by immediate filtration over Schleicher and Schuell glass fiber filters (presoaked in 0.1% polyethyleneimine) and then washed with 10 ml of ice-cold buffer. Filters were placed in plastic vials and 5 ml of Formula 989 (NEN) added. After 90 min, ^{3}H-nisoxetine radioactivity was counted by Liquid Scintillation Spectrometry, on a Beckman 3801 liquid scintillation counter at an efficiency of 50%. Competition experiments that determined the displacement of ^{3}H-nisoxetine (2.0 nM) by desipramine, a drug known to have high affinity for NE uptake sites, over 6 log units (21 points, 1.0 μM - 0.1 nM) were performed , and we found that ^{3}H-nisoxetine was labeling a single site in BAT as it does in the brain.

There were no effects of age, sex or prenatal treatment on the number or sensitivity of NE uptake sites (see Figure 9). Although these results do reflect an indirect measure, it does appear as if there are no differences in the number of functional axonal terminals in the sympathetic fibers innervating brown adipose tissue at 10 or 20 days of age.

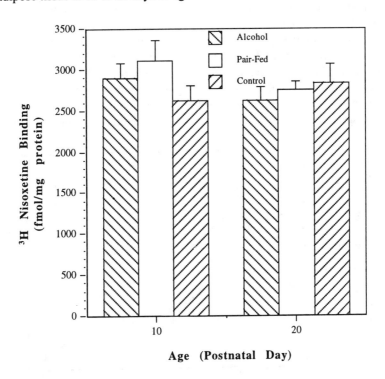

Figure 9. Mean concentration ± S.E.M. of ^{3}H-nisoxetine binding to norepinephrine transporter binding site in ten and twenty day old offspring (n's = 8-11/group) from each of three prenatal treatment group (Alcohol, Pair-fed or Control).

C. FETAL ALCOHOL EXPOSURE AND ADRENORECEPTORS

Another critical aspect in our investigation of the effects of prenatal alcohol exposure on the development of the sympathetic innervation of brown adipose tissue is the density and pharmacological properties of the receptors. Brown adipose tissue cells have both alpha and beta adrenergic receptors; the alpha receptors are thought to play only a minor role in thermogenesis.[49] In this next experiment, beta (β) adrenergic receptors were quantified. Brown adipose tissue was dissected and membranes prepared[74] from 1, 5, 10, and 20 day old male and female offspring from the three prenatal treatment groups.[75] For each age, 21 point competition studies comparing the displacement of ^{125}I-cyanopindolol (I-CYP; 50 pM) over 6 log units of propranolol, ICI 118,551 (a specific β_2 adrenoreceptor ligand), and ICI 89,406 (a specific β_1-adrenoreceptor ligand) were performed. These studies indicated only the presence of β_1- adrenoreceptors at any age tested. After this critical confirmation that propranol was binding to a single site, saturation studies to determine B_{max} were performed, with concentrations of the radioligand (^{125}I-CYP) ranging from 5-300 pM, in the absence and presence of propranolol (10 μM) to determine non-specific binding. All assays were run in triplicate; n's = 6 pooled samples/group/age.

Prenatal alcohol exposure did affect the number of β_1-adrenoreceptor binding sites (fmol/mg protein), as seen in Figure 10. There was a significant main effect of prenatal treatment group on the number of β_1-adrenoreceptor binding sites; the alcohol group differed significantly from the pair-fed and lab chow control groups, which did not differ from each other. There was also an age-related decrease in the number of β_1-adrenoreceptor binding sites.

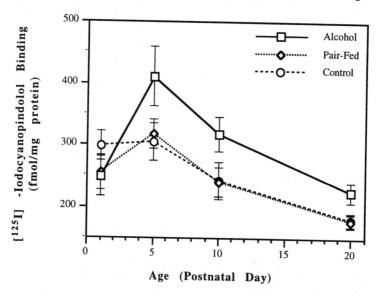

Figure 10. Mean concentration ± S.E.M. of beta1-adrenoceptor binding sites (fmol/mg protein) in brown adipose tissue for three prenatal treatment groups at 1, 5, 10 and 20 days of age. (From Zimmerberg, E. *et al.*, Alcohol 12, 71, 1995. With permission.)

Prenatal treatment did not affect the relative amount of protein in the tissue samples. This result is consistent with our two previous studies demonstrating that thermoregulatory deficits in alcohol-exposed offspring are not caused by substrate deficiencies in brown adipose tissue.[30,62]

These results are very interesting in light of the results from the norepinephrine concentration study discussed previously in Section A. During the first postnatal week, adrenergic receptors are present in advance of the incoming sympathetic fibers and are thought to play an important developmental role in establishing viable synaptic connections.[76-77] Prenatal alcohol exposure did not reduce the number of receptors available as a developmental signal on postnatal day one, the day after birth (before the arrival of the neurons). At five days of age, when the neurons are arriving and norepinephrine levels in alcohol-exposed subjects are 74% of controls, the number of β_1-adrenoreceptor binding sites is 129% of controls. This result suggests that the number of binding sites in alcohol-exposed brown adipose tissue cells continues to rise due to the absence of sufficient neurotransmitter, and reflects a delay in the arrival of SNS neurons.

During the second and third postnatal weeks, when norepinephrine concentrations are rising and reaching asymptotic levels, the number of β_1-adrenoreceptors in brown adipose tissue of control subjects is decreasing. This observation is consistent with a typical compensatory response in the number of receptors as the levels of neurotransmitter increases (a "downregulation"), and also suggests that the developmental role of these receptors is no longer necessary. Alcohol-exposed subjects, however, do not show a proportional downregulation. While norepinephrine concentration increases in alcohol-exposed subjects from 10 to 20 days of age (in contrast to the leveling off in controls), the number of β_1-adrenoreceptor binding sites decreases, but never reaches control levels. Thus, at 20 days of age, when norepinephrine concentration is 132% of control, the number of β_1-adrenoreceptor binding sites is still 125% of controls. Theoretically, receptor density should fall below control levels in alcohol-exposed subjects, since neurotransmitter concentration is higher than control levels. The expected compensatory "downregulation" response, therefore, may be altered in brown adipose tissue from subjects exposed to alcohol prenatally.

These results, however, are complicated by the recent discovery of a novel adrenoreceptor in brown adipose tissue. Although there was agreement that brown adipose tissue had an "atypical" receptor, there was some controversy regarding its exact nature.[78-80] The proposal of a β_3-adrenoreceptor in brown adipose tissue was based on pharmacological analyses of metabolic processes since binding studies were unable to characterize this "atypical" receptor.[78,81] Some investigators claimed that this receptor was unique to adipose tissue, but a very recent study of β_3-adrenoreceptor mRNA distribution in human adult autopsy material reported β_3-adrenoreceptor mRNA present in white and brown adipose tissue, gallbladder, heart, and colon, but not abdominal muscle, liver, lung, kidney, thyroid or lymphocytes.[82] Another recent study detected this β_3-adrenoreceptor mRNA in human neuroblastoma cells.[83] A β_3-adreno-receptor gene has now been cloned from human[84] and rat[85-86] brown adipose tissue. The human β_3-adrenoreceptor gene is 50% and 45% homologous with β_1 and β_2-adrenoreceptor genes, respectively.[87] Like the β_1-adrenoreceptor, the β_3-adrenoreceptor activates adenylate cyclase, but NE has 10- to 100-fold greater affinity for β_1 than β_3. The two receptors also have different phos-phorylation sites for regulatory kinases.[88]

The β_3-adrenoreceptor has been proposed to account for 70% of the adrenergic receptors in neonatal brown adipose tissue, and to be primarily responsible for inducing non-shivering thermogenesis.[89] It shows developmental changes in its functional activity, and will be recruited in adults under stressful conditions of cold or diet challenges. For example, β_3 adreno-receptor activation of adenylate cyclase predominates in 7 day old rat pups, while β_1 adrenoreceptor activation of adenylate cyclase predominates in 23 day old rat pups.[90] Although both β_1 and β_3 adrenoreceptors are critical for neonatal thermogenesis, it has been suggested that in adults, β_3 adrenoreceptors primarily mediate the NE-stimulated thermogenic response[78] while β_1 adrenoreceptors mediate the NE-stimulated hypertrophy and hyperplasia[91] during brown adipose tissue recruitment. There are no adequate radioactive ligands at present for good binding studies for the β_3-adrenoreceptor.[125] I-CYP does not bind to this site, and propranolol has a very low affinity for this AR. Repeated attempts under a variety of conditions to assess specific binding using ^{3}H-CGP and BRL 37,344 were completely unsatisfactory. There is agreement in the literature, however, that conventional receptor binding techniques are inadequate to quantify either number or sensitivity of this receptor because adequate high-affinity labeled ligands are not available and it is too difficult to detect β_3-adrenoreceptor receptors against the background of binding at high concentrations to β_1-adrenoreceptor and non-specific sites.[78,81] Thus, future investigations on adrenergic receptors are currently underway using a cDNA probe for the β_3-adrenoreceptor.

VI. CLINICAL IMPLICATIONS

Alterations in receptor density in response to changing concentrations of neurotransmitter at the synapse is one important mechanism underlying plasticity in the central nervous system. Using the sympathetic innervation of brown adipose tissue as a model system, we have demonstrated that prenatal alcohol exposure changes the functional status of the adrenergic synapse. The pattern of results in these studies suggest that the exposure of the SNS to alcohol during development will have long-term consequences for that neurotransmitter system both pre- and post-synaptically. Previous studies on other mechanisms of plasticity have also reported that prenatal alcohol exposure alters the normal response of neurons to damage or change in neural activity. For example, prenatal alcohol exposure resulted in a decrease in β_1-adrenoreceptor-mediated potentiation of several neurophysiological measures of long-term plasticity, including diminished long-term potentiation (LTP) in the hippocampus.[92] In addition, prenatal alcohol exposure was found decrease lesion-elicited dopaminergic neurons' responsivity in the olfactory tubercle;[93] however, prenatal alcohol exposure was also reported to enhance post-lesion axonal sprouting in the hippocampus.[94] Indeed, there may be age-related or region-specific changes in the effects of prenatal alcohol exposure on the ability of the nervous system to respond to environmental challenges.

Since the SNS is a critical component of the stress response, these results may also have implications for future studies in that area. Recent research in stress response has focused on alcohol's impairment of the hypothalamic-pituitary-adrenal (HPA) axis.[95-96] While the alcohol-exposed rat during the neonatal period has a suppressed adrenocortical response to stress,[33,97] alcohol-exposed adult rats have an exaggerated HPA axis stress response compared to controls.[19,37,98-100] In addition, there may be sex differences in alcohol-related birth effects on the HPA axis response to stress post-puberty.[37,101] Central hyperresponsiveness in adrenergic systems may also be affected by prenatal alcohol exposure. For example, the decrease in cortical and hypothalamic NE and the increase in hippocampal NE in response to stress is augmented in alcohol-exposed offspring.[102] The hyperresponsiveness of the HPA axis to stress seen in alcohol-exposed offspring in other laboratories[37,95-96,98-99,101] may reflect a more general pattern of hyper-responsiveness of the postsynaptic target cells of the SNS after prenatal alcohol exposure. A similar age-dependent pattern was seen in immune response; prenatal alcohol exposure initially suppresses the β-endorphin response to stress in neonates, but greatly enhances this stress response in three week olds. This pattern is remarkably parallel to our results described here.

If adrenergic receptors fail to downregulate in the presence of increased neurotransmitter, then stressful situations challenging the sympathetic nervous system may cause a relative hyperresponsiveness. An overactivation of brown adipose tissue thermogenesis might increase the risk of Sudden Infant Death Syndrome (SIDS). One of the striking findings in autopsies of children who die of Sudden Infant Death Syndrome (SIDS) is that they have abnormally retained their brown adipose tissue.[103-105] Histological abnormalities were also detected in brown adipose tissue from SIDS victims.[106] When the thermogenic capacity of BAT was measured in two cases of SIDS that were associated with fever, thermogenin content was elevated, and the authors conclude that inappropriate thermogenesis in a well-insulated, pyrexic infant might lead to fatal apnea or seizures.[107] SIDS victims have been noted to have abnormally high rectal temperatures even after death,[108] and histological changes in their small intestines identical to those found after heatstroke.[109] One model of

SIDS proposes death due to problems with thermoregulation, resulting in overheating, and aggravated by over-insulation, over-heated rooms and face-down position.[110] Interestingly, brown adipose tissue has also been found to bear responsibility for restraint stress-induced hyperthermia in rats.[111] Thus, stress, infection, or restraint may inappropriately trigger NST in BAT in SIDS cases leading to fatal hyperthermia.

Parallels exist between SIDS and FAS. SIDS infants are smaller at birth and show persistent growth retardation postnatally[112], as do alcohol-exposed newborns. SIDS victims are also reported to have had difficulties with respiration, feeding and temperature regulation:[113] they were "more breathless and exhausted during feeding, and had more abnormal cries." These reports sound remarkably similar to observations of infants exposed to moderate levels of maternal alcohol. Upper airway obstruction was observed in 3 FAS cases; the authors noted that it might lead to obstructive apnea or SIDS.[114] SIDS victims had previous prolonged periods of sleep apnea;[115] FAS infants also have periods of apnea.[116] Prenatal alcohol exposure has also been associated with hypoplastic lungs, which would contribute to hypoxemia.[117] Abnormal retention of BAT can be caused by chronic cold exposure, episodes of fever, or chronic hypoxemia.[118]

These similarities raise an intriguing question: is there any evidence that SIDS is increased in alcohol-exposed children? Although the relationship between maternal alcohol intake and SIDS has not been systematically investigated, it is listed as a "notable factor" in an Auckland post-neonatal mortality review.[119] According to the NICHD Cooperative Epidemiological Study of SIDS, 61.2% of the mothers of SIDS victims reported drinking during pregnancy.[120] However, they conclude that compared to their low birth weight control group, the SIDS odds is not increased (however, this study only used retrospective self-reporting of alcohol intake). Interestingly, this study did find that infant "hypothermia," "irritability," "poor feeding," and "droopy and listless appearance" were significant predictors of SIDS; again, these observations parallel similar observations about FAS infants.[1,121] One important clue may be that among all ethnic groups, Native Americans have the highest incidence of sudden infant death (SIDS) - 5.93 deaths per 1000 live births.[122] The incidence of FAS among Native Americans may be as high as 40 per 1000 births.[123] DiNicola[124] remarked on the similarity between the high incidence of alcoholism and the high incidence of SIDS among Native Americans, but could find no epidemiological studies on whether excessive maternal alcoholism was a risk factor for SIDS. A recent study reported that although the incidence of SIDS is twice as high among Native American infants in the Northwest and Alaska compared to Caucasian infants in the same regions, there is no ethnic difference in SIDS rates in the Southwest;[125] perhaps thermic stress in the more Northern climate accounts for this discrepancy. If alcohol-exposed neonates are less able to maintain an adequate body temperature during periods of cold stress, a compensatory increase in sympathetic activation of BAT thermogenesis might increase the risk of SIDS as the neonate develops and experiences sympathetic activation due to other stressors.

ACKNOWLEDGMENTS

This research was partially supported by a grant from the National Institute on Alcohol Abuse and Alcoholism, #AA08605. The experiments described in this chapter are the result of the excellent technical assistance of Mara E. Savacool, Carol D. Smith, Robert C. True, and Jacqueline M. Weider. Many thanks also to Nancy P. Piatczyc and Paul J. Schwartz for their invaluable assistance in preparing this manuscript.

REFERENCES

1. **Landesman-Dwyer, S., Keller, S., and Streissguth, AP.,** Naturalistic observation of the newborn: Effect of maternal alcohol intake, *Alc. Clin. Exp. Ther.,* 2, 171, 1978.

2. **Coles, C.D., Smith, I.E., Fernoff, P.M., and Falek, A.,** Neonatal ethanol withdrawal: Characteristics in clinical normal, nondysmorphic neonates, *J. Ped.,* 105, 445, 1984.

3. **Pierog, S., Chandavasu, O., and Wexler, I.,** Withdrawal symptoms in infants with the fetal alcohol syndrome, *J. Ped.,* 90, 630, 1977.

4. **Jones, K.L., Smith, D.W., Ulleland, C.N., and Streissguth, A.P.,** Pattern of malformation in offspring of chronic alcoholic mothers, *Lancet,* 1, 1267, 1974.

5. **Ioffe, S. and Chernick, V.,** Maternal alcohol ingestion and the incidence of respiratory distress syndrome, *Am. J. Ob. Gyn.,* 156, 1231, 1987.

6. **Sander, L.W., Snyder, P.A., Rosett, H.L., Lee, A., Gould, J.B., and Ouellette, E.M.,** Effects of alcohol intake during pregnancy on newborn state regulation: A progress report, *Alc. Clin. Exp. Res.,* 1, 233, 1977.

7. **Rosett, H.L., Snyder, P.A., Sander, L.W., Lee, A., Cook, P., Weiner, L., and Gould, J.,** Effects of maternal drinking on neonate state regulation, *Dev. Med. Child Neurol.,* 21, 464, 1979.

8. **Ioffe, S., Childiaeva, R., and Chernick, V.,** Prolonged effects of maternal alcohol ingestion on the neonatal electroencephalogram, *Pediatrics,* 74, 330, 1984.

9. **Avery, M. and Taeusch, H.,** *Schaffer's Diseases of the Newborn,* Saunders, Philadelphia, 1984, 50.

10. **Clarren, S. and Smith, D.,** The fetal alcohol syndrome, *N. Engl. J. Med.*, 298, 1063, 1978.

11. **Landesman-Dwyer, S.,** Drinking during pregnancy: Effects on human development, in *Biomedical Processes and Consequences of Alcohol Use; Alcohol and Health Monograph No. 2*, DHHS, Washington, DC, 1982, 335.

12. **Jones, K.L. and Smith, D.W.,** Recognition of the fetal alcohol syndrome in early infancy, *Lancet,* 2, 989, 1973.

13. **Miller, H.C. and Jekel, J.F.,** Incidence of low birth weight infants born to mothers with multiple risk factors, *Yale J. Biol. Med,* 60, 397, 1987.

14. **Cancalon, P.,** Influence of temperature on various mechanisms associated with neuronal growth and nerve regeneration, *Prog. Neurobiol.*, 25, 27, 1985.

15. **Zuckerman, B.S. and Hingson, R.,** Alcohol consumption during pregnancy: A critical review, *Dev. Med. Child Neurol.*, 28, 649, 1986.

16. **Zimmerberg, B., Ballard, G.A., and Riley, E.P.,** The development of thermoregulation after prenatal exposure to alcohol in rats, *Psychopharm.,* 91, 479, 1987.

17. **Zimmerberg, B., Beliveau, A.A., and Furniss, A.H.,** Effects of cross-fostering on thermoregulation development after prenatal alcohol exposure, *Soc. Neurosci. Abstr.*, 17, 1598, 1991.

18. **Abel, E.L., Bush, R., and Dintcheff, B.A.,** Exposure of rats to alcohol in utero alters drug sensitivity in adulthood, *Science,* 212, 1531, 1981.

19. **Taylor, A.N., Branch, B.J., Liu, S.H., Weichmann, A.F., Hill, M.A., and Kokka, N.,** Fetal exposure to ethanol enhances pituitary-adrenal and temperature responses to ethanol in adult rats, *Alc. Clin. Exp. Res.,* 5, 237, 1981.

20. **Taylor, A.N., Branch, B.J., Randolph, D., Hill, M.A., and Kokka, N.,** Prenatal ethanol exposure affects temperature responses of adult rats to pentobarbital and diazepam, alone and in combination with ethanol, *Alc. Clin. Exp. Res.*, 11, 254, 1987.

21. **Molina, J.C., Hoffmann, H., Spear, L.P., and Spear, N.E.,** Sensorimotor maturation and alcohol responsiveness in rats prenatally exposed to alcohol during gestational day 8, *Neurotoxicol. Teratol.*, 9, 121, 1987.

22. **Lancaster, F.E. and Spiegel, K.S.,** Voluntary beer drinking by pregnant rats: Offspring sensitivity to ethanol and preference for beer, *Alcohol*, 6, 207, 1989.

23. **Zimmerberg, B. and Mehr, S.T.,** Brown adipose tissue: Studies on SNS development in neonatal rats prenatally exposed to alcohol, presented at annual meeting of the International Developmental Psychobiology Society, San Diego, Nov. 1995.

24. **Zimmerberg, B. and Wang, G.J.,** Prenatal alcohol exposure alters the functional responsiveness of the SNS in brown adipose tissue, *Alc. Clin. Exp. Res.*, 19, 18, 1995.

25. **Alberts, J.R.,** Huddling in rat pups: Group behavioral mechanisms of temperature regulation and energy conservation, *J. Comp. Physiol. Psychol.*, 92, 231, 1978.

26. **Jans, J.E. and Leon, M.,** Determinants of mother-young contact in Norway rats, *Physiol. Behav.*, 30, 919, 1983.

27. **Hannigan, J.H.,** Alcohol exposure and maternal-fetal thyroid function: Impact on biobehavioral maturation, in *Alcohol and the Endocrine System*, Zakhari , S. Ed., NIH, Bethesda, MD, 1993, 313.

28. **Gilliam, D. and Kotch, L.,** Developmental thermoregulatory deficits in prenatal ethanol exposed long- and short-sleep mice, *Dev. Psychobiol.*, 25, 365, 1992.

29. **Al-Hilli, F. and Wright, E.A.,** The effects of changes in the environmental temperature on the growth of tail bones in the mouse, *Br. J. Exp. Pathol.*, 64, 34, 1963.

30. **Zimmerberg, B.,** Thermoregulatory deficits following prenatal alcohol exposure: Structural correlates, *Alcohol*, 6, 389, 1989.

31. **Zimmerberg, B., Broadhurst, K.M., and True, R.C.,** Sex-dependent effects of prenatal alcohol exposure on circadian rhythms of temperature and activity in rats, *Soc. Nsci. Abst.*, 18, 1072, 1992.

32. **Zimmerberg, B., Savacool, M.C., and Broadhurst, K.M.,** Sex-dependent effects of prenatal alcohol exposure on circadian rhythms of temperature and activity in rats, paper under review.

33. **Weinberg, J., Kim, C.K., and Yu, W.,** Early handling can attenuate adverse effects of fetal ethanol exposure, *Alcohol,* 12, 317, 1995.

34. **York, J.L. and Regan, S.G.,** Conditioned and unconditioned influences on body temperature and ethanol hypothermia in laboratory rats, *Pharm. Biochem. Behav.*, 17, 119, 1982.

35. **Melchior, C.L. and Allen, P.M.,** Temperature in mice after ethanol: Effect of probing and regain of righting reflex, *Alcohol,* 10, 17, 1993.

36. **Weinberg, J., Zimmerberg, B., and Sonderegger, T.B.,** Gender-specific effects of perinatal exposure to alcohol and other drugs, in *Perinatal substance abuse: Research findings and clinical implications*, Sonderegger, Y.B., Ed., Johns Hopkins, Baltimore, 1992, 51.

37. **Weinberg, J.,** Hyperresponsiveness to stress: Differential effects of prenatal ethanol on males and females, *Alc.Clin. Exp. Res.*, 12, 647, 1988.

38. **Satinoff, E.,** Developmental aspects of behavioral and reflexive thermoregulation, in *Developmental Psychobiology: New methods and changing concepts,* Shair, H.H., Barr, G.A. and Hofer, M.A., Eds., Oxford University Press, New York, 1991, 169.

39. **Fowler, S.J. and Kellogg, C.,** Ontogeny of thermoregulatory mechanisms in the rat, *J. Comp. Physiol. Psychol.,* 89, 738, 1975.

40. **Johanson, I.B.,** Thermotaxis in neonatal rat pups, *Physiol. Behav.,* 23, 871, 1979.

41. **Kleitman, N. and Satinoff, E.,** Thermoregulatory behavior in rat pups from birth to weaning, *Physiol. Behav.,* 29, 537, 1982.

42. **Zimmerberg, B., Khazam, C.D., and Riley, E.P.,** Prenatal alcohol exposure alters seizure susceptibility and thermoregulatory response to heat stress in neonatal rats, *Soc. Nsci. Abst.,* 13, 691, 1987.

43. **Gentry, G.D. and Middaugh, L.D.,** Effect of prenatal ethanol exposure on neonatal behavior, *Teratol.,* 41, 618, 1990.

44. **Zimmerberg, B., Tomlinson, T.M., Glaser, J., and Beckstead, J.W.,** Effects of prenatal alcohol exposure on the developmental pattern of temperature preference in a thermocline, *Alcohol,* 10, 403, 1993.

45. **Myers, R.D.,** Hypothalamic control of thermoregulation, in *Handbook of the hypothalamus,* Morgane, P.J. and Panksepp, J., Eds., Wiley-Liss, New York, 1980, 83.

46. **Satinoff, E.,** A reevaluation of the concept of the homeostatic organization of temperature regulation, in *Handbook of Behavioral Neurobiology,* Satinoff, R. and Teitelbaum, P., Eds., Plenum Press, New York, 1983, 443.

47. **Zimmerberg, B. and Shartrand, A.M.,** Temperature-dependent effects of maternal separation on growth, activity, and amphetamine sensitivity in the rat, *Dev. Psychobiol.,* 25, 213, 1992.

48. **Stone, E.A., Bonnet, K.A., and Hofer, M.A.,** Survival and development of maternally deprived rats: Role of body temperature, *Psychosomatic Medicine,* 38, 242, 1976.

49. **Himms-Hagen, J.,** Brown adipose tissue thermogenesis: Role in thermoregulation, energy regulation and obesity, in *Thermoregulation: Physiology and Biochemistry,* Schonbaum, E. and Lomax, P., Eds., Pergamon Press, New York, 1990, 327.

50. **Scarpace, P.J., Matheny, M., Borst, S., and Tumer, N.,** Thermoregulation with age: Role of thermogenesis and uncoupling protein expression in brown adipose tissue, *Proc. Soc. Exp. Biol. Med.,* 205, 154, 1994.

51. **Nicholls, D.G. and Locke, R.M.,** Thermogenic mechanisms in brown fat, *Physiol. Rev.,* 64, 1, 1984.

52. **Cannon, B., Hedin, A., and Nedergaard, J.,** Exclusive occurrence of thermogenin antigen in brown adipose tissue, *FEBS Lett,* 150, 129, 1982.

53. **Barnard, T., and Skala, J.,** The development of brown adipose tissue, in *Brown adipose tissue,* Lindberg, O., Ed., Elsevier, New York, 1970, 33.

54. **Saito, M., Minokoshi, Y., and Mihimazu, T.,** Ventromedial hypothalamic stimulation accelerates norepinephrine turnover in brown adipose tissue, *Life Sci*, 41, 193, 1987.

55. **Woods, A.J. and Stock, M.J.,** Biphasic brown fat temperature responses to hypothalamic stimulation in rats, *Am. J. Physiol.*, 266, R328, 1994.

56. **Thornhill, J., and Halvorson, I.,** Activation of shivering and non-shivering thermogenesis by electrical stimulation of the lateral and medial preoptic areas, *Brain Res.*, 656, 367, 1994.

57. **Egawa, M., Yoshimatsu, H., and Bray, G.A.,** Preoptic area injection of corticotropin-releasing hormone stimulates sympathetic activity, *Am. J. Physiol.*, 259, R799, 1990.

58. **Thornhill, J., Jugnauth, A., and Halvorson, I.,** Brown adipose tissue thermogenesis evoked by medial preoptic stimulation is mediated via the ventromedial hypothalmic nucleus, *Can. J. Physiol. Pharmacol.*, 72, 1042, 1994.

59. **Amir, S.,** Activation of brown adipose tissue thermogenesis by chemical stimulation of the posterior hypothalamus, *Brain Res.*, 534, 303, 1990.

60. **Druse, M.J.,** Effects of in utero ethanol exposure on the development of neurotransmitter systems, in *Development of the Central Nervous System: Effects of Alcohol and Opiates*, Miller, M.W., Ed., Wiley-Liss, New York, 1992, 139.

61. **Rudeen, P.K. and Weinberg, J.,** Prenatal ethanol exposure: Changes in regional brain catecholamine content following stress, *J. Neurochem.*, 61, 1907, 1993.

62. **Zimmerberg, B., Brown, A.P., Lee, H.H., and Slocum, R.D.,** Effect of prenatal alcohol exposure on uncoupling protein in brown adipose tissue in neonatal rats, *Alcohol,* 10, 149, 1993.

63. **Huttunen, P., Kortelainen, M.L., and Hivornen, J.,** Foetal and lactional exposure to alcohol increases oxidative capacity of brown adipose tissue in the rat. A possible relationship to cot death, *Br. J. Exp. Path.*, 70, 691, 1989.

64. **Bartolome, J., Lau, C., and Slotkin, T.A.,** Premature development of cardiac sympathetic transmission in the fetal alcohol syndrome, *Life Sci.*, 28, 571, 1981.

65. **Thadani, P.,** Effect of maternal ethanol administration on synaptic vesicles development in heart of rat offspring, *Neuropharm.*, 22, 931, 1983.

66. **Thadani, P. and Wells, M.,** Histoflourescence evaluation of sympathetic nerve fibers in hearts of developing rats exposed to ethanol during gestation, *Neuropharm.*, 23, 1075, 1984.

67. **Gottesfeld, Z., Christie, R., Feltin, D.L., and LeGrue, S.J.,** Prenatal ethanol exposure alters immune capacity and noradrenergic synaptic transmission in lymphoid organs of the adult mice, *Neurosci.*, 35, 185, 1990.

68. **Johnson, M.I. and Covey, R.D.,** Ethanol stimulates axonal growth but reduces Schwann cell numbers in cultures of rat sympathetic neurons, *Alc. Clin. Exp. Res.*, 17, 484, 1993.

69. **Wigal, S.B.E., Amsel, A. and Wilcox, R.E.,** Fetal ethanol exposure diminshes hippocampal β-adrenergic receptor density while sparing muscarinic receptors during development, *Dev. Brain Res.* 55, 161, 1990.

70. **Zimmerberg, B., Carson, E.A., Kaplan, L.J., Zuniga, J.A., and True, R.T.,** Role of noradrenergic innervation of brown adipose tissue in thermoregulatory deficits following prenatal alcohol exposure, *Alc. Clin. Exp. Res.,* 17, 418, 1993.

71. **Tejani-Butt, S.M.,** [3H]Nisoxetine: A radioligand for quantification of norepinephrine uptake sites by autoradiography or by homogenate binding, *J. Pharm. Exp. Ther.,* 260, 427, 1992.

72. **Tejani-Butt, S.M., Yang, J., and Zaffar, H.,** Norepinephrine transporter sites are decreased in the locus coeruleus in Alzheimer's disease, *Brain Res.*, 631, 147, 1993.

73. **De Oliveira, A.-M., Schoemaker, H., Segonzac, A., and Langer, S.Z.,** Differences in the temperature dependence of drug interaction with the noradrenaline and serotonin transporters, *Neuropharm.*, 28, 823, 1989.

74. **Langin, D., Portillo, M.P., Saulnier-Blache, J.S., and Lafontan, M.,** Coexistence of three β-adrenoreceptor types in white fat cells of various mammalian species, *Eur. J. Pharm,* 199, 291, 1991.

75. **Zimmerberg, B., Smith, C.D., Weider, J.M., and Teitler, M.,** The development of β-adrenoreceptors in brown adipose tissue following prenatal alcohol exposure, *Alcohol*, 12, 71, 1995.

76. **Duman, R.S. and Alvaro, J.D.,** Developmental expression of adrenergic receptors in the central nervous system, in *Receptors in the Developing Nervous System Vol. 2*, Zagon, I.S. and McLaughlin, P.J., Eds., Chapman & Hall, London, 1993, 1.

77. **Slotkin, T.A.,** Endocrine control of synaptic development in the sympathetic nervous system, in *Developmental Neurobiology of the Autonomic Nervous System,* Gootman, P.M., Ed., Humana Press, Clifton, NJ, 1986, 97.

78. **Arch, J.R.S.,** The brown adipocyte β-adrenoreceptor, *Proc. Nutr. Soc.*, 48, 215, 1989.

79. **Granneman, J.G.,** Norepinephrine and BRL 37344 stimulate adenylate cyclase by different receptors in rat brown adipose tissue, *J. Pharm. Exp. Ther.*, 254, 508, 1990.

80. **Zaagsma, J. and Nahorski, S.R.,** Is the adipocyte β-adrenoreceptor a prototype for the recently cloned atypical β3-adrenoreceptor?, *Trends Pharmacol.,* 11, 3, 1991.

81. **Tavernier, G., Galitsky, J., Bousquet-Melou, A., Montastruc, J.L., and Berlan, M.,** The positive chronotropic effect induced by BRL 37344 and CGP 12177, two beta-3 adrenergic agonists, does not involve cardiac beat adrenoreceptors but baroreflex mechanisms, *J. Pharm. Exp. Ther.,* 263, 1083, 1992.

82. **Krief, S., Lonnqvist, F., Raimbault, S., Baude, B., Van Spronsen, A., Arner, P., Strosberg, A.D., Ricquier, D.,** Tissue distribution of β3-adrenergic receptor mRNA in man, *J. Clin. Invest.,* 91, 344, 1993.

83. **Esbenshade, T.A., Han, C., Theroux, T.L., Granneman, J.G., and Minneman, K.P.,** Coexisting β1 and atypical β-adrenergic receptors cause redundant increases in cyclic AMP in human neuroblastoma cell, *Mol. Pharmacol.,* 42, 753, 1992.

84. **Emorine, L.J., Marullo, S., Briend-Sutren, M.M., Patey, G., Tate, K., Delavier-Klutchko, C., and Strosberg, A.D.,** Molecular characterization of the human β3-adrenergic receptor, *Science,* 245, 1118, 1989.

85. **Granneman, J.G., Lahners, K.N., and Chaudhry, A.,** Molecular cloning and expression of the rat β3-adrenergic receptor, *Mol. Pharmacol.,* 40, 895, 1991.

86. **Muzzin, P., Revelli, J.P., Kuhne, F., Gocayne, J.D., McCombie, W.R., Venter, J.C., Giacobino, J.P., and C.M., F.,** An adipose tissue-specific β-adrenergic receptor, *J. Biol. Chem.,* 266, 24053, 1991.

87. **Emorine, L.J., Feve, B., Pairault, J., Briend-Sutren, M.M., Nahmias, C., Marullo, S., Delavier-Klutchko, C., and Strosberg, A.D.,** The human β3-adrenergic receptor: Relationship with atypical receptors, *Am. J. Clin. Nutr.,* 55, 215, 1992.

88. **Granneman, J.G. and Lahners, K.N.,** Differential adrenergic regulation of β1- and β3- adrenoreceptor messenger ribonucleic acids in adipose tissues, *Endocrinology,* 130, 109, 1992.

89. **Zhoa, J., Unelius, L., Bengtsson, T., Cannon, B., and Nedergaard, J.,** Coexisting b-adrenoceptor subtypes: Significance for thermogenic process in brown fat cells, *Am. J. Physiol.,* 267, C969, 1994.

90. **Chaudhry, A., Lahners, K.N., and Granneman, J.G.,** Perinatal changes in the coupling of beta1- and beta3 adrenergic receptors to brown fat adenylyl cyclase, *J. Pharm. Exp. Ther.,* 261, 633, 1992.

91. **Bronnikov, G., Houstek, J., and Nedergaard, J.,** β-adrenergic, cAMP-mediated stimulation of proliferation of brown fat cells in primary culture, *J. Biol. Chem.,* 267, 2006, 1992.

92. **Stanton, P.K., Bommer, M., Heinemann, U., and Noble, E.P.,** *In utero* alcohol exposure impairs postnatal development of hippocampal noradrenergic sensitivity, *Neurosci. Res. Commun.,* 1, 145, 1987.

93. **Gottesfeld, Z., Garcia, C.J., Lingham, R.B., and Chronister, R.B.,** Prenatal ethanol exposure impairs lesion-induced plasticity in a dopaminergic synapse after maturity, *Neurosci.*, 29, 715, 1989.

94. **Dewey, S.L. and West, J.R.,** Direct evidence for enhanced axonal sprouting in adult rats exposed to ethanol *in utero*, *Brain Res. Bull.*, 14, 339, 1985.

95. **Taylor, A.N., Branch, B.J., Nelson, L.R., Lane, L.A., and Poland, R.E.,** Prenatal ethanol and ontogeny of pituitary-adrenal responses to ethanol and morphine, *Alcohol*, 3, 255, 1986.

96. **Weinberg, J.,** Prenatal ethanol exposure alters adrenocortical development of offspring, *Alc.Clin. Exp. Res.*, 13, 73, 1989.

97. **Angelogianni, P. and Gianoulakis, C.,** Prenatal exposure to ethanol alters the ontogeny of the β-endorphin response to stress, *Alc.Clin. Exp. Res.*, 13, 564, 1989.

98. **Nelson, L.R., Taylor, A.N., Lewis, J.W., Poland, R.E., Redei, E., and Branch, B.J.,** Pituitary-adrenal responses to morphine and footshock stress are enhanced following prenatal alcohol exposure, *Alc.Clin. Exp. Res.*, 10, 397, 1986.

99. **Taylor, A., Branch, B., Liu, S., and Kokka, N.,** Long-term effects of fetal ethanol exposure on pituitary-adrenal response to stress, *Pharm. Biochem. Behav., 16, 585, 1982.*

100. **Weinberg, J. and Gallo, P.V.,** Prenatal ethanol exposure; Pituitary-adrenal activity in pregnant dams and offspring, *Neurobehav. Toxicol. Teratol.*, 4, 515, 1982.

101. **Weinberg, J.,** Prenatal ethanol exposure alters adrenocortical response to predictable and unpredictable stressors, *Alcohol*, 9, 427, 1992.

102. **Rudeen, P. and Weinberg, J.,** Prenatal ethanol exposure: Changes in regional brain catecholamine content following stress, *J. Neurochem.*, 61, 1907, 1993.

103. **Naeye, R.,** Hypoxaemia and the sudden infant death syndrome, *Science*, 186, 837, 1974.

104. **Naeye, R.L.,** Sudden infant death, *Scientific American,* 242, 52, 1980.

105. **Valdes-Dapena, M., Gillane, M., and Catherman, R.,** Brown fat retention in sudden infant death syndrome, *Arch. Pathol. Lab. Med.*, 100, 547, 1976.

106. **Stephenson, T.J. and Variend, S.,** Visceral brown fat necrosis in postperinatal mortality, *J. Clin. Pathol.*, 40, 896, 1987.

107. **Lean, M.E. and Jennings, G.,** Brown adipose tissue activity in pyrexial cases of cot death, *J. Clin. Pathol.*, 42, 1153, 1989.

108. **Sunderland, R. and Emery, J.L.,** Febrile convulsions and cot death, *Lancet*, 2, 176, 1981.

109. **Stanton, A., Scott, D., and Downham, M.,** Is overheating a factor is some unexpected infant deaths?, *Lancet*, 1, 1954, 1980.

110. Nelson, E.A.S., Taylor, B.J., and Weatherall, I.L., Sleeping position and infant bedding may predispose to hyperthermia and the sudden infant death syndrome, *Lancet*, 1, 199, 1989.

111. Shibata, H. and Nagasaka, T., Contribution of nonshivering thermogenesis to stress-induced hyperthermia in rats, *Jap. J. Physiol.*, 32, 991, 1982.

112. Hoffman, H.J., Damas, K., Hillman, L., and Krongrad, E., Results of the National Institute of Child Health and Human Development SIDS cooperative epidemiological study, *Annals N.Y. Acad. Sci.*, 533, 13, 1988.

113. Naeye, R.L., Messmer, J., Specht, T., and Merrit, T.A., Sudden infant death syndrome: Temperament before death, *J. Pediatr*, 88, 511, 1976.

114. Usowicz, A.G., Golabi, M., and Curry, C., Upper airway obstruction in infants with fetal alcohol syndrome, *Am. J. Dis. Children*, 140, 1039, 1986.

115. Steinschneider, A., Prolonged apnea and the sudden death syndrome: Clinical and laboratory considerations, *Pediatrics*, 50, 646, 1972.

116. Rosett, H.L. and Weiner, L., *Alcohol and the Fetus: A Clinical Perspective*, Oxford, NY, 1984.

117. Inselman, L.S., Fisher, S.E., Spencer, H., and Atkinson, M., Effect of intrauterine ethanol exposure on fetal lung growth, i, 19, 12, 1985.

118. Guntheroth, W.G., *Crib Death: the Sudden Infant Death Syndrome*, Futura, Mount Kisco, 1982.

119. Mitchell, E.A., Hassall, I.B., and Becroft, D.M.O., Postneonatal mortality review in Aukland: Two years experience, *N.Z. Med. J.*, 100, 269, 1987.

120. Hoffman, H., Damas, K., Hillman, L., and Krongrad, E., Risk factors for SIDS: Results of the National Institute of Child Health and Human Development SIDS Cooperative Epidemiological Study, *Annals N.Y. Acad. Sci.*, 533, 13, 1988.

121. Streissguth, A.P., The behavioral teratology of alcohol: Performance, behavioral and intellectual deficits in prenatally exposed children, in *Alcohol and Brain Development*, West, J.R., Ed., Oxford University Press, New York, 1986, chap. 3.

122. Kaplan, D., Bauman, A., and Krous, H., Epidemiology of sudden infant death syndrome in American Indians, *Pediatrics*, 74, 1041, 1984.

123. May, P.A. and Hymbaugh, K.L., Epidemiology of fetal alcohol syndrome among American Indians of the Southwest, *Soc. Biol.*, 30, 374, 1983.

124. DiNicola, A., Might excessive maternal alcohol ingestion during pregnancy be a risk factor associated with an increased likelihood of SIDS?, *Clin. Pediatr.*, 24, 659, 1985.

125. **Bulterys, M.,** High incidence of sudden infant death syndrome among Northern Indians and Alaska Natives compared with southwestern Indians: Possible role of smoking, *J. Community Health*, 15, 185, 1990.

Chapter 15

ALCOHOL WARNING LABELS:
INFLUENCE ON DRINKING

Janet R. Hankin

I. BACKGROUND

In response to concerns about the adverse effects of alcohol, the Congress of the United States[1] passed the Federal Beverage Labeling Act in 1988. The law requires that all containers of alcoholic beverages display the following warning:

> **Government Warning**: (1) According to the Surgeon General, women should not drink alcoholic beverages during pregnancy because of the risk of birth defects. (2) Consumption of alcoholic beverages impairs your ability to drive a car or operate machinery and may cause health problems.

Public Law 100-160 applies to all containers sold or distributed in the United States on or after November 18, 1989. This chapter compares the impact of the alcohol warning labels on self-reported drinking of younger versus older gravidas, and tests the hypothesis that older women are less attentive to the warning label. Given data that the risks for Fetal Alcohol Syndrome and Alcohol Related Birth Defects increase with age,[2-4] it is important to understand the response of older women to the warning label.

II. PREVIOUS RESEARCH ON THE WARNING LABEL

The Eighth Report to Congress on Alcohol and Health concluded, as of mid-1990, many people had not noticed the existence of the warning label.[2] Data collected from a nationally representative sample in 1990 showed that 37% of adults knew about the warning label.[5] Gallup Polls of cross-sectional national samples of adults from 1991, 1992, and 1993 found that the percent of persons aware of the label for each year was 49.8%, 45.6%, and 55.0% respectively.[6-7]

Data from a sample of African American gravidas seeking prenatal care in Detroit, Michigan, showed a four month lag between the implementation of the label law and a significant increase in label warning awareness. While implemented in November, 1989, awareness did not increase until February, 1990.[8] Time series analysis on this sample of gravidas indicated a decrease in

0-8493-7685-8/96/$0.00+$.50
© 1996 by CRC Press, Inc.

self-reported drinking during the post-label period, but only among non-risk drinkers (defined as women drinking less than 0.5 ounce absolute alcohol per day). This decrease did not occur until July, 1990, seven months after the law was implemented.[9]

This chapter extends previous analyses and examines the hypothesis that older gravidas would not decrease their drinking in the post-label period, while younger gravidas would decrease alcohol intake after the label was implemented. Based on previous research,[10] a multivariate model was used to estimate drinking during pregnancy as a function of time (pre- versus post-label), awareness of the warning label, and attitudes about drinking during pregnancy. Drinking at the time of conception and maternal characteristics (gravidity and weeks' gestation) were used as control variables in the model. These controls were necessary in order to separate out the impact of the warning label from changes in the patient population that may have occurred from the pre- to the post-label period.

III. METHODS

A. SAMPLE

The sample included 9,767 African American gravidas who sought care at the Hutzel Hospital prenatal clinic between May 22, 1989 and June 30, 1994. The clinic is located in Detroit, Michigan and is affiliated with the Detroit Medical Center and the Wayne State University School of Medicine Department of Obstetrics and Gynecology. The clinic serves a low income population, and 85% of the women are on welfare. Hutzel Hospital delivers half of all babies born in the City of Detroit and is a tertiary referral center for high risk pregnancies.

B. DATA COLLECTION

As part of the Fetal Alcohol Research Center at Wayne State University, every woman was interviewed at her first prenatal visit to the clinic, for most women, during the second trimester of pregnancy. After checking in at the desk, women were directed to the interviewers who were employees of the research center and not part of the clinical staff. This part of the clinic visit was perceived by the clinical staff and patients as a routine event proceeding the physical examination. Patients were told that the interview was voluntary and the decision to participate would not affect the care received. Informed consent was obtained. The response rate for the interview was 99%.

Data were obtained on maternal characteristics, including weeks' gestation (age of the fetus in weeks at the time of the interview), birthdate of mother, gravidity, self-reported alcohol consumption, awareness of the warning label, and attitudes about drinking during pregnancy. Details about the measurement of drinking, label awareness, and attitudes are described below.

C.   SELF-REPORTED DRINKING

Women were asked about their drinking during the one week around the time of conception (*periconceptional drinking*) as well as drinking during the two weeks prior to the first prenatal visit (*antenatal drinking*). The shorter time period used for periconceptional drinking was in part a function of the long lag time between conception and the first prenatal visit (on average, about 22 weeks). Using questions developed by Sokol *et al.*,[11] women were asked if they had anything to drink each day, and if so, the type and amount of beverage consumed (See Hankin *et al.*[10] for the wording of the daily drinking history questions). For both antenatal and periconceptional drinking, the amount of absolute alcohol consumed per day (AA/D) was calculated using standardized methods.[11-12] Liquor contains 40% alcohol, wine contains 20%, wine cooler 5% and beer 4%. The ounces consumed were multiplied by these weights, and the amount of absolute alcohol was totaled. In order to obtain the daily average amount of absolute alcohol consumed, the total was divided by 7 for periconceptional drinking and by 14 for antenatal drinking.

Several studies demonstrate the reliability and validity of the drinking measures. For example, Hankin *et al.*[10] examined data from 20,948 interviews of women seen at the Hutzel prenatal clinic between 1986-1992. They found a correlation of .82 between reports of antenatal drinking one week and two weeks prior to the first prenatal visit. Ernhart *et al.*[13] reported a correlation of .67 between antenatal drinking reported in the prenatal clinic and retrospective reports of drinking during pregnancy obtained five years later. In another comparison of clinic interviews at the first prenatal visit and retrospective reports of drinking obtained 13 months postpartum, Jacobson *et al.*[14] found a correlation of .60 between the two reports. The measure has predictive validity for alcohol related birth defects.[11]

Periconceptional drinking served as a control variable in the analysis. It represented the average amount of absolute alcohol consumed before the confirmation of the pregnancy. It is unlikely that the warning label impacted on periconceptional drinking, since four-fifths of the pregnancies among women using the Hutzel clinic were unplanned. During the course of the study, there was evidence that the population shifted toward heavier drinkers. To account for this change, and to avoid masking the impact of the label law, the analyses incorporated periconceptional drinking as a control variable.

D.   AWARENESS OF THE WARNING LABEL

Women were asked, "Is there a health warning on alcoholic beverages (something that says alcohol may affect your health)? Would you say, Yes, No, or Don't Know?" This measure of awareness was crude, since we did not ask the women about the specific wording of the warning label. Women who responded "Yes" were coded as "1" (aware of the label), while women who responded "No" or "Don't Know" were coded as "0" (unaware of the label).

E.   ATTITUDES ABOUT DRINKING DURING PREGNANCY

Subjects were also asked two questions to ascertain their attitudes about drinking during pregnancy:

- •"What are the chances a baby will be okay if a mother drinks a lot of alcohol during pregnancy?" (Reported as a percentage from 0-100%.)
- •"How often do you think it is safe for a woman to drink during pregnancy? Would you say daily (=1), weekly (=2), monthly (=3), less than once per month (=4), never (=5)?"

F.   TRANSITIONAL PERIOD FOR IMPACT OF LABEL

Although the warning label was implemented on November 18, 1989, it was hypothesized that there would be a transitional period. Old stock was not required to be labeled, so until it cleared the shelves, consumers could still purchase unlabeled containers of alcohol after November 18th. Indeed, there was evidence that several months passed before the labels penetrated retailers' shelves. In May and June, 1990, six retail stores in the Detroit inner city were visited, and 18,888 alcoholic beverage containers were examined. Six months after the law was implemented, the small survey indicated that 86% of beer containers, 69% of wine cooler containers, 34% of wine bottles, and 30% of liquor bottles were labeled.[8] Beverages with shorter shelf lives were more likely to be labeled than those with longer shelf lives. These results suggested the need to incorporate a lag time before any label impact could be ascertained. Using time series analysis of antenatal drinking among 12,026 Hutzel Hospital gravidas, Hankin et al.[9] determined that July, 1990 was the first month where antenatal drinking by Hutzel patients showed a response to the warning label. In the analyses described below, July 1, 1990 was used as the date to indicate the post-label period. Women initiating prenatal care after that date were coded "1" on the post-label variable, while women starting care prior to that date were coded "0."

G.   STATISTICAL METHOD

Tobit analysis was used to predict reported antenatal drinking. This method uses maximum likelihood estimation and adjusts for the skewness of the distribution of the dependent variable.[15] Since the percentage of nondrinkers was quite large (at the time of the first prenatal visit, 80% of the women said they were abstaining from alcohol, so antenatal drinking = 0), the distribution of antenatal drinking was skewed. When interpreting the results, t-ratios are used to determine the significance of each predictor variable.

Separate equations were estimated for three different age groups: 1) women aged 11-20 years old, 2) women aged 21-29 years old, and 3) women aged 30-46 years old. The age groups were constructed using the following rationale. Underage drinkers (less than 21 years old) represent a unique group. They are drinking illegally, and may be differentially affected by the warning label. In addition, there is a higher probability that they are nulliparous. On the other hand, women aged 30 and over are more likely to be multiparous and have high risk pregnancies. These older women presumably were warned about the risks of drinking during pregnancy with each succeeding pregnancy, so the warning label may not offer any new information. Women aged 21-29 logically comprise the third group for the data analysis.

To compare the three equations in greater detail, elasticities were calculated.[15] While the tobit coefficients are unstandardized, elasticities allow the comparisons of a variable's impact across equations. Elasticities have the additional advantage of allowing one to compare the impact of the warning label for all women versus the subgroup of women who drank during pregnancy. Elasticities represent the percentage change in the dependent variable (in this case, antenatal drinking) elicited by a 1% change in the independent variable (i.e., the probability of being seen after the label date, July 1, 1990).

Bonferroni (Dunn) T-tests were used for pairwise comparisons between women under 21 versus those 21-29 and between women under 21 versus gravidas over 29 years of age. The critical value of T used was 2.34, p < .05. Given the large number of women in each group, even small differences between the age groups may be statistically significant.

IV. RESULTS

A. SAMPLE CHARACTERISTICS

Table 1 shows the means of the variables for the entire sample, as well as the three age groups and the results of the Bonferroni T-tests. The average woman was 23.74 years old, and the age range was 11-46 years old. Eighty-three percent of the women entered care after July 1, 1990 (post-label), and 60% said there was a warning label on alcoholic beverages. The average woman entered care in the second trimester, when the fetus was almost 22 weeks old. The mean gravidity for the sample was 1.25 previous live births.

The average woman said a woman should not drink during pregnancy (frequency = 5) or should drink less than once a month (frequency = 4). On average, women thought there was a 26% chance that the baby would be okay if the mother drank a lot while pregnant.

The mean for periconceptional drinking was .30 AA/D, or about .75 ounce liquor, 1.5 ounces wine, 6 ounces of wine cooler, or 7.5 ounces of beer. By the time of the first prenatal visit, reported alcohol consumption dropped to .04 AA/D.

Table 1

Variable Means and Standard Deviations

Variable	Entire Sample		Age ≤ 20		21 ≤ Age ≤ 29		Age ≥ 30	
	Mean	S.D.	Mean	S.D.	Mean	S.D.	Mean	S.D.
Post-Label	0.83	0.37	0.84	0.37	0.83	0.38	0.83	0.37
Gravidity	1.25	1.53	0.45	0.73	1.38*	1.37	2.56†	1.98
Age of Fetus	21.89	9.09	22.53	8.78	21.31*	9.29	21.92	9.15
Periconceptional Drinking	0.30	1.09	0.14	0.59	0.33*	1.23	0.53†	1.40
Aware of Label	0.60	0.49	0.65	0.48	0.60*	0.49	0.50†	0.50
Chances Baby OK	26.26	24.06	25.02	24.08	26.77*	23.6	27.57†	24.95
Frequency Safe to Drink	4.63	0.81	4.73	0.69	4.61*	0.83	4.47	0.96
Antenal Drinking	0.04	0.28	0.01	0.06	0.04*	0.28	0.12†	0.48
Age	23.74	6.17	17.94	1.70	24.37*	2.59	33.79†	3.27
N	9767		3684		4226		1857	

* $p > .05$ Comparing the 20 and under Age Group to the 21 to 29 Age Group
† $p > .05$ Comparing the 20 and under Age Group to the 30 and over Age Group

B.   COMPARISONS ACROSS AGE GROUPS

There were significant differences across the age groups on almost all of the variables used in the model. As expected, gravidity was significantly and positively related to age (See Table 1). While younger women had .45 previous deliveries, older mothers averaged 2.56. Younger women entered prenatal care significantly later than the middle age group, but there was no difference between the youngest and oldest groups on weeks' gestation.

Younger women drank significantly less at conception and also at the time of the first prenatal visit compared to the other two age groups. For example, the oldest group of women drank 12 times more than the youngest group at the first prenatal visit (.01 antenatal AA/D versus .12 AA/D). In terms of periconceptional drinking, the difference between the youngest versus oldest groups was smaller, but statistically significant (.14 periconceptional AA/D versus .53 AA/D).

It is important to note that the average woman 30 and over drank at risk levels (defined as consuming more than .50 AA/D), and thus increased the probability that her baby would have slower reaction times,[16] slower rate of growth,[17] and poorer performance on the Bayley Mental Developmental Index.[4]

Younger women were significantly less likely to feel that the baby would be okay if the mother drank a lot during pregnancy (25.02%) compared to the older age groups (26.77% and 27.57%). Younger women were significantly more likely to feel a pregnant woman should drink infrequently compared to the older women (4.73 versus 4.61 and 4.47). On average, 65% of the youngest women were aware of a warning label, compared to 60% of women aged 20-29 and 50% of women over age 30 (p < .05).

C.   TOBIT REGRESSIONS

Table 2 shows the maximum likelihood estimates from the Tobit regressions to predict antenatal drinking, separately for each of the age groups. The log likelihood function is much smaller for the youngest group, suggesting a better fit for the model compared to the fit for the other two age groups. All else equal, the warning label had a significant, negative impact on antenatal drinking *only* for the youngest age group. Thus, after July, 1990, younger women decreased their drinking in response to the implementation of the warning label. The label date variable was not significant for women aged 21-29 and those 30 years old and over.

For the youngest and oldest age groups, awareness of the warning label predicted antenatal drinking. Women who were aware of the warning drank more than those who were not aware of the warning label. However, awareness did not reach significance for women aged 21-29. Attitudes predicted drinking for all three age groups. Women who cited higher chances that the baby would be okay if the mom drank a lot while pregnant also reported higher alcohol consumption. Respondents who said women should never drink when pregnant or should drink less than once a month (frequency variable coded as "5" or "4") tended to drink less than other women. There is thus evidence of consistency between attitudes and behavior.

Table 2

Tobit Regression to Predict Antenatal Drinking

Age ≤ 21			
	Coef	S.E.	t-ratio
Post-Label	-0.0594	0.0218	2.73**
Gravidity	0.0399	0.0102	3.90***
Age of Fetus	-0.0030	0.0010	3.11***
Periconceptional Drinking	0.0647	0.0082	7.87***
Aware of Label	0.0711	0.0193	3.69***
Chances Baby OK	0.0009	0.0003	2.60**
Frequency Safe to Drink	-0.0783	0.0099	7.95***
Constant	-0.0061	0.0538	0.11
N	3684		
Log-Likelihood	-582.16		
21 ≤ Age ≤ 29			
	Coef	S.E.	t-ratio
Post Label	-0.0327	0.0393	0.83
Gravidity	0.0242	0.0105	2.32*
Age of Fetus	0.0000	0.0016	0.02
Periconceptional Drinking	0.1658	0.0100	16.61***
Aware of Label	0.0533	0.0310	1.72
Changes Baby OK	0.0025	0.0006	4.14***
Frequency Safe to Drink	-0.1730	0.0155	11.19***
Constant	-0.0334	0.0871	0.38
N	4226		
Log-Likelihood	-1741.9		
Age ≥ 30			
	Coef	S.E.	t-ratio
Post-Label	-0.0203	0.0693	0.29
Gravidity	0.0346	0.0130	2.67**
Age of Fetus	0.0056	0.0029	1.90
Periconceptional Drinking	0.2763	0.0149	18.58***
Aware of Label	0.2033	0.0525	3.87**
Changes Baby OK	0.0029	0.0010	2.88**
Frequency Safe to Drink	-0.2087	0.0241	8.66***
Constant	-0.2108	0.1443	1.46
N	1857		
Log-Likelihood	-1114.7		

* p<.05 / ** p<.01 / ***p<.001

Table 3

Elasticities for Label Date

Age	All Women	Women Drinking During Pregnancy
< 21	-0.444	-0.065
21 - 29	-0.083	-0.016
30	-0.036	-0.008

Other predictors of drinking included gravidity, weeks' gestation, and periconceptional drinking. Women with higher gravidity drank more than those with lower gravidity. Among the youngest age group only, gravidas entering prenatal care later drank less. Periconceptional drinking was one of the strongest predictors of antenatal drinking. Women who drank more around the time of conception tended to drink more during pregnancy.

D. ELASTICITIES

Table 3 shows the elasticities for the tobit regressions. For the youngest age group, the elasticity of the label date variable is -.444, that is, a 1% change in the probability of being seen after July 1, 1990 resulted in a .444% decrease in drinking. Among the subsample of underage drinkers who actually drank during pregnancy, a 1% change in the probability of being seen post-label resulted in a .065% decrease in alcohol consumption. Note that among the two older age groups, the elasticities are much smaller. For example, among women who drank during pregnancy, the elasticities are -.016% for the 21-29 year olds, suggesting that the label had a very small impact on drinking. Among women 30 and over, the elasticity was close to zero (-.008%).

V. DISCUSSION

A. SUMMARY OF RESULTS

The results suggest that the implementation of the alcohol beverage warning label was related to a modest reduction in drinking only for underage drinkers, pregnant women under the age of 21. Older gravidas did not respond to the warning label.

While at least half of the sample were aware of the warning label, knowledge was highest in the underage drinkers. A counterintuitive finding was the positive relationship between antenatal drinking and label awareness among the youngest and oldest gravidas. It appears that heavier drinkers had greater exposure to the warning label and were thus more likely to know of its existence.

For the entire sample, attitudes about drinking during pregnancy were consistent with antenatal alcohol consumption. However, compared to older women, younger ones were more likely to cite lower probabilities that a baby would be okay if the mother drank a lot. In addition, younger women were more likely to say that a pregnant woman should abstain from alcohol, while older women suggested that gravidas could safely drink some alcohol.

B.   EXPLAINING THE RESULTS

Why did younger women heed the warning label while older women ignored it? There are several possible explanations, which are described below:
   • The novelty of the warning for the underage drinkers,
   • Higher perceived vulnerability of the fetus among younger gravidas,
   • Decreased willingness to take risks among younger women.

1. Novelty

Younger women were more likely to have lower gravidity and parity than older women. Thus, they had less exposure to the message about the dangers of drinking during pregnancy. The warning was new to them. On the other hand, older women may have heard the warning so many times that they became immune to it.

2. Perceived Fetal Vulnerability

The data indicate that older women, compared to younger ones, cited higher percentages in response to the question, "What are the chances the baby will be okay if the mother drinks a lot of alcohol during pregnancy?" While the differences were not large, they were statistically significant, and suggest that the older woman felt the fetus was less vulnerable to alcohol than her younger counterpart. When interpreting the response to this particular question, it is important to note that while only one in ten of heavy drinkers will have a baby with Fetal Alcohol Syndrome,[18] the risk of Alcohol Related Birth Defects among heavy drinkers is much higher.

Prior experience with pregnancy is an important element in perception of fetal vulnerability and the risks from antenatal drinking. The older gravida may have consumed alcohol during previous pregnancies, and felt that it did not hurt her other children. Thus, she may be inclined to cite lower rates of harm, discount the warning, and continue drinking during the current pregnancy. On the other hand, the underage drinker may be a nulliparae and have no prior experience with infants. This lack of experience may encourage her to heed the warning. The obvious question is whether the observed results are a function of parity, age, or a combination of both.. It is difficult to sort out the relative contribution of these variables, and further research is necessary to answer this question.

3. Risk Taking

It is possible that older women are more likely to take risks than younger women. They may understand the dangers of drinking during pregnancy, but feel that it will not happen to *them*. They prefer to take their chances and drink heavily during pregnancy rather than abstain from alcohol. The older gravidas may enjoy gambling and tempting fate, and may feel that the benefits of drinking outweigh the 10% chance of having an FAS baby. Younger women may be unwilling to take any chances of having a baby with birth defects.

In addition, younger women may be more concerned about having a healthier baby than older women. Given that this may be the first child, the underage drinkers may be more anxious about the outcome of the pregnancy and more willing to follow health care providers' advice. Older women may be less worried about the pregnancy and more likely to discount the warning message.

C.   LIMITATIONS OF THE RESEARCH

There are several limitations to this research. The sample is comprised of inner city African American gravidas, and the results are not generalizable to a wider population group. The measures of alcohol consumption are self-reports, and may not be as valid as more objective measures, such as blood alcohol levels. Some under-reporting of alcohol use may have occurred. The measure of label awareness is crude, since women were not asked the specific wording of the warning label. Finally, while the analysis controls for changes in the population over time, the causal link between the drop in alcohol consumption by younger gravidas and the warning label can be questioned. It is important to note that the Detroit area did not launch any other public health campaigns to decrease drinking during pregnancy during 1989-1994. There were no major media campaigns, there were no warning signs in bars or liquor stores, there were no billboards warning pregnant women not to drink. However, it is possible that other unmeasured factors, besides the warning label, may have contributed to the observed decline in alcohol consumption among underage drinkers.

D.   IMPLICATIONS

The results from this study suggest that older gravidas, who are at highest risk for Fetal Alcohol Syndrome and Alcohol Related Birth Defects, have not heeded the alcohol beverage warning label. For a variety of reasons, this public health intervention has not reached this group of women. On the other hand, the good news is that underage drinkers have listened to the warning message.

It appears that older pregnant women need to be targeted for special prevention efforts. Such efforts might emphasize that their risk for FAS increase with age, and while they were lucky with previous pregnancies, the next pregnancy is at increased risk for FAS and other Alcohol Related Birth

Defects. The message should be clear and concise: In order to prevent FAS and ARBDs, a pregnant woman should never get drunk or high, because when she drinks, she drinks for two.

ACKNOWLEDGMENTS

I would like to thank J.J. Sloan for his assistance with computer programming. This work is supported in part by the National Institute of Alcohol Abuse and Alcoholism grant nos. AA08561 and AA07606.

REFERENCES

1. **US Congress,** Alcohol Beverage Labeling Act of 1988, *Public Law* 100-690, 27, 201, 1988.
2. **National Institute of Alcohol Abuse and Alcoholism,** *Eighth Special Report To The US Congress on Alcohol and Health.* Government Printing Office, Washington, D.C., 1994.
3. **Abel, E.L. and Hannigan, J.H.,** Maternal risk factors in Fetal Alcohol Syndrome: Provocative and permissive factors, *Neurotox. Teratol.,* 17, 445, 1995.
4. **Jacobson, J.L., Jacobson, S.W., Sokol, R.J., Martier, S.S., Ager, J.W., and Kaplan-Estrin, M.G.,** Teratogenic effects of alcohol on infant development, *Alc. Clin. Exp. Res.,* 17, 174, 1993.
5. **Kaskutas, L. and Greenfield, T.,** First effects of warning labels on alcoholic beverage containers, *Drug Alcohol Depend.,* 31,1, 1992.
6. **Mazis, M.B., Morris, L.A., and Swazey, J.L.,** Awareness, recall, and acceptance of alcohol warning labels, *Public Health Reps,* in press.
7. **Greenfield, T.K. and Hilton, M.E.,** Warning labels on alcoholic beverage containers in the US. Paper presented at the 38th International Institute on the Prevention and Treatment of Alcoholism: International Council on Alcohol and Addictions, Prague, June 6-10, 1994.
8. **Hankin J.R., Sloan, J.J., Firestone, I.J., Ager, J.W., Sokol, R.J., Martier, S.S., and Townsend, J.,** The alcohol beverage warning label: When did knowledge increase? *Alc. Clin. Exp. Res.,* 17, 428, 1993.
9. **Hankin, J.R., Sloan, J.J., Firestone, I.J., Ager, J.W., Sokol, R.J., and Martier, S.S.,** A time series analysis of the impact of the alcohol warning label on antenatal drinking, *Alc. Clin. Exp. Res.,* 17, 284, 1993.

10. Hankin, J.R., Firestone, I.J., Sloan, J.J., Ager, J.W., Goodman, A.C., Sokol, R.J., and Martier, S.S., The impact of the alcohol warning label on drinking during pregnancy, *J.Pub. Pol. Mar.*, 12, 10, 1993.

11. Sokol, R.J., Miller, S.I., Debanne, S., Golden, N., Collins, G., Kaplan, J., and Martier, S., The Cleveland NIAAA Prospective Alcohol-In-Pregnancy study: The first year, *Neurobehav. Toxicol. Teratol.*, 3, 203, 1981.

12. Bowman, R.S., Stein, L.I., and Newton, J.R., Measurement and interpretation of drinking behavior, *J. Stud. Alcohol*, 36, 1154, 1975.

13. Ernhart, C.M., Morrow-Tlucak, M., Sokol, R.J., and Martier, S.S., Underreporting of alcohol use in pregnancy, *Alc. Clin. Exp. Res.*, 12, 506, 1988.

14. Jacobson, J.L., Jacobson, S.W., Sokol, R.J., Martier, S.S., and Ager, J.W., Prenatal alcohol exposure and neurobehavioral function in infancy: Evidence for threshold and differential vulnerability, *Am. J. Obstet. Gynecol.*, 166, 346, 1992.

15. Maddala G.S., Limited dependent and qualitative variables, in *Econometrics*, Cambridge University Press, New York, 1983.

16. Jacobson, S.W., Jacobson, J.L. , and Sokol, R.J., Effects of fetal alcohol exposure on infant reaction time, *Alc. Clin. Exp. Res.*, 18, 1125, 1994.

17. Jacobson, J.L., Jacobson, S.W., and Sokol, R.J., Effects of prenatal exposure to alcohol, smoking, and illicit drugs on postpartum somatic growth, *Alc. Clin. Exp. Res.*, 18, 317, 1994.

18. Hankin, J.R. and Sokol, R.J., Identification and care of problems associated with alcohol ingestion in pregnancy, *Sem. Perinat.*, 19, 286, 1995.

INDEX